WB18PAL

NOTES FOR THE MRCGP

...rned on or before
. stamped below.

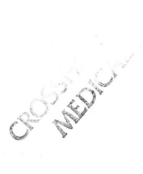

Notes for the MRCGP

K. T. PALMER
MA BM BCh MRCGP MFOM DRCOG

THIRD EDITION

ell

© 1988, 1992, 1998 by
Blackwell Science Ltd
Editorial Offices:
Osney Mead, Oxford OX2 0EL
25 John Street, London WC1N 2BL
23 Ainslie Place, Edinburgh EH3 6AJ
350 Main Street, Malden
  MA 02148 5018, USA
54 University Street, Carlton
  Victoria 3053, Australia
10, rue Casimir Delavigne
  75006 Paris, France

Other Editorial Offices:
Blackwell Wissenschafts-Verlag GmbH
Kurfürstendamm 57
10707 Berlin, Germany

Blackwell Science KK
MG Kodenmacho Building
7–10 Kodenmacho Nihombashi
Chuo-ku, Tokyo 104, Japan

The right of the Author to be
identified as the Author of this Work
has been asserted in accordance
with the Copyright, Designs and
Patents Act 1988.

All rights reserved. No part of
this publication may be reproduced,
stored in a retrieval system, or
transmitted, in any form or by any
means, electronic, mechanical,
photocopying, recording or otherwise,
except as permitted by the UK
Copyright, Designs and Patents Act
1988, without the prior permission
of the copyright owner.

First published 1988
Reprinted 1989 (twice), 1990
Second edition 1992
Reprinted 1993, 1994, 1996
Third edition 1998
Reprinted 1999

Set by Excel Typesetters Co.,
  Hong Kong
Printed and bound in Great Britain by
  MPG Books Ltd, Bodmin, Cornwall

The Blackwell Science logo is a
trade mark of Blackwell Science Ltd,
registered at the United Kingdom
Trade Marks Registry

For further information on
Blackwell Science, visit our website:
www.blackwell-science.com

DISTRIBUTORS

Marston Book Services Ltd
PO Box 269
Abingdon
Oxon OX14 4YN
(Orders: Tel: 01235 465500
          Fax: 01235 465555)

USA
 Blackwell Science, Inc.
 Commerce Place
 350 Main Street
 Malden, MA 02148 5018
 (Orders: Tel: 800 759 6102
                 781 388 8250
          Fax: 781 388 8255)

Canada
 Login Brothers Book Company
 324 Saulteaux Crescent
 Winnipeg, Manitoba R3J 3T2
 (Orders: Tel: 204 837-2987)

Australia
 Blackwell Science Pty Ltd
 54 University Street
 Carlton, Victoria 3053
 (Orders: Tel: 3 9347-0300
          Fax: 3 9347-5001)

A catalogue record for this title
is available from the British Library

ISBN 0-86542-777-1

Library of Congress
Cataloguing-in-Publication Data
Palmer, K.T.
    Notes for the MRCGP /
K.T. Palmer.–3rd ed.
        p.   cm.
      Includes bibliographical
references and index.
      ISBN 0-86542-777-1
      1. Medicine.   2. Family
    medicine. I. Title.
R130.P35 1998
610—dc21   97–46538
                                 CIP

For further information on
Blackwell Science, visit our website:
www.blackwell-science.com

Contents

Preface to the Third Edition

Year on year general practice changes at a frenetic pace. In the second edition of this book I described the first new national contract for GPs in 40 years; a new fundholding scheme that doctors regarded with great suspicion; and several major changes to the College's Membership examination. A mere 5 years on, half the population is covered by practices who hold budgets; computers sit on most GPs' desktops; and doctors have organised themselves into purchasing consortia and out of hours co-operatives that run their own emergency centres. The vocational training programme has a new, exacting exit requirement; while the MRCGP examination has changed thrice more, most significantly to encompass videotape assessment of performance in the surgery.

No respite can be expected. A government bill has introduced a choice of contractual terms for GPs, allowing those who prefer to work the national contract, and others to set local terms — to be salaried and employed, to manage bigger units, or to retain the long cherished status of the independent contractor. Fundholding will soon be replaced by commissioning and Primary Care Groups. Performance indicators for GPs and practice league tables are in the early stages of discussion. Change is all around. A GP who had spent the last decade abroad would no doubt find on his return that the landscape had changed beyond recognition. The author sympathises with his plight! Relatively few sections of this book have escaped revision, reflecting the new topography.

However, some things do not change, such as the timeless requirement for concise but comprehensive revision material in the run-up to an examination. I hope that this third edition of *Notes for the MRCGP* will enable MRCGP candidates to find their way and press onwards to exam success.

Preface to the First Edition

The MRCGP examination is one of the fairest of postgraduate examinations, and given reasonable preparation candidates stand a good chance of success in it. The chief challenge arises from the breadth of the syllabus, which draws on many areas of medical practice — clinical, psychological, social, administrative, interpersonal, legal and ethical. In preparing for my own examination I became aware that while there were several excellent books on each aspect and several study books that worked their way through sample examination papers, there was no concise revision text that tried to encompass the whole broad canvas of the syllabus. This is not really surprising when you consider the limitless scope the examiners have and the wide range of reading material available. Nevertheless, examination candidates in the latter stages of their preparations often express a need to have a fact-packed concise revision source around which to formalise their thoughts. I hope this book will meet their needs.

Adopting the 'short notes' format leaves an author open to the accusation that his coverage is superficial, arbitrary or dogmatic. Brevity naturally promotes a didactic style and I hope I will be excused this failing in the cause of a greater good. Certainly the 'facts' and opinions in this book are not written on tablets of stone and candidates should be sensitive to the eternal cycle of debate and change which characterises general practice.

In selecting my material I have deliberately concentrated on those aspects of practice which are non-clinical — the running of a business, communication and couselling, the social and legal aspects, the 'wider issues' — almost to the exclusion of 'pure' clinical medicine. There are two major reasons for this: first, most candidates by this stage already have a strong foundation in clinical matters from their hospital training, and to duplicate this material would make the book unnecessarily cumbersome; second, experience suggests that the non-clinical areas pose a greater obstacle to candidates, a fact examiners recognise in setting their questions. The book concludes with some useful statistics, further reading, and the examination itself: the syllabus, the format and my personal ideas and suggestions on examination technique. I hope this approach will help the candidate to steer a steady course to examination success. Happy navigating!

Acknowledgements

In the preparation of this book I found the following to be valuable sources of information: *Running a Practice*, R.V.H. Jones, K.J. Bolden, D.J. Pereira Gray & M.S. Hall, Croom Helm; *Practising Prevention*, BMA publication; *Preventive Medicine in General Practice*, eds M. Gray & G.H. Fowler, Oxford Medical Publications; *Sociology as Applied to Medicine*, eds D. Patrick & G. Scambler, Baillière's Concise Medical Textbooks; *Common Dilemmas in Family Medicine*, ed. J. Fry, MTP; *Common Diseases*, J. Fry, MTP; various editorials and articles from the *Journal of the Royal College of General Practitioners*, notably those by A. McPherson (May 1985), C. Freer (June 1985), J. Cohen (Sept. 1985) and D. Tant (Nov. 1985); and the *Update Clinical Debate* series (1985). The series *Trainee's Guide to Practice Management* by Dr M. Mead proved especially helpful in the writing of Section 1.3 and I am indebted to him: his discussion of practice record-keeping is so expert and comprehensive that little extra of value has been or need be added.

The chapter on epidemiology and statistics would not have proved possible but for the lucid teachings of Dr R. McNamee on behalf of Manchester University's Distance Learning Course for occupational physicians. Thanks are due in special measure to her for all that is good in this chapter. The failings, if failings there be, are mine alone.

I would also like to thank my former tutors for their advice in the book's first edition and in particular Dr R. Coles for his helpful suggestions. Thanks are also due in large measure to my father-in-law for his knowledge and to my wife for her fortitude and forbearance.

1 Practice Matters

1.1 THE BUILDING

Types of ownership
Premises are in two major categories:

1   Owner-occupied (i.e. owned by one or more partner or a close relative).
2   Rented.

Each category can be subdivided according to the premises' origins:

   (a) purpose-built (i.e. newly built as a surgery or a substantially altered existing property not previously used for medical practice);
   (b) adapted (i.e. not originally intended for medical purposes but now approved for them by the Health Authorities (HAs)).

The capital costs of practice premises
In the case of *rented* premises the capital cost is borne by the owner and not the GP. Purpose-built rented premises are usually Health Centres — now the responsibility of Community Trusts and built specifically to rent to GPs; alternatively private developers or the General Practice Finance Corporation (GPFC) may do the same with HA agreement.

In *owner-occupied* premises the capital is raised by the partner(s), either from private funds or a loan from the GPFC, High Street banks or building societies. The interest on the loan for purpose-built premises is usually covered by the cost-rent scheme (see below).

The running costs of practice premises
In rented premises
The 1966 GP Charter undertook to provide rent and rate reimbursements to GPs. In Health Centres this is essentially a formality: a rent is charged and fully reimbursed, making it a book transaction only.

In other rented premises a 100% reimbursement is also available, provided that the rent charge is 'reasonable'. An employee of the Inland Revenue called the *district valuer* determines what is 'reasonable' by inspecting and comparing it with the current market rent charged on comparable properties in the same area.

In owner-occupied premises
If these are purpose-built under an approved cost-rent scheme, the rent and rates are again entirely reimbursed. If the premises are adapted, the owner-doctor is compensated for the capital he or she has tied up in bricks and mortar by the payment of a notional rent, i.e. although he pays no actual rent, he receives an annual payment comparable to the current market rent of similar local property (the sort of

rent he could have received himself if the premises were used other-wise). The value of the notional rent is set by the District Valuer and reassessed every 3 years or when any change occurs. (GPs who dispute the District Valuer's assessment can employ an independent valuer to argue their case, and can ultimately appeal to the Secretary of State.)

Note that the GP's Terms of Service (see Section 7.12) impose the responsibility of providing 'adequate' surgery premises and HAs can withhold reimbursements if premises are substandard.

Running costs other than rent and rates are *not* reimbursable although they are tax-deductible—GPs in Health Centres pay a quar-terly consolidated service charge (covering use of heat, light, cleaning services, etc., in proportion to their overall use of the building), and other GPs pay their own service expenses as they arise.

The cost-rent scheme

This scheme is controlled by the HA and covers the cost of three categories of purpose-built premises:
1   the building of completely new premises;
2   substantial modification of existing practice premises;
3   the acquisition of premises 'for substantial modification'.

The *principle* is that the partners raise the capital and the HA meets the interest payments on the loan. Several *practical* points apply:
1   In all cases, prior HA approval and consultation are needed as well as planning permission. The HA has discretion to accept or reject a scheme, depending on their budget and priorities.
2   Strict Red Book schedules exist regarding allowable expenditure, e.g. acceptable building costs per square metre, architects' fees, plan-ning consent costs, etc.
3   The final rent reimbursed is called the *cost-rent* and is calculated from the capital costs of the project and the interest rate charged. (This interest rate is linked to the GPFC's rate and the loan may be at a fixed or variable interest rate.)
4   As the cost-rent is a scheduled percentage of the building cost, there comes a time when the revalued notional rent exceeds it. At the next triennial review the practice can then opt to switch from cost-rent to notional rent.

This area of practice finances is due for overhaul. In 1990 strict cash limits were imposed on the scheme, and a civil service report labelled it 'archaic and complex'. The White Paper, *Primary Care: Delivering the Future* (1996) proposes new arrangements in which doctors will be allowed to plough back their budget savings into surgery improve-ments; and HAs will be empowered to loan grants that help GPs to buy out of leases on substandard buildings. Private finance schemes are to be encouraged; and more flexibility will be allowed on permis-sible size and floor space, to accommodate practices that work collaboratively (e.g. share primary care budgets or operate out-of-hours emergency centres).

Improvement grants

These are available from the Department of Health (DOH) provided that:
- there is prior HA approval;
- work is on facilities for patients (and not primarily on doctors' accommodation);
- the grant is to improve 'what already exists' and not to provide new premises.

Projects should normally comply with the standards of accommodation in Para. 56/Schedule 1 of the Red Book. Payments may be up to two-thirds of the total cost, but there is:
- a minimum project cost;
- an overall cost limit and maximum grant per doctor;
- a condition that tax relief claims are forfeit on capital costs met by grant (Para. 56/Schedule 1 of the Red Book).

A cost-rent is also available (assuming the usual conditions of the cost-rent scheme are satisfied).

Some HAs are applying the rules flexibly to enable improvements in building facilities and equipment, e.g. to provide security alarms, central heating, ramps for the disabled and extra switchboard capacity.

Part of the grant is repayable if premises are no longer used as an NHS surgery within 3 or (depending on grant level) 4 years.

Pros and cons of Health Centre and owner-occupied premises
See Table 1.1.

Branch surgeries

Many practices, especially those in rural areas, have branch surgeries; these often arise from the historical amalgamation of separate practices.

Advantages
1   The major advantage is to patients in rural areas who have shorter distances to travel, and do not have to depend on infrequent rural bus services to see doctors.
2   Home visiting to this group of patients is reduced by encouraging them to attend a surgery.
3   GPs in rural areas are able to sustain a higher list size, with consequent increase of profits.

Disadvantages
1   Facilities are often primitive compared with the main surgery.

Table 1.1 Pros and cons of Health Centre and owner-occupied premises.

		Health Centre	Owner-occupied
1	Initial financing	By the community trust; the GP only invests minimally in practice equipment	By the partners; this means capital is needed early in a GP's career, and may cause problems in expensive areas with high housing prices
2	Capital growth	None for the doctors	Appreciable long-term investment (especially since the cost-rent scheme effectively grants an interest-free loan)
3	Control of premises	Limited: (a) consultation on the initial design may be limited; (b) it may prove difficult to make substantial alterations (funds come from the community trust's budget and compete directly with other community services: delays in decision-making and the 'drying up' of funds are common problems); (c) maintenance and redecoration are the trust's responsibility; unless covered by prior agreement the timing can be a source of dispute between GPs and their landlord	Design is in the hands of the GP and his architect; Alterations are easier to make (and can be covered by improvement grants and the cost-rent scheme); Maintenance decisions are in the hands of the Principals
4	Staff employment	Staff may be shared with the community trust by joint appointment or entirely employed by the practice. If they are on the trust payroll, the administrative burden of calculating and paying salaries is borne by the trust, but the GPs sacrifice control over their activities and may find themselves in dispute with the trust over shared staff	The GP hires and fires his own staff and has control over their wage levels and work activities
5	Running costs	A service charge is set by the trust; this varies considerably and GPs may find themselves in dispute over the level set	These are more directly under the control of the GPs and dependent on their management policies. They are usually higher than those of average Health Centres
6	Allowed use of premises	At present virtually unrestricted, except that if private work comprises more than 10% of total income, reimbursements are reduced in proportion and stopped if 50% is private. However, since the property is not owned by the partners it is conceivable that further conditions could be placed upon its use	As for Health Centres (although security of future use is possibly greater)

2 There is a duplication of administrative and running expenses which drains practice profits (unless GPs dispense from branch surgeries the net result is usually a financial loss).

3 Various practical problems are posed, e.g.:

(a) the security of largely unattended premises with drug stocks and confidential records;

(b) how to run an appointment system and staff the premises;

(c) where to house paper clinical records.

4 They cannot be closed save by permission of the HA. Since branch surgeries are jealously defended by consumers and local communities, it often proves difficult for doctors to terminate this responsibility once they have undertaken to provide it.

1.2 THE PEOPLE

Recruiting staff

When a vacancy occurs, the following steps need to be taken:

1 A *review*—does the post need to be filled?

2 The preparation of:

(a) a *job description* (main function, task and scope of job);

(b) a *profile* of the person required (e.g. qualifications and experience, potential, personal qualities, commitment).

3 A search for applicants—this can be:

(a) by word of mouth (this is cheap and simple, and draws in candidates with local ties and loyalties, but may pose problems if dismissal or confidentiality become issues);

(b) by advertisement (e.g. local newspaper);

(c) by checking with local colleges and career services. (Application forms add to administrative costs and lengthen the selection procedure but do allow direct comparison of applications.)

4 *Short-listing*—should someone carry out a preliminary sift?

5 The *interview*—establish beforehand:

(a) Who is on the interview panel?

(b) What points do they want to clarify/cover?

(c) Who will ask the questions?

Avoid interruptions, insufficient time and repetition of questions. The London Business School recommends a formal approach:

- draw up a checklist of desirable qualities;
- allocate particular questions pertaining to this list to particular interviewers in advance;
- ask candidates similar questions, at least some of the time, so that the answers can be directly compared;
- score the candidates' answers as they are given: this allows some objective comparison to be made.

6 *After the interview*—if in doubt, defer the appointment. Otherwise:

(a) confirm the job offer by letter (stipulating the starting date and the main headings of the contract to follow);

(b) plan an induction period and an induction plan for the new employee;

(c) produce a contract (as outlined below).

Employees' rights

Contracts

1 More than 50% of GPs fail to issue their employees with a contract, presumably because they forget, or it takes too much time, or they feel it is formal and intrusive.

2 Legally, as employers, they should provide for any employee working more than 8 hours per week a written statement of the main employment terms within 2 calendar months of commencement.

3 The contract must include certain items, including:

(a) the names of the parties;

(b) the job title;

(c) the date of commencement and continuity of contract;

(d) the place of work;

(e) a statement of hours, pay and holiday;

(f) a statement of sick pay and pension;

(g) a statement of notice, grievance and disciplinary procedures.

4 Even where there is no legal obligation to provide a contract it is still advisable, in anticipation of possible future labour management disagreements.

5 Where no *written* contract exists, the law may still deem a *verbal* contract to exist and interprets its conditions on the basis of precedence and practice.

Employment law

This is a very complex field, with frequently changing legislation. The *principles*, however, change more slowly, and are described in Table 1.2.

Staff finances

Reimbursements

The Red Book makes provision for the reimbursement of the major part of the expense of employing staff. Prior to 1990 the following costs were reimbursed for qualifying staff (an approved quota performing approved duties):

1 70% of salary paid (less any Statutory Sick Pay paid);

2 100% of the employer's National Insurance (NI) contributions;

3 contributions paid by the employer to the NHS or certain private superannuation schemes;

4 70% of the costs incurred in approved extra-practice training of staff.

Following changes to GPs' contractual terms these reimbursement

Table 1.2 The main principles of employment law.

		Rights	Conditions
1	Notice	To receive a minimum period of notice	After 4 weeks' employment: also an employee's obligation after 4 weeks to serve a minimum notice
2	Contract	To receive a contract	Within 2 months (if employed for $\geqslant 8\,$h/week)
3	Pay statement	To receive an itemised pay statement, including all deductions	
4	Time off	To have reasonable time off for: (a) approved trade union duties; (b) certain public duties; (c) to look for a new job if redundancy is impending; (d) antenatal care	Unpaid Unpaid After a minimum period of employment Employers can demand certification of pregnancy (form FW8), and proof of antenatal appointments
5	Discrimination	The right not to be: (a) discriminated against on grounds of sex or race; (b) unfairly dismissed; (c) discriminated against because of union activities (or to be forced to join a trade union)	
6	Redundancy	To receive redundancy pay	After 2 years (if employed $\geqslant 8\,$h/week). Pay is based on a statutory formula. (The employer can claim a rebate of half this from the State Redundancy Payment Fund and the balance from the HA)
7	Maternity	The right to: (a) keep one's job;	No dismissal on grounds of pregnancy or childbirth alone, irrespective of length of service or weekly working hours
		(b) receive maternity leave;	Minimum leave of 14 weeks with benefits of employment preserved Claimants must furnish written notice of maternity leave and a certificate of expected confinement (form Mat BI)
		(c) receive maternity pay;	Statutory Maternity Pay is payable for 18 weeks to women with 26 weeks of continuous service who have made qualifying NI contributions. The cost can be recovered from the DSS. (Employers can pay more than the statutory rate if they choose)
		(b) return to work after maternity	The same conditions as for (b) above. In addition: • 3 weeks' written notice of intention to return; • a postnatal time limit of 29 weeks (for those employed at least 2 years)

Continued on p. 8

Table 1.2 *Continued*

		Rights	Conditions
8	Safety	Health and safety at work rights place on the employer several obligations:	
		(a) to display a statement of safety policy;	If five or more ancillary staff are employed
		(b) 'so far as reasonably practicable' to ensure a safely maintained workplace;	
		(c) to notify certain categories of accident to the Health and Safety Executive;	e.g. hospital admission for more than 24 h and major fractures
		(d) to keep an accident book;	
		(e) to take out insurance against accidents to staff, and to display the insurance certificate. (The Health and Safety Executive inspectors have the power to enter and inspect premises to ensure they comply with the Health and Safety at Work Act)	
9	Statutory Sick Pay (SSP)	Employers are responsible for paying SSP to employees who have made qualifying class 1 National Insurance contributions	For first 28 weeks
10	Pensions	Obligatory to offer full-time employees either the State Pension Scheme or an approved private one	Part-time staff rarely qualify for an occupational pension; state entitlement depends on qualifying NI contributions

arrangements exist only for staff who were in post on 1 April 1990. For replacements and new appointees fresh conditions apply. Reimbursements are still available in these cost categories, as well as for redundancy payments and absences for 'reasonable' holiday, sickness, maternity leave and training. But:

1   The extent of approval and degree of reimbursement are at the discretion of the HA, and are said to depend on the HA's:

   (a) perception of need;

   (b) own development strategies, budget and priorities;

   (c) evaluation of the proposed job description (role, objectives, contractual and training needs) and job candidates (minimum qualifications and experience).

2   Decisions on these discretionary reimbursements can be reviewed at intervals of no less than 3 years.

All GP principals are eligible (whether part-time or full-time). No quota system operates, nor is there a stipulation regarding the type of staff or their activities, other than that there should be local approval.

Prior to these changes, the subsidy was underused (in 1984 each GP in the UK employed the equivalent of only 1.06 full-time ancillaries against a quota maximum of 2 per head). The removal of qualifying restrictions was trumpeted as a move to encourage more staff and a wider range of duties while at the same time targeting more precisely according to need and in the light of local job markets. However, indications at the first 3-year review were that the converse had transpired: reimbursements had fallen because of competing claims for limited funds.

Salaries
1   A good guide to the minimum acceptable pay levels is provided by the appropriate Whitley Council rates paid to HA employees doing the same jobs. (Arguably the rate should be higher, since HA employees receive an index-linked pension, and a good sick pay scheme, whereas relatively few GPs make these provisions for their staff.)
2   As an employer, the GP is obliged to deduct income tax and class 1 NI contributions before giving employees the balance of their pay. The deduction is calculated using NI contribution and tax tables; then, on or before the 14th day following the end of the month, a cheque is submitted to the tax collector including total tax and staff and employer's NI contributions. The reimbursement of salary and employer's NI contributions is claimed quarterly from the HA.

The health visitor
Qualifications and training
1   Always SRN.
2   Often state-certified midwife as well.
3   Must possess:
    (a) an approved obstetric certificate;
    (b) a health visitor's certificate (obligatory).
4   Must undertake a year's full-time study in preventive and social medicine and human development to obtain the health visitor's certificate.

Employers
•   Employed by the HA and accountable to the nursing managers.
•   Attached to nearly all practices (Cartwright & Anderson 1981).

Possible roles
The health visitor has a very broad potential brief, which includes some *statutory* duties.
1   Postnatal home visiting: this is a statutory duty from the day the midwife stops attending (usually the 10th day), and follow-up usually continues until the child attends school; the function is to educate and support the mother in basic baby care, common postnatal

problems and minor childhood illness and developmental milestones. Similar advice is offered at child health clinics.

2   Child developmental and screening work, undertaken in the
home or at the child health clinic, and including simple tests of sight,
hearing and development.

3   Case work — the specific surveillance and support of at-risk
groups, e.g.:

  (a) single-parent families;
  (b) cases of potential non-accidental injury;
  (c) the handling of children with emotional and behavioural
  problems, or physical and mental handicap;
  (d) marital counselling.

4   Preventive work and health education:

  (a) immunisations;
  (b) health education (including antenatal/parentcraft and relaxation classes, weight-watching groups, etc.);
  (c) visiting/screening the elderly;
  (d) family planning advice.

5   Advisory and liaison work:

  (a) advice on local resources, e.g. mother and toddler groups, day
  nurseries, self-help groups;
  (b) advice on home safety, home helps, welfare benefits; liaison
  with GP and social worker.

Workload

In practice the work is mainly with the *young* and much less with the
elderly; for example in one study:

- 65% of the clientele were under 5 years old;
- 13% were over 65 years old;
- although these two groups commanded nearly 80% of the health
visiting caseload, they represented only 20% of the practice
population.

There is, however, a new and growing breed of health visitor with
a special interest and expertise in the elderly, the geriatric health
visitor, whose role may have to expand to meet the needs of the
increasing elderly population.

The community nurse

Qualifications and training

1   Usually RGN or District EN.

2   RGNs require a Degree in District Nursing, although many practising community nurses hold a Diploma under earlier qualifying
arrangements.

3   DENs require the National Certificate in District Nursing (DEN).

Employers

- Employed by the HA and accountable to the nursing managers.

- More recently community fundholding budgets have enabled practices to directly employ their own community nurses.
- *Attached* to nearly all practices (Cartwright & Anderson 1981).

Possible roles

There is a broad potential overlap with other members of the primary health care team but the natural training and experience of the district nurse favour clinical nursing in the community above other roles.

1 General nursing care including:
    (a) prevention of pressure sores;
    (b) bowel care and catheter care;
    (c) treatments, e.g. injections and dressings;
    (d) venepuncture;
    (e) rehabilitation, etc.

2 A special role in the care of the elderly, disabled and terminally ill. In addition to general nursing care (above) this includes:
    (a) psychological support to patients and family;
    (b) mobilisation of resources, e.g. incontinence aids, commodes, ripple beds, night nursing and bath nurses, etc.

3 Assessment, referral and liaison work:
    (a) with GP, health visitor and social worker;
    (b) advice to patients on local resources and voluntary associations.

4 Preventive work, e.g.:
    (a) monitoring at-risk groups by home visiting;
    (b) health advice;
    (c) influenza vaccinations.

5 Assistance in the surgery's treatment room (with any of the tasks listed below under **The practice nurse**).

Workload

In practice 95% of the community nurse's time is spent in practical nursing and only 5% in educational work. Much of the caseload comprises the elderly, chronically sick and severely disabled.

The practice nurse

Qualifications and training

There is no fixed or standard requirement. The practice, as the employing body, can choose according to its own needs and from the local material available. However, the specialty of practice nursing has recently been recognised by the UK Central Council for Nursing, Midwifery and Health Visiting, and there now exists a Degree in Practice Nursing. Most practice nurses are experienced RGNs who value part-time work, fixed hours and general practice-based responsibilities. Many now have family planning training.

Employers

Employed by practice principals.

Possible roles

The role of the practice nurse depends in part on personal interests, confidence and experience, and also on the degree of responsibility and freedom encouraged by the GP employers. At one extreme is the nurse-practitioner, who sees and vets minor illness, provides an alternative appointment system for the patient and refers to the GP at her discretion. Whatever the degree of freedom allowed, the GP remains ultimately responsible for the practice nurse's decisions and must take steps to ensure that:

- the nurse is adequately trained for the job;
- the boundaries of responsibility are defined and understood.

The most commonly performed tasks are:

1 Basic nursing procedures, e.g. dressings, venepuncture, injections, immunisations, basic observations (weight, blood pressure, urine testing), suture removal, ear syringing, taking swabs, etc.

2 The management of minor accidents.

3 The management of minor illness.

4 Special clinics (e.g. wart clinics, diabetic clinics, hypertensive and well-woman clinics).

5 Pill checks and taking cervical smears (family planning trained nurses).

6 Assistance with various procedures (e.g. intrauterine device fitting, minor surgery, insurance medicals, ECG recordings).

7 Regulation of treatment room stock and other paperwork (e.g. filling in item-of-service claims).

8 Health promotion and advice.

9 New patient consultations and over 75s assessments (see p. 44).

10 Limited prescribing. Recent regulations allow suitably qualified nurses to prescribe prescription-only medicines from the *Nurses' Prescribing Formulary*, provided that they have attended an ENB-run nurse prescribing course. Pilot exercises are planned in some 500 practices in 1998.

Advantages of employing a practice nurse

1 The service is relatively inexpensive. Part of the salary may be reimbursable and the remainder allowable against tax. Increased income from item-of-service work undertaken in the treatment room and health promotion and disease management clinics may help to pay the difference.

2 Nurses are said to be better than GPs in following clinic protocols, and may thus achieve more by running them.

3 It saves the GP's time, leaving him free to do other work.

4 Patients express a high level of satisfaction with the facility and appreciate it (e.g. Murray *et al.* 1993).

5   The service can be very effective. Marsh *et al.* (1995) trained their nurse to manage minor illness, and offered an appointment with her to patients requesting same-day consultations. Eighty-nine per cent of those seen in the ensuing 6 months were dealt with by the nurse alone; and 79% did not present again through the same illness episode. It was concluded that a lot of minor illness in general practice can be managed by an appropriately trained nurse.

Disadvantages
1   Practice nurses need adequate training which the GP may have to provide, especially when the nurses are asked to take on new responsibilities.
2   There is a problem in defining the boundaries of responsibility—a GP who delegates must live with the possibility that he may, at some time, be answerable for someone else's error. GPs are liable for the acts and omissions of their staff, and mishap arising from ill-considered delegation may be punished by the General Medical Council (GMC). It is difficult to provide a fail-safe referral policy that covers all possible circumstances. The GP must also satisfy himself that the correct decisions are being made without appearing to question his colleague's professional competence — this is a difficult balance to achieve and the relationship hinges on it.
3   The facility may generate more work when its convenience is appreciated. In particular, patients may use the practice nurse to bypass the appointment system, then causing the GP's surgery to be interrupted because it transpires a doctor's opinion was required.
4   If a practice nurse is employed, this generally means (because of the limited quota of reimbursable salaries) that one fewer receptionist is employed.

Trends
Through the 1980s an expansion was seen in the number of practice-employed nurses because they held two clear advantages over community nurses in the treatment room:
1   The GP had tighter control over their activities when he was the employer than when they were answerable to the HA.
2   It circumvented the awkward problem of asking HA-paid nurses to undertake item-of-service work, the profits of which went to the practice.

The introduction of the 1990 GP Contract fuelled extra demand, as doctors were hard pressed to meet the various health promotion targets and well-person assessments. In consequence between 1985 and 1991 the number of practice nursing whole-time equivalents rose six-fold.

Some authorities believe the trend should continue, and that the practice nurse's role should be expanded, to offset current recruitment difficulties amongst the doctors. In future, according to some views, nurse-practitioners will be widely employed in a triage model of primary care: filtering out and treating minor illness, and referring more serious or difficult cases to their GP manager. The least that can be said is that the role of the nurse in primary care is evolving rapidly.

The practice manager
Qualifications and training
In the past, qualifications and training for practice managers have been ill defined but there are now three bodies — the Association of Medical Secretaries, Practice Administrators and Receptionists (AMSPAR); the Association of Health Centre and Practice Adminis-trators (AHCPA); and the Guild of Medical Secretaries—who provide recommendations on training. AMSPAR and AHCPA also organise diploma courses in practice administration. In general, however, it is left to the partnership's discretion to select someone of managerial pedigree. Broad requirements are:
- personal qualities such as innovative thinking, tact and sensitivity, patience and persuasiveness;
- administrative skills;
- training and experience in managing personnel, books and record-keeping, and the business side of general practice.

Pre-employment and in-service training are reimbursable (see Para. 52.8 of the Red Book).

Responsibilities
Responsibilities can and often must be delegated, but the practice manager retains overall control of six broad categories of administra-tion — staff, finances, administrative work, premises and supplies, future planning and liaison.

1 Staff:
   (a) hiring and firing;
   (b) induction and training;
   (c) rotas and holidays;
   (d) contracts;
   (e) grievances and problems.
2 Finances:
   (a) monitoring (and maximising) all sources of income;
   (b) monitoring (and controlling) all outgoings;
   (c) paying staff salaries, pensions, NI, outside bills, petty cash;
   (d) record keeping, accounts preparation, cash-flow analysis, interpreting the Red Book, etc.
3 Administration:
   (a) ensuring all forms are completed and submitted to the HA as required;
   (b) organisation of basic administrative tasks concerning records, filing, appointments, repeat prescribing, the age–sex register,

reception and office procedures, HA returns, item-of-service claims, etc.

4 Premises and supplies:
(a) stock control—stationery, forms, bottles, etc.;
(b) purchase and maintenance of equipment;
(c) maintenance of decorations, building, fixtures and fittings.

5 Future planning:
(a) monitoring activity statistics and current practices—to anticipate change or improvement;
(b) ensuring that the practice is developing towards its goals;
(c) reviewing journals for new ideas;
(d) investigating new equipment and approaches, e.g. computers, commissioning.
(e) helping to plan building changes.

6 Liaison work:
(a) consultation with staff and doctors;
(b) arranging meetings, minute-taking, circulating information, notifying others about policy changes;
(c) liaison with accountants, workmen, drug company representatives, the HA and other agencies;
(d) handling staff and public complaints (public relations work).

Computer literacy is now a prerequisite for many of these managerial tasks.

The reception staff
Qualifications and training
There are no statutory qualifications; again, personal qualities (e.g. manner, aptitude, motivation, flexibility) and experience/clerical ability are the only guidelines. Staff job descriptions are available from the Guild of Medical Secretaries and training courses through the Association of Medical Secretaries.

Responsibilities
Approximately 40% of the work involves direct patient contact. The main responsibilities are:

1 Reception duties:
(a) making new and repeat appointments;
(b) receiving and directing patients, and answering their enquiries;
(c) taking visit requests.

2 Telephone duties:
(a) answering the telephone and taking messages;
(b) operating the switchboard.

3 Filing and record duties:
(a) locating patient records for surgeries and re-filing them after use;

(b) dealing with the post;

(c) filling in claim forms and collecting fees for different certificates;

(d) registering new patients, obtaining their records from the HA and returning obsolete records;

(e) updating clinical and computer-held records (commonly one member of staff is given special responsibility in this area);

(f) administering the repeat prescribing system.

4 Numerous *general duties*, e.g.:

(a) handling waiting room problems and tidying the waiting room;

(b) maintaining and distributing stationery stocks;

(c) opening and closing the premises;

(d) delivering messages, etc.

5 Specialist secretarial duties, e.g.:

(a) shorthand dictation and typing;

(b) maintaining files and indexes;

(c) taking agendas and minutes of meetings;

(d) organising clinics and patient recall;

(e) liaison work — transport, social services, community nurse, private appointments, etc.

The social worker

Qualifications and training

Various training paths can be followed by those wishing to become social workers: courses are through colleges and universities, and are open to graduates, non-graduates and post-graduates; relevant degrees may shorten the training period; field experience is also required.

The Central Council for Education and Training in Social Work (CCETSW) currently recognises two qualifications: the Diploma in Social Medicine and the Certificate of Qualification in Social Work (CQSW) (although the latter examination has now been phased out).

Employers

Social workers are employed by Local Authority Social Services, i.e. they are independent professionals, not answerable to HAs or GPs. Their caseload therefore includes public self-referrals.

Workload

The four basic areas are:

1 Individual casework, e.g.:

(a) counselling those individuals and families with financial and personal problems;

(b) marital and bereavement counselling;

(c) counselling disturbed children and their families;

(d) follow-up and support for the mentally ill.

2 Advice and allocation of resources:
(a) home helps and meals-on-wheels;
(b) social service day-centre places;
(c) advice to the impoverished, disabled and homeless (to whom a wide range of support resources are available — home adaptations, telephone installation grants, welfare benefits, legal housing rights, voluntary and self-help groups, etc.).

3 Statutory responsibilities (and work with legal implications):
(a) supervision of children in care;
(b) supervision of adoption, fostering, childminding and day nurseries;
(c) the management of child abuse cases;
(d) the compulsory admission of mentally ill patients under the Mental Health Act (1983);
(e) responsibilities for disabled people under the Disabled Persons Act (1970).

4 Liaison work, e.g. between clients and primary care, social services, hospitals and occupational therapists.

Social work and general practice

1 There is a wide overlap in the caseloads of primary care and the Social Services Department (many patients have social and emotional problems, while many of the Social Services clientele have physical or psychological problems).

2 Despite this overlap, the relationship between social workers and GPs is infamous for its hostility and antagonism.

3 This has been explained in terms of the obvious differences of age, training and knowledge, ideology and priorities.

4 It is said that the typical GP has a stereotyped impression of social workers as: young and unqualified; constrained by bureaucracy; lacking energy and effectiveness; lacking a general practice perspective and loyalty.

The typical social worker, by contrast, perceives the average GP to be: resistive to change and blinkered in outlook; arrogant; overpaid and overrated; a prescriber when he really should be a counsellor; lacking a social worker's perspective!

5 Various attempts have been made to improve relations, basically by adopting one of two possible strategies:
(a) *attachment schemes*—in which the social worker takes referrals from GPs using practice premises as base; the social worker's commitment to practice policies outweighs his other Social Services Department commitments;
(b) *liaison schemes*—social workers visit practices at certain times and collect referrals or discuss cases; their work for the practice is second in priority to the Department's needs.

Surveys indicate that more than 50% of local authorities participate in these schemes. The liaison system is preferred by all parties because it promotes more effective communication and mutual trust and education.

6   The disadvantages of these schemes are:

(a) *to the social worker*: the risk of professional isolation, divided loyalties and abuse by GPs who refer inappropriately or use the social worker to offload their problems;

(b) *to the team*: time must be found for regular structured meetings;

(c) *to the GP*: there is a problem with confidential information — should social workers have access to clinical records?

Despite these disadvantages social workers have important skills to contribute to the GP's daily practice, so it is to be hoped that these liaison schemes will flourish.

1.3 THE RECORDS

The current state of records in general practice

Standards have traditionally been *poor*, e.g.:

1   Tulloch (1976) reviewed 400 incoming records over a 6-year period:

(a) more than 50% were not in chronological order;

(b) there was no attempt to highlight important information in 85%;

(c) less than 5% had any form of indexing;

(d) only 33% of patients taking the contraceptive pill had this fact recorded and up to 25% of records missed essential information (including open heart surgery, deep venous thromboses, renal failure and hysterectomies!).

2   Moulds (1985) reviewed 1000 new patient records coming into the practice:

(a) only 92 had letters/reports in chronological order and only nine had *all* notes in order;

(b) only 15 had summary cards;

(c) only eight had drug cards in the notes.

3   Other criticisms of records include the following:

(a) vague and firm data are mixed and diagnoses recorded without evidence;

(b) objectives are seldom noted;

(c) there is a failure to assemble all relevant factors (especially family and social histories).

Requirements of a record system

The traditional *functions* of clinical notes are several:

1   *To improve patient care*, e.g. to:

(a) make diagnoses clearer;

(b) make management decisions clearer;

(c) make follow-up more systematic, especially in chronic illness;

(d) avoid simple errors (e.g. drug interactions and sensitivities, unnecessary repetition of investigations, prescribing that is inappropriate to the patient's past history).

2   To aid communication:

(a) between doctors (especially in large group practices and those without personal list systems);

(b) in the primary care team (e.g. by keeping immunisation cards);

(c) with outside agencies (medical reports, referral letters, legal correspondence, etc.).

3   As an *aide-mémoire*:

(a) of main events in the patient's life (physical, psychological, social) and of his family;

(b) of what was said and done at the last consultation.

4   *As a tool* in:

(a) audit, research, epidemiology;

(b) teaching;

(c) planning of patient services.

5   *As a medico-legal record* (important in a climate of increasing litigation).

6   *As a means of maximising income,* by recording when items of service are undertaken and when claims are due.

Some authorities have questioned GPs' reasons for note-taking — *not* for others to read if they are largely illegible and *not* to record the consultation accurately when they often write initial remarks rather than balanced conclusions. Are these notes idiosyncratic? Are they just a personal habit?

The requirements of a good record system are:

1   A complete database.
2   Information recorded at the level of certainty.
3   Important information indexed and highlighted.
4   Clear progress notes (in order!) recording objectives.

Improving clinical records

Many doctors now feel that the minimum requirements are:

1   Continuation cards in chronological order—treasury-tagged.
2   Hospital letters and reports arranged likewise.
3   Pruning of irrelevant, duplicated and illegible material.
4   A summary card.
5   A drug record card for patients on repeat prescriptions.
6   An immunisation/vaccination card.
7   Tagging of the record envelopes with colour-tags, e.g.: blue — hypertension; brown—diabetes; yellow—epilepsy; red—drug sensitivity; green—tuberculosis; white—long-term maintenance; black—attempted suicide; chequered—measles.

Useful additions to the notes include:

1 A card to summarise the patient's personal, social and family history.

2 Flow sheets for specific conditions (e.g. graphical records of blood pressure or blood sugar control on hypertensive or diabetic record cards; cards covering the geriatric, new registration and periodic medicals).

3 Highlighting of investigations and diagnoses (e.g. by writing investigations in red and marking diagnoses with a box).

Increasingly more of this information is transferred to, and retrieved from, the practice computer rather than written down, although manual and electronic systems are bound to coexist for some time to come.

The different record systems
Traditional: Lloyd George records (FP5/6)
Introduced in 1911. The commonest system. The records are the property of the Secretary of State.

1 Advantages:
  (a) pocket-sized:
  - easy to carry around on visits;
  - require less shelf storage space;
  - may encourage brevity;

  (b) it is the status quo—any change involves thousands of records and is a big administrative undertaking.

2 Disadvantages:
  (a) lack of space — leads to cramped illegible entries which may end up too brief;

  (b) hospital letters, now A4, must be folded. This leads to bulky records and a reluctance to unfold, read and refold them in consultations.

A4 records
In 1973 the DHSS agreed in principle to conversion of records to A4 but progress has been slow.

1 Advantages:
  (a) plenty of space to make entries;
  (b) better layout:
  - space for summary cards, flow sheets, etc.;
  - indexing is easy;
  - hospital letters can be filed unfolded and hence may be read more easily;
  - facilitates research and audit.

2 Disadvantages:
  (a) storage space (A4 records occupy $1^1/_2$ times more space; and almost half of GPs could not be able to accommodate them without building changes);

(b) secretarial costs of transfer (approximately one full-time secretary per principal for 2 years);

(c) the cost of stationery (£2000 for 3000 folders) has to be met by the GP (FP5/6s are free);

(d) in the transition period there would be difficulty in transferring records between practices using different systems;

(e) A4 records, by definition, do not slip readily into the pocket;

(f) more writing space may encourage verbosity!

Problem-orientated medical records (POMRs)

Proposed by Lawrence Weed (1969). There are three main ingredients:

1   Problem list (active and inactive, medical and social).

2   Background information package:

(a) fixed information, e.g. sex, date of birth, personal and family history, immunisations, etc.;

(b) changing information, e.g. marital status, job, address, screening tests, etc.

3   Progress notes (mnemonic—SOAP):

(a) *subjective*—the patient's observations;

(b) *objective*—the doctor's observations and tests;

(c) *analysis*—the doctor's understanding of the problem;

(d) *plans* — goals, further information needed, action, advice to patient.

- Advantages:

(a) encourages logical thought and approach; information is recorded at the level of understanding;

(b) makes records much clearer to other readers;

(c) records can easily be audited and are a better research and teaching tool;

(d) the database is more comprehensive;

(e) orderly notes allow planning of preventive care.

- Disadvantages:

(a) space and time (really needs A4 record space to avoid bulkiness);

(b) SOAP is long-winded and inappropriate for straightforward problems;

(c) it makes sensitive information clearer as well, raising worries about confidentiality.

The age–sex register

What is it?

The age–sex register formerly consisted of a series of cards (blue for males, pink for females) for every patient on the list. Each card recorded the patient's name, date of birth, address, date of entry into the register and anything else desired (e.g. last cervical smear date). The cards were filed, males and females separately, alphabetically under the year of birth. The same process is now performed more quickly, more accurately and more informatively by computer.

Uses of the age–sex register
There are four main categories of use:

1 *Screening and recall*, e.g. planning a child health surveillance clinic, an over-40s blood pressure screening clinic, home visiting for the over 75s, etc.

2 *Improving practice income*—by identifying patients who qualify for items of service separately payable. Examples might include over-25's cervical cytology or immunisations at key ages (pre-school, school entry, school leaving, rubella vaccination of all 10-year-old girls). An age–sex register also allows you to check that HA capitation payments are in accordance with the age profile and list size of the practice.

3 *Research*, e.g.:
   (a) easy to generate age–sex-matched controls, and
   (b) to identify at-risk groups by age and sex.

4 Planning, e.g. identifying changes in the age–sex structure of the practice and hence its changing needs.

Morbidity registers
Constructed to identify groups with special needs for chronic care, e.g. all practice diabetics, all patients on maintenance thyroxine.

Simple morbidity registers can be constructed:
* using tagged notes;
* from partners' memories;
* from repeat prescription cards;
* opportunistically (records passed on to the secretary for entry after the patient attends for something else);
* by manual search of all records (laborious, but obviously faster if there are summary cards);
* by computer search (the preferred method and increasingly used).

More elaborate registers include the E book. This is a loose-leaf ledger, filled in after every consultation with a code number corresponding to the diagnosis. When analysed the ledger provides comprehensive local and national morbidity statistics that assist research and planning.

Advantages
1 They allow the audit of prescribing, compliance and other measures of standards in primary care.
2 They allow the planning and implementation of change in services (e.g. by identifying special-risk groups who could benefit from preventive activities).
3 They greatly simplify research.

Disadvantages
1   Time involved (for doctors and secretarial staff).
2   The need for a high level of motivation and co-operation — they need to be maintained and all new diagnoses (hospital or surgery) need to be entered or amended.
3   Unless run on a computer system there is often a limit to the number of conditions for which registers can be set up, stored and maintained.
4   Registers cannot be guaranteed to be accurate: diagnoses are often tentative or simply wrong.

Computerised records
Because of its unique ability to shuffle and re-sort information rapidly the computerised record system is considerably more flexible than its manual counterpart. Nowadays nearly all general practices enjoy this benefit.

Uses
1   As a clinical *prompt*:
    (a) in opportunistic screening;
    (b) in long-term maintenance.
For example, appointment lists can be printed with reminders that cervical smears, blood pressure checks, tetanus vaccinations, digoxin levels, thyroxine levels or glycosylated Hbs are overdue; surveillance clinics can be organised and word-processed letters printed; geriatric home visiting lists can be drawn up, etc. Furthermore, computers can sort into 'degree of overdueness' so that with limited resources a start can be made according to priority.
2   As a source of *information*:
    (a) drug formulary information;
    (b) warning of drug interactions or contraindications;
    (c) a guide to the Red Book;
    (d) a word processor and printer of patient information pamphlets.
3   In record-keeping, e.g.:
    (a) summary cards;
    (b) age–sex registers;
    (c) morbidity registers;
    (d) patient lists.
4   As an *administrative* tool, e.g.:
    (a) computer-run repeat prescribing systems;
    (b) accounts and workload analysis;
    (c) as a claim prompt;
    (d) as a check of HA returns;
    (e) as a fundholding tool.
5   In *audit*, *research* and *epidemiology*.

Disadvantages

1   Capital costs are fairly high, although help is available from the Government (see Table 1.6, pp. 56–61).

2   Cost-effectiveness in strict financial terms has been questioned — although new stricter performance-related payments increase the computer's attractions.

3   The administrative work needed to transfer patient records on to a computer is considerable (especially since many records are not orderly to begin with).

4   Staff must be trained to use the new equipment.

5   Confidentiality of records is a source of concern. Access must be keyword protected to prevent unauthorised access; and users must be registered with the Data Protection Registrar.

6   Concern has been expressed, as practices gradually shift towards paperless processes (10% are already in this position), that electronic records may not be admissible in medico-legal proceedings. For example, a computer record could be challenged, unless unalterable or supported by an audit trail enabling alterations to be traced.

7   GPs' terms of service still require them to keep records on the forms provided by the DOH. However, duplication of records appears a wasteful effort.

8   There are also worries that technological changes are rapid and today's equipment may be tomorrow's 'white elephant', or that power cuts in an influenza epidemic may paralyse a practice, or that operator error may erase vital records!

These problems notwithstanding, the computer has become an integral feature of modern general practice. It has also had an impact on the way consultations are transacted. Sullivan and Mitchell (1995) reviewed the evidence, and concluded that consultations now tend to take longer, and result in more health promotion and doctor-initiated contact time; but in rather less social and patient-initiated contact time.

The practical considerations of choosing a computer system are considered in Section 1.4.

Access of patients to their records

Patient access to records came to the fore because of bodies like Campaign for Freedom of Information and a climate of increasing litigation and accountability. The Data Protection Act gave patients access to computerised health records, and the Access to Health Records Act 1990 accorded similar rights in the case of manual health records (see Section 7.8, p. 225).

Advantages
Advantages include:

1   Open, 'nothing to hide' approach may help patient's confidence.

2   It may improve the doctor–patient relationship (patients are on a more equal footing).

3   It may provide reassurance.
4   It may act as a reinforcing cue to the doctor's advice. ('It must be important, since he's written it in the notes.')
5   Shared understanding and more patient involvement may improve compliance.
6   Casual, prejudicial remarks are less likely to appear in the notes.
7   Factual errors can be corrected by means of mutual co-operation.
8   The Act's proponents would argue in an open society that it should be a patient's right.

Disadvantages/possible consequences
1   More questions will be raised and a lot of time used in additional explanation.
2   Patients may misinterpret the record.
3   The doctor–patient relationship may be harmed if the patient resents what is written.
4   Alternatively honest notes and honest impressions may not get written down. Doctors may feel less secure under threat of public scrutiny (and possible litigation), but lack of frankness in the notes may be to the ultimate disservice of a patient if those notes are used by another doctor.
5   The notes may create unnecessary alarm, e.g. early speculations about multiple sclerosis.
6   Problems arise with sensitive information that doctors feel it is not in their patients' best interests to read, e.g. mention of cancer.
7   Sometimes loyalties are divided — is it right that patients should read medical insurance reports without the permission of the insurance company?

Case for patient-held records
Finally, patient-held records have their advocates because:
1   up to 10% of doctor-held records get lost;
2   doctors often fail to locate notes when they most need them (e.g. out-of-hours calls, temporary residents, new registrations, soon after hospital discharge);
3   50% of patients leaving hospital do not understand their discharge diagnosis and 30% cannot name their treatment!

Repeat prescribing
The scale of repeat prescribing
Each GP issues 13 000 scripts per year (a budget per doctor of £120 000 per year). Of these, 30–50% are repeats and a majority are for the elderly, psychotropics making up a third of these drugs.

Problems
Problems with repeat prescribing include:
1   Failure to review patients properly:

(a) the drug may be inappropriate or the diagnosis questionable;
(b) the patient's needs may have changed;
(c) side-effects, interactions and problems of compliance cannot be assessed;
(d) the *illness* for which the drug was given may require review.

2 The doctor–patient boundary may be widened.
3 Repeat prescribing is time-consuming.
4 Scripts written by ancillary staff may contain errors.

Advantage

The main advantage is convenience to patients and doctors, especially in chronic illness where repeated consultations may be unnecessary.

Requirements of a good repeat prescribing system

1 Patients should receive scripts promptly, e.g. within 24 h.
2 Scripts should be accurate and error-free.
3 The system should be simple and cheap.
4 It should have a built-in recall system, clear to all.
5 It should be auditable.
6 A doctor using the records should know what the patient is taking and when last supplied.
7 A doctor should be able to gauge compliance and/or abuse.

Systems of repeat prescribing

The commonest system for repeat prescribing employs a card which the patient keeps. Pitfalls are that:
- the cards often fail to make clear how many repeats are allowable;
- patients lose their cards or turn up without them;
- points 6 and 7 above are not covered unless a duplicate record is kept in the notes.

Many practices therefore include a separate drug card in the clinical records and mark both cards when each script is issued.

There are several alternatives to this commonly used system:
1 *Computers*. Now an extremely popular option. These will:
  (a) print scripts;
  (b) indicate recall frequency;
  (c) check compliance;
  (d) carry out automatic audit;
  (e) update the records;
  (f) minimise written errors and free staff time;
  (g) warn of drug interactions and contraindications;
  (h) enable budget holding and dispensing practices to monitor drug expenditure more closely.
2 *Repeat registers* — a ledger kept at the front desk. This is easily adapted to audit and recall and is acceptable to staff (as it saves time extracting and refiling the notes) but the doctor still needs a duplicate record when he consults.

3 *Abolish repeat prescribing altogether* and see all patients. Scott (1985) and others have tried this approach and commend it. Extra consultations are needed initially, but this is partly offset by those instances in which unnecessary medication can be stopped. In appropriate cases large prescriptions (e.g. a 6-month dose) are issued each time, which actually saves the NHS money on container and dispensing fees. (Some doctors have reservations about prescribing such large stocks of drugs to patients, who could misuse them.)

Audit

There is some confusion over the expressions people use to discuss quality of care: various terms such as 'audit', 'peer review' and 'assessment' are used, and a distinction is often drawn between audit and 'research'.

Mourin (1976) defined audit as an enumeration of past events or items. According to this definition audit is essentially a counting exercise (the number of patients screened for hypertension in the last 5 years; the percentage of the target population vaccinated, etc.). In *Working for Patients* the Government defined audit as: 'the systematic critical analysis of the quality of medical care, including procedures used for diagnosis and treatment, the use of resources and the resulting outcome and quality of life for the patients'. This implies a process more active than mere counting — there should be self-improvement through standard-setting, measurement, change and remeasurement.

The scope of audit

Two major categories of activity are of consummate interest:

1 Audits of *process* (examining records, appointment books, immunisation records, to see *how* patients are being treated).

2 Audits of *outcome* (mortality, morbidity, patient satisfaction — looking at the *results* of treatment).

The exercise often takes one of several popular forms:

(a) periodic random review of clinical records (with peer group discussion);

(b) the enumeration of process variables (workload, diagnosis, referral rates, waiting times, visiting rates, use of investigative facilities) and analysis of their trends;

(c) adverse outcome reviews (a post-mortem on cases with undesirable outcomes, to see if a better result could have been achieved);

(d) outcome surveys;

(e) patient satisfaction surveys;

(f) peer group structured practice inspections (of the sort undertaken for training approval).

The principal steps of the audit cycle

The essential steps in performing an audit are to:

1 Define objectives (what needs to be measured and why).
2 Agree ideal performance standards (these may come from the consensus statements and guidelines of expert bodies or, where available, the conclusions of formal clinical trials).
3 Define methods (how the data are to be collected and analysed).
4 Perform the audit.
5 Compare the outcome with performance criteria.
6 Agree and implement change—to bring expected and actual performance closer together.
7 Repeat steps **4–6**, remeasuring and improving until the agreed standards are achieved.

This is the so-called virtuous cycle (Fig. 1.1). Steps **4–7** are essential to 'close the feedback loop' and to effect beneficial change. In theory this should be continuous and never-ending.

Audit comes of age

Doctors generally accept and the Government now requires that self-improvement through self-examination should be an everyday part of medical practice. More specifically:

• the GMC document *Duties of a Doctor* describes audit as an essential professional responsibility;
• the Royal Colleges and Faculties require evidence of audit when accrediting posts for specialist training;
• Medical Audit Advisory Groups (MAAGs) exist to assist the process (see Chapter 9).

Cost, benefits and problems of audit in general practice

There are some basic problems with general practice research:

• GPs deal in small patient numbers;
• studies tend to be descriptive rather than fundamental;
• scientific controls are often not possible;
• insufficient knowledge of natural history, placebo effects and clinician bias lead to shortcomings when audit is compared with more formal research.

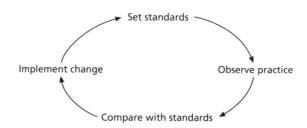

Set standards

Implement change

Observe practice

Compare with standards

Figure 1.1 The audit cycle.

Critics have complained that audit is limited, local and parochial. Patterson (1985), however, points out in its defence that — provided honest, cautious and realistic conclusions are drawn — it shares in common with formal research important beneficial characteristics:
- the promotion of logical thought;
- the need for a rational and controlled approach;
- the quest for rational policies;
- the opportunity to define a starting point for wider thought.

In practice several other benefits have been forthcoming, e.g.:
- improved standards of medicine;
- improved morale;
- improved income;
- improvements in practice management and planning of patient services.

Several costs need to be counted as well. Audit demands:
- time and effort;
- commitment (which may not be shared equally in a partnership);
- a willingness to be inspected;
- a receptive attitude to constructive criticism and the flexibility to change.

Notwithstanding these points, over the last 25 years research and audit in primary care have helped to fill in many gaps in our knowledge, and have fostered in GPs a new willingness to improve by self-examination. The Royal College of General Practitioners has been an instrumental force in this spirit of change.

The problem of measuring quality of care is considered in Section 4.11 and the ethical aspects of medical research are covered in Section 7.11.

1.4 THE EQUIPMENT

In the MRCGP exam viva, reference may be made to the equipment the candidate's practice possesses. Note that you are expected not only to be familiar with your own practice's selection and the use made of it, but with the full range of possibilities and what other practices do. Also be critical of its value—does it really make a difference to your management? If your practice were to be given a lump sum by a local charity, which equipment purchase would receive priority?

An example: ECG machine
Many practices have an ECG machine, which may be used for:
- the diagnosis of acute chest pain;
- the assessment of an irregular pulse or palpitations;
- screening hypertensives for left heart strain;
- investigating confusional states, shock, collapse or breathlessness.

Its advantages appear to be:

- high patient convenience (rapid access to a service in their own surgery);
- savings to the overworked local ECG department (and NHS budget);
- doctor satisfaction: more complete personal care and preservation of previously acquired skills through use.

However, there are disadvantages as well:

- high capital expense;
- machines that are either not robust enough or that are robust but bulky and non-portable;
- running costs (ECG paper, servicing);
- ECGs are time-consuming for doctors or practice nurses to take;
- expertise is needed to read ECGs — could a GP be liable if he missed something important? Does he do enough to maintain his skills?

Does an ECG alter management?

1 In myocardial infarctions? In chest pain at home this is open to some question, since machines are not very portable, delays in transfer to hospital may be unacceptable and decisions can be made on clinical probability (10% of myocardial infarctions do not show typical ECG changes anyway) and the clinical state of the patient. One notable exception may be in the confirmation of diagnosis prior to early thrombolytic therapy. However, the decision on whether to administer such treatment in the community or to transfer the patient speedily to hospital is itself the subject of debate and study (see Section 4.7), and may depend on whether or not hospital care is close at hand.

2 In hypertension? — certainly, evidence of end-organ damage would make treatment more important. Also ECGs are more sensitive than chest X-rays in detecting left ventricular hypertrophy (and this is much cheaper for the NHS if practices do them). However, the yield may be small and largely confined to difficult cases bound for the outpatient department anyway.

3 In arrhythmias? Assuming a doctor has the expertise to read these difficult ECGs and then the expertise to treat them, a practice ECG machine is valuable. It may also be easier for patients with paroxysmal arrhythmias to get to a practice machine at the time than to a hospital one.

The pros and cons of possessing a practice ECG machine can be debated. Other equipment should also be considered critically, especially for the purposes of an exam viva.

Computers

The following points should be considered in selecting and installing a computer system:

1 *Requirements*. With several suppliers to choose from, the General

Medical Services Council (GMSC) has emphasised that doctors should think carefully before taking the plunge:

(a) is there the capacity to extend the system if requirements grow?

(b) is the supply company of adequate financial standing?

(c) does it provide a suitable after-sales service?

(d) will the system satisfy the demands of fundholding and item of service targets?

Broadly speaking it should be able to:

(a) check capitation lists;

(b) identify populations attracting target payments;

(c) monitor immunisation, cytology and new-patient registration take-up;

(d) operate a repeat prescribing system (ideally monitoring prescribing patterns);

(e) log practice activities (referrals, investigations, admissions) to assist in audit and compilation of the practice report;

(f) generate word-processed correspondence.

The support software for computers in fundholding practices need to meet qualifying standards which are re-examined annually.

2 *Selection.* The Government intends soon to limit reimbursements to computer equipment systems that comply with national guidelines, it wishes to establish an NHS-wide linked network, and inevitably selection will be influenced by this consideration. However, in practical terms partners should:

(a) decide on what functions are required;

(b) short-list systems matching their criteria;

(c) obtain a demonstration (or visit other practices with computers already installed);

(d) establish what training, support and updating facilities are available;

(e) obtain quotes and investigate financial options (bank loans, leasing, rental, HA reimbursements, etc.);

(f) select a system and agree an installation date.

Each HA has a computer facilitator who can provide useful advice.

3 *Installation:*

(a) identify sites which are clean and dry, ventilated, not subject to extremes of temperature and humidity, out of direct sunlight, yet accessible to a power source and convenient to staff;

(b) provide adequate desk space;

(c) remember that central processing unit-based tasks (disk housekeeping) need peace and quiet, whereas terminals need to be in the midst of the action;

(d) make provision for insurance and security;

(e) consult and train the staff at every stage (experts recommend appointing a computer key worker with special responsibilities);

(f) establish a working database:

- either manually from Lloyd George envelopes (very time-consuming);
- or by down-loading computerised HA age–sex data on to the computer (quicker, but the HA register is believed to have an error rate of up to 25% and needs to be checked against the practice age–sex register). This step is very labour-intensive.

4 *Reimbursements* — part of the cost of installing new computer equipment may be reimbursed (see Section 1.6).

Other equipment

1 *Nebulizers* are unquestionably valuable but are they safe in all circumstances? Their indications and disadvantages need to be defined.

2 *Glucometers* are quite expensive and their accuracy, when compared with a laboratory blood sugar, is very much dependent on reproducible technique: can a practice process enough samples on a regular basis to obtain meaningful results? (The same can be said of haemoglobinometers.)

3 *Audiology equipment* — many practices that possess audiometers and ECG machines find that they use the former more often (although if home thrombolytic treatment becomes fashionable the situation may change).

4 *Peak flow* meters—simple, cheap and very useful, e.g.:
   (a) to establish a diagnosis of reversible airways disease;
   (b) to establish the severity;
   (c) to establish the benefits of treatment;
   (d) to monitor daily patterns (and hence assess night-time control and the occupational element);
   (e) to alert patients at an early stage to the need to see a doctor.
But peak flow meters have some limitations as well, e.g.:
   (a) they cannot be used by young children and often not in the elderly;
   (b) even after careful instruction some patients cannot master the technique and give unreliable readings;
   (c) the more mobile mini-meters are not quite as accurate and not so durable.

In conclusion, if your practice has equipment, ask how it is used, whether it helps and whether there are any shortcomings, pitfalls or problems with it. Be aware of what others do too.

1.5 THE MANAGEMENT

Management and teamwork
Principles of teamwork
According to Gilmore the characteristics of teamwork are:

1 The members *share a common purpose* which binds them together and guides their actions.
2 Each member understands his own function, the contribution of other professions and their common interests.
3 The team works by pooling knowledge, skills and resources, and shares the responsibility for outcome.

Other authors also emphasise the importance in effective teamwork of:

- Pooling;
- Delegation;
- Specialisation of function;
- Multidisciplinary discussion and peer group support.

Advantages and disadvantages

In principle the patient should gain from the co-ordinated action of specialists with a common plan, and effective teamwork should bring harmony, order and a group of self-supporting workers. However, there are practical problems as well:

1 Teamwork needs time and frequent meetings. This may encroach on the time needed for face-to-face patient care.
2 It requires commitment and agreement.
3 There is a danger that no one person will accept overall responsibility (the so-called 'collusion of anonymity' described by Balint 1957); alternatively, if one member assumes overall charge (primacy) there is a danger that personal status and pecking order will diminish the team's harmony and effectiveness.
4 There is a problem of size: large teams contribute more skills and viewpoints, but dilute and delay decision-making and make communication more difficult.
5 Primary health care teams suffer the problems common to any group of workers—jealousies, prejudices, fears of exploitation or discrimination, peer group rivalry and competition. In particular, differences in training, status and remuneration have traditionally been a disruptive influence. Good will and a desire to get on are the most important elements of teamwork.

Management models

Management models vary between two possible extremes:

1 In the *egalitarian* model primacy and pecking order are minimised and equality of personal status is encouraged.
2 In the *hierarchical* model primacy is clear-cut and the chain of authority is clearly and rigidly defined.

Both extremes (and shades in between) exist in general practice; both have their advocates and may be appropriate in different contexts. A hierarchical management system is commonest in practice, because under his Terms of Service the GP assumes the ultimate responsibility for outcome.

Certain ground rules aid the task of management:

1   The decision-making process should be clearly defined and not haphazard.
2   Important rules (and the reasons for them) should be known to all.
3   The processes of information-sharing, feedback and grievance-airing should be encouraged.

Practice meetings

It is all too easy for busy doctors to concentrate on clinical problems while neglecting longer-term plans. Practice meetings serve several purposes:

1   To ensure that necessary decisions are made.
2   To review policies and agree standards of care.
3   To improve communication and morale.
4   To review budgetary provisions.
5   To make contact with team members.
6   To educate and inform (e.g. by holding journal clubs).

Regular meetings are especially important when the team is large or has a lot to discuss.

The steps involved in organising a practice meeting are:

1   to define its purpose;
2   and hence its agenda and participants;
3   then to make decisions, draw conclusions and communicate them effectively;
4   to identify necessary action and those responsible for doing it. Then to give feedback to the next meeting on the outcome.

Experienced campaigners advocate a formal agenda, such as: apologies for absence; minutes of the previous meeting; matters arising; items for discussion; any other business. Someone should act as chairperson and someone should record the minutes.

There are potential benefits from this chore:
• groups in discussion often reach better decisions than an individual would acting alone;
• communication is more efficient and complete, avoiding the piecemeal approach.

Increasingly GPs have to host or attend meetings that involve outside parties (e.g. in co-operatives, multifunds or purchasing consortia). Clear communication and a systematic approach assume even greater importance when the agenda is complex, the participants know one another only slightly and the decisions difficult to make!

Personal lists?

At present the majority (more than three-quarters) of GPs adopt a shared or combined list system. Under this system, while the patients' wishes are accommodated wherever possible and doctors try to follow up illness episodes themselves, patients have the freedom to choose a new doctor at every consultation and the practice has the freedom to direct patients and visits to doctors in a way that spreads the workload and speeds the throughput.

In personal list systems, by contrast, the aim is for patients to stay with the same doctor as closely as the system will allow and on a long-term basis.

The merits of the two systems have been much debated and the principal arguments are summarised below.

Advantages
1   To the patient:
(a) he sees the same doctor each time — he can therefore get to know him and to choose a doctor whose qualities suit and inspire confidence in him;
(b) he also feels the doctor knows and understands his particular problems; unnecessary repetition is avoided; polypharmacy and outright errors are minimised;
(c) the patient is more likely to receive consistent information, and the doctor to implement a consistent plan—this may facilitate compliance;
(d) patients who call late or have a difficult problem or personality are not passed around from partner to partner.
2   To the doctor:
(a) he gets to know the patient and his problems and this eventually saves time; he is more likely to understand the real reason for consultation and to judge the urgency/necessity of visit requests;
(b) he does not inherit patients who are 'shopping around', or patients who have been managed by a colleague in a way that he finds he disagrees with;
(c) assuming similar list sizes, it encourages approximate equality of workload;
(d) the doctor gets more feedback on his performance, which may promote higher standards and professional satisfaction;
(e) personal care may promote a better doctor–patient relationship and more mutual tolerance (and hopefully less complaint and litigation!).
3   To ancillary staff: they know which doctor to speak to; responsibility is clearly defined and there is no argument.

Disadvantages
1   To the patient:
(a) it makes it harder to 'sample' all the doctors and make an informed choice;
(b) it removes his choice in individual appointments—in practice patients may wish to take particular problems to a member of their own sex; some prefer to take an embarrassing problem to a strange doctor and others to a familiar one: should they not have this choice?

(c) doctors may get stuck in a groove and a second opinion occasionally helps; sometimes different doctors within a practice offer different skills and referral to a partner who, for example, injects varicose veins, may save an outpatient visit;

(d) waiting times for appointments may be lengthened. This is frustrating to a patient with a straightforward problem and no particular doctor preference.

2 To the doctor:

(a) the vagaries of demand may mean an uneven workload, day-to-day, with one doctor inundated with appointments and visits, and another empty-handed;

(b) to be effective:

- a doctor must make himself personally available as much as possible, e.g. he should field the late calls that could go to the duty doctor in a combined list system;
- he should minimise all outside commitments, e.g. assistantships, committee posts, etc.

This represents some sacrifice of personal freedom and ties doctors to a telephone.

(c) personal-list doctors are less aware of their colleagues' working patterns and will learn less from them; their experiences can only be shared in general terms; practice policies are harder to implement; professional isolation may be increased.

3 To the ancillary staff:

(a) personal lists sometimes mean uneven waiting times for puzzled and therefore irate patients—the brunt of this is borne by the receptionist;

(b) it is difficult for training practices to provide trainees with a personal list.

Recent changes in general practice (such as out-of-hours co-operatives, minor surgery and paediatric lists, chronic disease clinics and the tendency within practices of partners to develop specialist interests) have made it more difficult to sustain the personal list ideal, as the present structure of general practice is more item-centred than patient-centred.

Out-of-hours services

The demand for out-of-hours (evening, night and weekend) visits in general practice is rising. Between 1967 and 1976 the national rate of night visit claims rose from 4.3 per 1000 population to 10.1 per 1000 (Buxton *et al.* 1977); and by 1981 in one health district had reached 15.5 per 1000 (Sheldon *et al.* 1984). In parallel, casualty departments have seen an approximate doubling in new attendance rates, with many primary care problems presenting directly to them.

Over this period GPs typically spent less time on call. In a 1989 national survey nearly a third reported no regular personal night cover duties (Hallam 1992), and deputies carried out 46% of all night visits.

In 1992 the GMSC conducted a ballot on out-of-hours arrangement. Among 23 000 respondents, 82% felt it should be possible to opt out of 24-h patient responsibility, and three-quarters expressed a wish to do so. (The problem of an ever-growing out-of-hours workload was held to be of primary importance in the low morale and recruitment problems reported by GPs.)

Discussions with the Department of Health eventually led to an agreement that GPs could transfer their out-of-hours responsibility to another GP on the HA's list, if they could find a substitute. The responsibility for errors and omissions could be passed on too (formerly GPs could be held responsible for the mistakes of their deputies). The DOH recognised that new patterns of out-of-hours care provision were needed, and it established a 'development' fund to encourage innovative solutions (see below).

By 1996 two-thirds of GPs were no longer regularly doing their own night and weekend work. The most common alternative arrangements were:

- deputising services (44% of GPs); and
- out-of-hours co-operatives (35% — 11 000 GPs in some 120 co-operatives).

Deputising services

Traditionally doctors have entertained mixed views about these services:

1 Some studies indicate that 80% of users have found care 'satisfactory'.

2 But in 1981 at least 52% of doctors felt deputising to be a *disadvantage* to patients (Cartwright and Anderson).

The public image of deputising services is poor:

1 In the past some deputising services have clearly employed staff with inadequate experience.

2 Medical disasters involving deputising services have been given prominent press coverage, causing the public to react with predictable concern.

3 A questionnaire by Sawyer and Arber (1982) tried to quantify feelings:

    (a) 94% of patients were satisfied if seen by their own doctor;

    (b) 91% were satisfied if seen by a doctor who knew the practice;

    (c) 58% were satisfied when deputising was used.

Recurring worries were:

    (a) lack of relationship, trust and familiarity;

    (b) concern that their past medical history was not known;

    (c) greater difficulty in contacting deputies;

    (d) deputies with a poor command of English.

4   Other surveys of the time also indicated a preference for non-deputising arrangements.

Advantages

1   The personal freedom of doctors to enjoy a social life out of hours and escape the pressures of work at antisocial times. This creates less personal and family strain in a profession already showing signs of it (higher than average rates of alcoholism, drug abuse and suicide).

2   (Arguably) a better standard of care in the 97–99% of daytime consultations since doctors are fresh, alert, motivated and refreshed by a break.

3   Deputies who start the night-shift fresh may make better decisions than tired doctors who have already worked a full day.

4   The personal availability of deputising doctors is high: surveys suggest they are likely to respond to a call by visiting, while the GP is more likely to give telephone advice.

5   Deputies can provide cover under difficult practice circumstances (e.g. for the single-hander in need of an annual holiday; prolonged sickness in a small practice).

Disadvantages

1   Patients mistrust and are dissatisfied with deputising (and this may affect their compliance).

2   There is a risk of inadequately qualified deputies.

3   There is no continuity of care—patients are all unfamiliar and there is limited or no access to their notes. It has therefore been suggested that deputies:

   (a) make more errors;

   (b) refer and treat inappropriately;

   (c) have a tendency to visit, prescribe and refer more when patients are unknown—this involves unnecessary repetition and may also encourage patients to be less independent in the longer term; it also overuses hospital resources;

   (d) because they lack personal knowledge of the patient, deputies often fail to appreciate the hidden agenda—the real reason for the call—so the problem is deferred but not resolved.

4   Deputising incurs some sacrifice of earnings.

5   Many bodies oppose deputising on principle. The standing of general practice may be damaged if others believe, rightly or wrongly, that standards are being compromised.

The facts on deputising

Relatively few studies have been done:

1   They confirm deputies visit more often.

2   Deputies do not necessarily treat inappropriately, e.g. Stevenson (1982) revisited 57 of his patients after a deputy and judged their care was satisfactory.

3   Studies suggest that most deputising services reply fairly promptly.

4   Studies from Portsmouth Hospital, where a whole-town extended rota operates, found referrals to be no more frequent and no more inappropriate from the deputising service than from practices outside the scheme (Bain 1984).

GP co-operatives

The most popular alternative to deputising is to work in organised co-operatives and shared rotas. Co-operatives can be large enterprises (up to 180 doctors) with a central administration, remote answering services and special facilities such as chauffeured transport for visiting doctors or a staffed night-time emergency centre that patients are encouraged to attend.

Co-operatives share a number of pros and cons in common with deputising services. However:

1   The membership of a co-operative is locally determined and drawn from a pool of local principals. To this extent a tighter control may exist over standards;

2   Members can offset the cost of getting someone else to do their night visiting by taking a turn in the rota themselves; and better organisation and facilities may permit fewer doctors to provide the necessary cover, further defraying costs;

3   To be effective, co-operatives require a carefully thought-out organisational infrastructure—the degree of cover, the competency of its members, and the arrangements for prioritising care requests and transferring clinical details back to the patient's own doctor must all be addressed.

4   In many locations deputising services do not operate and a co-operative offers the main alternative to doctors accepting that they have to be on call more often.

Many co-operatives assembled in haste lack adequate legal agreements; and GPs withdrawing from co-operatives have found themselves in dispute over their share of its assets, including development money.

Development fund

The Government has provided an annual fund so that doctors can claim reimbursement of expenses related to the delivery of out-of-hours care. Allowable expenses include:

•   the cost of communication equipment (pagers, mobile phones, switchboard equipment, fax machines, call diversion facilities, etc.);

•   some of the costs of belonging to a co-operative rota or subscribing to a deputising service (those relating to altered premises, new equipment and non-medical staff, so long as the expense can be justified for out-of-hours care); and

- locum costs for isolated GPs.

The effect of this development money has been to promote the delivery of emergency care by doctors other than the patient's chosen one, with all the attendant advantages and disadvantages. In a relatively short period this has become the established pattern of care.

Appointment systems

In a 1951 survey 2% of practices used an appointment system. In Cartwright and Anderson's survey of 1981 the figure had changed to 88%.

Advantages

The principal advantage is efficient use of time, space and resources but there are others:

1   Patients know when they will be seen and (hopefully) do not suffer an unpredictably long wait. (This in turn may encourage them to come to the surgery rather than request a home visit.)

2   Doctors know their timetable: they do not experience unpredictable surges of demand and troughs of idleness. Their workload is spread, regulated and adjusted to fit their personal timetable; follow-ups can be planned around their duty and leave rota.

3   In practices that favour shared lists, the appointment system allows the workload to be spread.

4   An efficient use of limited consulting-room space may be planned.

5   Less waiting-room space is needed (only about five seats per GP consulting).

6   Where appropriate, consultations can be planned so that relevant team members (e.g. practice nurse or health visitor) can attend.

7   Consultation lengths can be planned in some instances according to their needs (e.g. cervical smear or coil-fitting appointments; double appointment space for counselling).

None of this advanced planning is possible if demand is not spread and GPs do not know with any certainty when their surgeries will begin and end.

Disadvantages

1   The administrative workload increases: staff are needed to run the system and they, in turn, need training and salaries.

2   In some branch surgeries consultations may be too few to justify the system.

3   Appointments are not convenient for some customers, e.g.:

   (a) the elderly, who have to make separate trips to a telephone and to the surgery;

   (b) rural patients who rely on infrequent bus services.

Inevitably there are other patients who abuse the system and do not 'play ball'.

4 Most important of all is the worry that appointment systems are perceived as an extra barrier between patient and doctor. Rigid and inflexible systems may deny access in cases of true urgency, while inefficient systems may result in extra delay before an appointment is secured.

Running an appointment system
When patients are balloted by their doctors on proposed changes to the system they tend to prefer the status quo (appointments if they already have them, open access if they do not).

Practices running appointment systems need to review them periodically:
- How long do patients have to wait for non-urgent consultations?
- How often are patients denied the right to see a doctor the same day when they request it?
- Do appointments run to time?
- Are enough consultations on offer, or do surgeries always run over because of 'extras'?
- What provision is made to allow urgent cases to be seen promptly?

Length of appointment
What effect does the length of the appointment have on its outcome? To what extent is this determined in turn by list size? A study where booked time was used as an experimental variable has helped to clarify the benefits of longer consultations (Morrell *et al.* 1986, Roland *et al.* 1986). This study compared patients allocated at random to surgeries booked at 5-, 7.5- and 10-min intervals, respectively, using taped consultations. In 5-min appointments patients were no less likely to be examined, and no more likely to receive a prescription, be referred to hospital or asked to return again, but in longer consultations the doctor did:
- identify more problems;
- carry out more preventive procedures;
- spend more time listening and explaining. Patients were more satisfied.

Risdale *et al.* (1992) have reported that doctors and patients ask more questions when more time is available; and that patients express their views more freely.

Others have found that doctors offering longer appointment times:
- pay more attention to lifestyle and screening (Wilson 1992);
- devote extra time to psychosocial issues (Howie *et al.* 1989) and long-term health problems (Howie *et al.* 1991);
- feel less job stress (Wilson *et al.* 1991).

Several sources indicate that when doctors have smaller lists their patients consult more often and spend more booked time with their doctor.

Some doctors have experimented with allowing patients to choose their own length of appointment. This has the advantage that patients share with their doctor from the outset an idea of the amount of time available, and have had a say in setting it. Published studies suggest that patients are generally good at estimating their requirements and do not request overlong appointment times (Lowenthal & Bingham 1987). Furthermore, a system based on patient-determined booking times offers the chance to cut patient waiting times at little extra cost (Harrison 1987).

Home visiting
Current figures
The average number of home visits per patient per year is 0.5. According to Cartwright and Anderson (1981), 81% of patients require none and 10% require one. More than 75% of the visits are to patients aged over 75 or under 1 year.

Variation between doctors
The variation between doctors is striking and not entirely explained:
• Fry (1973) found a 32-fold variation in a study of 14 doctors;
• a Birmingham GP research group (1978) found a 26-fold variation between 22 doctors.

Trends
There has been a dramatic decline in home visiting rates. For example, Fry found from his personal records that there were 60% fewer visits per person per year in 1971 than in 1949; and the average proportion of consultations conducted at home fell further, from 22% in 1971 to 10% in 1994 (General Household Survey 1994).

The decline in home visiting has been viewed with dismay by some doctors and with approval by others.

This trend has been explained in a variety of ways:
1 Improved community health (e.g. fewer serious childhood illnesses through effective immunisation and sanitation policies).
2 Changes in the attitudes of doctors and patients:
  (a) general practice is perceived more as a business, with the emphasis on efficiency: patients are under pressure to justify their request;
  (b) patients have telephones and cars, and (either through goodwill or coercion) tend to use them;
  (c) patients and doctors expect higher standards of diagnosis and treatment in the surgery;
  (d) changes in working arrangements (appointment systems with less waiting time; more hospitable premises; doctors' attempts to be flexible) have encouraged patients to come to the surgery;

(e) possibly patients are more knowledgeable and more self-reliant;

(f) possibly the primary health care model has resulted in more delegated visiting (by nurses or health visitors for example).

Advantages

1 *Public relations.* Home visiting is a good public relations exercise and helps to cement rapport in the doctor–patient relationship. These benefits are intangible but real.

2 *Humanitarian and screening benefits.* It is kinder to the elderly and infirmed, and allows surveillance of 'at-risk' patients who might not otherwise attend and 'waste the doctor's time'.

3 *Fuller assessment.* It allows whole-patient assessment — the chance to see the family together in the home environment may provide important social information that could not be gathered in the surgery. It also allows compliance to be gauged (drawers full of untouched pills tell a useful tale!).

4 It is the safest option:

(a) serious conditions cannot easily be excluded by telephone;

(b) patients are poor judges of serious and trivial illness;

(c) 'failure to visit' is one of the more successful complaints that patients bring against doctors in Service Committee hearings.

5 It may be the only option when the patient appears unfit to travel.

Disadvantages

1 *Time.* The average surgery consultation lasts 5–6 min but a home visit needs at least 15 min from the surgery and perhaps 30 min from home. Time spent in a car travelling is at the expense of other patients — through their taxes, through the loss of surgery services they could have had (e.g. extra clinics) and through fewer of the 'efficient' surgery appointments on offer per day.

2 *Standards.* Poor lighting, low beds, lack of diagnostic facilities and equipment potentially lower the standard of care.

3 *Costs.* These are not readily calculated. At the simplest level there are travelling expenses, but more home visiting may actually mean that the exchequer employs more GPs, which is clearly expensive to the NHS (who wish to pay doctors to consult, not travel!).

4 *Inconvenience.* Many patients who request home visits do so either on social grounds (lack of transport, difficulty getting an appointment, lack of baby-sitter, bad weather), *or* through erroneous medical beliefs (e.g. fear that a febrile child will catch a chill en route). A smaller proportion are genuinely not fit to visit the surgery or are elderly and infirm. If the visit is in the former category, who should bear the inconvenience—the patient, who sees a doctor on average 3–5 times a year, or the doctor, who runs a business, has 2500 other clients and conducts between 22 and 76 other consultations each day?

5 *The fostering of incorrect attitudes.* More motivation and self-reliance might follow if doctors rationed their visits to genuine emergencies.

6 *Risk of personal injury.* Doctors who visit disreputable areas at night-time run some risk of personal injury. The surgery is a safer environment.

Telephone advice

The burgeoning requirement for out-of-hours care has caused doctors to consider the role of the telephone as an alternative to home visiting. While 95% of patients who seek help want a doctor to visit (Dixon & Williams 1988), some doctors think that more than half of cases may be managed without detriment by giving advice over the telephone (Marsh *et al.* 1987). If so, differences between public and medical perceptions need to be reconciled.

Medical assessments

General Practitioners are required by their Terms of Service to perform two particular kinds of medical assessment:

1 *The new registration medical*:

    (a) *Offered* to all newly registered patients over the age of 5 years;

    (b) *Format of the offer*: in writing, or if verbal, confirmed in writing (the date of invitation should be recorded in the notes);

    (c) *Timetable of the offer*: the appointment must be offered within 28 days of registration. Patients can refuse the invitation. In order to attract payment it must be performed within 3 months of registration, except:

        • where a large number of patients are inherited at once, giving grounds for deferment;

        • when all reasonable efforts were made and the medical was performed as soon as possible.

(No registration fee can be paid unless the patient actually undergoes the consultation).

    In fulfilling this obligation, the GMSC recommends that practices should:

    (a) develop a standard invitation for each registration;

    (b) include a simple questionnaire with the written invitation, to be completed prior to consultation;

    (c) delegate wherever possible or incorporate appointments into a well-person clinic.

2 *Patients aged over 75*:

    (a) *Offered* annually to all patients over 75;

    (b) *The format of the offer* is similar to that for new registrations, except that a domiciliary visit must be offered.

The content of these medicals is described in Table 8.2 (p. 242); their clinical merit is examined in Section 3.3.

It used to be a requirement (until 1993) to offer additional health checks to patients not seen by any doctor in the previous 3 years. Patients can still request such a check under the Patient's Charter rights, and practices and HAs are required to publicise the entitlement.

Leaflets, reports and directories
Practices are required by their Terms of Service to produce leaflets and annual reports, and HAs to maintain accurate local directories on their principals.

Practice reports
Required annually by HAs. The minimum content is dictated in GPs' Terms of Service (Table 1.3).

Many doctors regard this scheme with suspicion, fearing that information on referrals and prescribing will be used to contain NHS costs rather than to improve quality of care. However, annual reports in some form have been advocated and produced by enthusiasts for a number of years prior to this contractual obligation. Keeble *et al.* (1989) have emphasised its potential as the hub of objective setting and performance review, and the dissemination of information throughout the practice. Others accept that vital statistics must be collected before the health service can be planned, justified or improved, and can be useful educationally.

Discretionary information that some practices produce for internal use includes:
1 Demographic data:
   (a) number of list patients;
   (b) age–sex structure;
   (c) morbidity profiles.

Table 1.3 Ingredients of the annual practice report.

Employed staff
Number, individual principal duties, hours worked, qualifications and relevant recent training

Surgery
Changes (introduced or imminent) in floor space, design and quality

Referral data
A breakdown of total numbers referred, as inpatients and outpatients, with reference to specialty and to hospital; also self-referrals the doctors learns about

Outside work
Posts held and work undertaken as a medical practitioner (annual hourly commitment)

Patient feedback
The nature of arrangement set up to receive patients' comments

Prescribing
Doctors' repeat prescribing (and where applicable, dispensing) arrangements; whether a practice formulary is in operation

2 Workload figures:
   (a) numbers of consultations;
   (b) numbers of visits (and night visits);
   (c) numbers of telephone calls;
   (d) numbers of temporary residents seen.
3 Performance data:
   (a) numbers failing to attend;
   (b) screening uptake;
   (c) prescribing figures;
   (d) clinical outcomes.
4 Statements of practice policy and practice objectives.
5 The results of specific audit projects.

Local directories

Since 1990 HAs have compiled and published a local directory of family doctors. The intention is to provide patients with the information needed to make an informed choice of doctor. The directory is revised annually and sent free to community health councils, libraries and citizens' advice bureaux.

Principals are listed alphabetically with details of:
* their sex;
* registrable qualifications;
* age (or date of first full registration);
* normal surgery hours and special clinics;
* other relevant aspects of their practice (e.g. employment of other staff, assistants, trainees or deputies).

Supplementary information can be provided on a voluntary basis, for example other languages spoken and doctors' special clinical interests.

Practice leaflets

The minimum content of the practice leaflet is now prescribed by GPs' Terms of Service (Table 1.4). All principals must make this information available to the HA and to their list patients, and update it annually as appropriate. Some doctors have taken the opportunity to include general health information and advice on self-management of minor ailments; others have sought and obtained commercial sponsorship, including advertisements, in their leaflet.

Fundholding

The NHS and Community Care Act 1990 made it possible for general practitioners to hold and control a budget to fund primary care services. The scheme was introduced on a voluntary basis, but pressure exists to involve all GPs in fundholding or commissioning.

Despite initial opposition one practice in three was involved in the scheme by 1995/6 and half the population was covered by it. Fund-holders accounted for 7% of all NHS expenditure on hospital and

Table 1.4 Ingredients of the practice leaflet.

Doctor details
Name, sex, registered medical qualifications, date and place of first registration

Working arrangements
Consulting hours and appointment arrangements
How to obtain non-urgent and urgent appointments
How to obtain non-urgent and urgent domiciliary visits
Out-of-hours arrangements
Repeat prescribing and dispensing arrangements
Practice area (defined by sketch or plan)
Arrangements for receiving patients' comments

Services and facilities offered
Maternity services
Contraception
Child health surveillance
Minor surgery
Special clinics (purpose and time of operation)
Access for the disabled

Practice structure
Employed staff (numbers and roles)
Whether a partnership is in operation
Whether trainees, medical students and assistants are likely to be in attendance

community services, receiving £232 million in management and administration costs. The average fundholding practice managed an annual budget of £1.7 million (£140–170 per patient).

Fundholding has fallen into political disfavour following a change of Government, and it has been announced that the scheme will be disbanded in 1999, to be replaced by a system of universal commissioning. It is presented here, however, because it still has currency and because a number of the ideas are pertinent to the scheme that will succeed it.

Principles
Fundholding involves:
1 Negotiating a budget with the HA to cover a range of:
   (a) hospital care (such as outpatient appointments and planned surgery);
   (b) NHS medicines;
   (c) practice staff costs and extra practice administrative costs (e.g. computing).
2 Negotiating 'best buys' for medical care with chosen providers.
3 Administering the system by:
   (a) checking providers' bills andmonitoring prescribing costs;
   (b) switching funds between the three general areas of drugs, staff and hospital services;
   (c) maintaining a budget account with monthly reports and an annual statement to the HA;

(d) allowing accounts to be inspected by the Audit Commission.

At the scheme's inception certain services were specifically excluded (emergency treatments; inpatient medical care; maternity services; certain screening and direct-access services; and 'expensive' patient care (more than £6000 in a year)).

For most fundholders this still represents the position, but since 1994 a number of pilot exercises are have been conducted in 'total purchasing', i.e. inclusive of emergency and inpatient care.

Eligibility

Future access to the fundholding scheme has been frozen given its imminent demise. However, recent eligibility has depended on:

1 *List size* at least 5000 patients for standard budget-holding; and no minimum size for *community budget-holding* (a scaled down version in which the budget covers community and practice, but not hospital purchasing powers). Some smaller practices have grouped together to meet the main size requirement, and some *'multifunds'* are operating under common management.

2 *Ability*—practices were first assessed by the HA who considered their performance standards, computer support provisions and general competence.

Potential benefit

1 *Financial*:

Hitherto several financial incentives have been provided to encourage fundholding, and a number of potential advantages to the NHS touted in favour of the scheme:

(a) fundholders have been able to charge administrative costs (e.g. computer costs, new equipment, management time) to the budget. Allowances have included:
- a basic fixed allowance (£28 000 in 1996);
- a per capita supplement (for general, but not community, fundholding);
- a group allowance (for practices who share a budget);
- a site allowance (for major branch surgeries); and
- a start-up allowance in the preparatory period.

(b) they also have the opportunity to use budgetary savings for approved uses (additional staff or hospital services; improved premises; better patient facilities—but not personal income);

(c) And it has been argued that doctors who are made more aware of the financial consequences of their clinical behaviour may generate efficiency savings for the NHS. (The drug bill for fundholders has risen more slowly than for non-fundholders. However, the Audit Commission reported that the £206 million of savings that had been generated up to 1994/5 was outweighed by £232 million paid towards the scheme's management. In addition HAs were spending an extra £6000 per year and trusts employing two to three extra staff to run the scheme at their end.)

2   *Administrative and professional* — budget-holders may be able to exercise more control over their own affairs, improving the quality of their patients' care. For example, they may:

(a) Negotiate shorter waiting times for non-urgent operations and outpatient appointments

(b) Improve the quality and timeliness of discharge information from hospitals;

(c) Exert more influence over the availability and standard of local services. Eighty per cent of fundholders specify quality standards in their contract. Also fundholding has enabled practices to introduce consultant clinics into their surgeries, bringing services closer to the patient; and to exert leverage over local problems, such as the courtesy and convenience of services.

(d) Take on staff with new skills (for example, fundholding practices employ a physiotherapist twice as often as non-fundholding practices);

(e) Offer their patients more choice. Fundholding has made it easier in some cases to refer outside a HA's boundaries (extra-contractual referrals).

3   *Efficiency gains*:

Fundholders have an incentive to cut waste, benefiting the NHS as a whole. They may, for example:

(a) negotiate lower cost care (e.g. day surgery, rather than inpatient care);

(b) switch contracts to lower cost providers (published tariffs vary two-fold between providers);

(c) limit unnecessary repeat procedures (e.g. 20% of fundholders place a review limit on the number of outpatient attendances);

(d) prescribe in a more cost-effective way (see Chapter 2);

(e) avoid hospital overheads by hosting services within the practice. (Some surgeries have evolved into polyclinics, offering procedures normally only available in hospitals.)

Potential problems

1   *Financial* — Balancing a large budget is a complex operation. According to Enthoven (1989) that a list size of 11 000 (the original minimum size) would be too small to cope with random fluctuations in demand and yet keep within the 5% budget. Some fundholders have since overspent their budgets, with risk of sanction.

2   *Administrative and professional* — The volume of work necessary is considerable, involving frequent practice meetings, extensive doctor and accountancy time, reporting, phoning and negotiating, collecting and endorsing receipts, and so on.

3   *Legal and ethical*:

(a) from the doctor–patient viewpoint: a patient's trust and confidence could be undermined if the doctor were thought to have a pecuniary interest in the outcome of the consultation;

(b) from the partnership's viewpoint: budget-holding represents a fundamental change in contractual terms between partners, and requires unanimous agreement legally and in the interests of practice harmony. Budget-holding practices have been subject to intense external scrutiny — from HAs, auditors and patient consumer groups

(c) from the point of view of society:

- the cheapest service may not be the best one;
- general practice may become cash-limited;
- doctors' attention may be deflected from their primary clinical role;
- the existence of two types of practice favours a two-tier system, in which those with greater purchasing power exert more influence. A *Which?* survey confirmed that two-thirds of GPs are of this opinion, and there is also evidence to support it e.g. in at least one region the per capita funding was reported to be more generous for fundholding than non-fundholding practices (Dixon *et al.* 1994). There have been reports of shorter waiting times for appointments and non-urgent operations in patients of fundholders; of a greater willingness to accommodate their patients around critical planning periods for the provider—such as its financial year-end; of more flexibility in offering direct referral services, such as radiology; and of greater willingness to accept ECRs from them;
- GPs with limited experience, training and resources may not be best placed to manage a complex budget. The Audit Commission (1996) reported a failure among many fundholders to maximise efficiency savings (they recommended training in commissioning);
- the Audit Commission also reported a general failure among HAs to monitor the wisdom of fundholders' judgements, and to provide them with information on their comparative performance.

Of these various concerns, the accusation of two-tierism has the greatest political fallout. The new Labour Government has banned preferential access to health care for fundholders' patients and announced plans to disband the scheme altogether.

The model that will replace it has emerged from attempts by some fundholders to address the chief concerns. These doctors entered into local alliances (fundholding consortia and multifunds) for logistic reasons, but these large local consortia hold out prospects to:

- restore equity in local access to medical care;
- allow the recruitment of high calibre professional management;
- share out the administrative burden;
- exert more influence over local services (through their enhanced purchasing power);

- encourage closer ties between practices and better co-ordination of community services.

Commissioning

However, in Nottingham 200 non-fundholding GPs went a step further and joined together in liaison with their purchasing authority to provide a low cost, equitable system of health care commissioning (Black *et al.* 1994), and others have followed. Some 9000 GPs now belong to local commissioning groups, the Government's intended alternative to fundholding.

A National Association of Commissioning General Practices has also emerged, and by 1999 all GPs in England and Wales will be required to belong to a local commissioning (primary care) group (PCG).

Many of the principal advantages of fundholding (collective muscle, local innovation, etc.) apply equally to commissioning schemes. In addition, it is argued that these schemes are more openly democratic, more community-focused, and better for collective planning of service provision. Against this, a more elaborate (bureaucratic) management structure may be required, and the incentives, which are one step further removed from practices and patients, may be diluted.

Three main structural models of commissioning are proposed:

1 an advisory body to the HA,
2 a budgetary subunit under HA control; or
3 a free-standing commissioning body (primary care trust).

In each case funds will come from a single cash-limited budget, administered through the HA, and will need to cover all aspects of local health care (including primary and secondary care services). The management boards of PCGs will include GPs and representatives of nursing and social services, and will be financially and publicly accountable. HAs will have to draw up 'Health Improvement Programmes' which will form the basis of contractual agreements with the PCGs, while two new Government bodies, a National Institute for Clinical Excellence and a Commission for Health Improvement, will facilitate standard setting and compliance monitoring.

At the time of writing many details have not been established, and the implications of the proposals are unclear. Nonetheless, they clearly represent a massive shift in the framework of general practice governance and funding, and important future ramifications appear likely.

Big bang pilot schemes

At the time of writing, GPs still work the nationally agreed 1990 contract as self-employed independent contractors, but legislation in the wake of the White Paper *Choice and Opportunity — Primary Care: The Future* offers a choice of employment terms, including:

- *a salaried contract*, held for example with an NHS trust, practice partnership or other body;
- *a practice-based contract*, held between HAs and the practice team

(including managers and nurses, as well as doctors), perhaps involving a single amalgamated budgetary agreement covering secondary as well as primary care services;

- new contracts with HAs to provide *extra non-core services* for extra remuneration.

Participation in the new arrangement is voluntary: doctors who prefer can continue to work within the contractual framework described in Tables 1.6 and 7.2. But for interested parties the NHS Executive has published guidance on the alternatives. GPs must first apply to run a pilot scheme on a trial basis. These will be agreed locally and vetted centrally (a national advisory body, the National Consultative Group for Choice and Opportunity for Pilots (CHOPPS), is advising the Government on proposals). Applications:

1   must:
   (a) relate to a defined list of patients;
   (b) appear to offer some advantages over existing provision (improved skill mix, cost-effectiveness, improved services, etc.);
   (c) incorporate the full range of general medical services (GMS), including out-of-hours care;
   (d) involve all members of a partnership in the same arrangement
2   will result in a local contract with the HA, rather than a national contract; and
3   will be one of two main types:
   (a) a local contract covering GMS ('PMS'); or
   (b) a similar contract with additional hospital, community and/or non-core services ('PMS' plus);
4   may, under some conditions, require transfer of surpluses for those in the fundholding scheme;
5   may be supported by HA funding

The NHS (Primary Care) Bill was intended to encourage innovative proposals for the delivery of primary care services, and the new arrangements offer some potential advantages, for example, to:

- ease recruitment problems in inner city and isolated areas;
- allow doctors who wish to relinquish the administrative duties of running a business;
- allow young principals to enter practice without having to commit capital early on in their career;
- allow a more flexible employment arrangement between practices and principals, facilitating job mobility;
- amalgamated budgets may allow ambitious GPs to extend their role by taking control of cottage hospitals, employing hospital consultants or other GPs on a sessional basis, or even founding primary care trusts:

There is an opposite side to the coin. For example, the new arrangements may:

- permit cash-strapped community and hospital trusts to gain access to primary care budgets; or

- limit employed doctors' professional freedom, requiring them to refer in-house (to own-trust providers); and to work according to the employers' dictates (effectively side-stepping the issue of non-core services.)

The scheme is in its earliest stages, and its take-up and form remain unclear. However, the potential now exists for radical structural change in general practice.

The effect of practice size on practice matters

There is no ideal size for a practice but the character, facilities and organisation are strongly influenced by the number of principals. In Table 1.5 a large group practice (four or more doctors) is compared with a single-handed practice to illustrate this. The current trend is towards ever bigger practices, with all the attendant pros and cons.

Dispensing

Eligibility to dispense

1   When the drug/appliance is supplied and personally administered by the prescribing doctor. This includes:

Table 1.5 The effect of practice size on practice matters. (Figures from Cartwright & Anderson's 1967 study.)

Aspect	Group practice (≥4 doctors)	Single-handed practice
Patient care	1 More equipment and facilities, e.g.: • ECG machine (60% cf. 13%); • peak flow meter (81% cf. 64%); • treatment room (92% cf. 47%) 2 More services (e.g. diabetic and well-woman clinics) 3 From the patient's point of view, more choice of doctor	1 Personal care of patients with: • good rapport; • better knowledge of the patient; • consistent advice 2 From the doctor's point of view patients who know where they are and who they will see; who cannot 'shop around' and abuse the system
Doctors	1 On call less often—less personal and family strain; less use of deputising services 2 Fewer problems in covering sickness and holidays, or coping with epidemics 3 More opportunity for research, audit, teaching, study leave and sabbaticals (44% train, cf. 20% of single-handers)	1 Own boss. No one else to get on with 2 Fewer problems with communications and organisation and no decision-making by committee 3 Other problems can be avoided (e.g. shared rota with another practice)
Staff	1 More likely to have attached staff, e.g.: • district nurse (71% cf. 27%); • health visitor (96% cf. 74%); • social worker, community psychiatric nurse, etc. 2 More likely to employ: • practice nurse (56% cf., 27%); • practice manager, caretaker, etc.	
Financial	1 Capital costs of the building are shared 2 More contributors to the pool when expensive practice equipment is bought	1 No dilution of the profit when capital appreciation occurs

(a) emergency injections;
(b) anaesthetics;
(c) diagnostic reagents;
(d) intrauterine devices, caps and diaphragms;
(e) vaccinations;
(f) certain pessaries and suture materials.
(Separate regulations for oxygen.)

2   For patients (or temporary residents) who live more than a mile away from the nearest chemist. These patients form the dispensing list. (Note that it is feasible, indeed common, to dispense to patients on the dispensing list from surgery premises less than a mile from the nearest chemist: it is the distance from the patient's *home* that matters!)

Scale of payments

Dispensers receive:

1   The *basic price* of the drug or appliance (as defined in the Drug Tariff, and less a discount laid out in Para. 44/Schedule 1 of the Red Book);
2   An *on-cost allowance* of 10.5% of the basic (pre-discount) price;
3   A *container allowance* (currently 3.8p per script);
4   A *dispensing fee* (laid out in Para. 44/Schedule 2 of the Red Book—it depends on the volume of dispensing);
5   A *VAT allowance*.

Claims

All prescriptions, for dispensing and administering doctors, must be noted and sent with a complete FP 34D to the Prescription Pricing Authority (not later than the 5th day of the month following issue of the prescription).

Benefits

1   GPs make a profit on the basic cost of the drug by bulk purchase and also pocket the container fee and dispensing allowance, so dispensing is fairly lucrative and compensates rural practices for their lower lists and higher travel costs. (Profits on dispensing range from about 10 to 17% of the gross turnover of the dispensary.)
2   It also provides a good service to patients, who can find doctor and drugs under a single roof and do not have to make a separate visit to the chemist. Doctors visiting rural patients, the elderly and infirmed can dispense the prescription in the same visit—a valuable service.
3   It imposes the discipline of limited list prescribing on the principals and forces them to examine carefully their prescribing habits and rationale. It also brings home the real cost of their prescribing.
4   It is an interesting and stimulating exercise.
5   Dispensing doctors can offer a wider range of drugs out of hours.

Costs

1   Inevitably choice will be limited. It is not possible to stock every

prescribable item. Practical problems are more likely to arise for prescriptions arising through hospital directives.

2   It involves extra security precautions, as the dispensary may attract would-be burglars.

3   Other costs include:

(a) insurance of drug stock;

(b) a capital cost to incoming partners (who must purchase a share of this stock);

(c) a small capital risk (investment in drugs that may be discredited/withdrawn from use);

(d) the extra administrative burden, extra commitment of staff time and extra staff responsibilities.

Many dispensing practices employ a pharmacist (qualified dispensers are reimbursed at the higher clerical officer rate in the Whitney Council scale of salaries). There is no legal obligation to employ a qualified dispenser. Nevertheless the legal obligations to dispense accurately, safely and in accordance with the various Drug Acts still apply and so responsibility for the service rests with the dispensing doctor.

1.6 THE FINANCES

Income

The three broad categories of a GP's income are:

1   Private medical work.

2   Income from the NHS.

3   Personal (non-medical) income.

Private income

Income from private medical work depends on the level of commitment to extra-practice activities, the opportunity for private work and the practice's policy towards private patients.

Sources of private income are numerous and include:

•   insurance examinations and reports;

•   other private medical exams and certificates (fitness to start a job, HGV licence applications, fitness to dive, etc.);

•   solicitors' reports; court witness;

•   cremation fees;

•   industrial appointments;

•   local authority appointments, e.g. police duties, developmental or family planning clinics; school medical officers;

•   hospital appointments (assistantships or practitioner posts);

•   lecturing.

Income from the NHS

Under present arrangements income from the NHS comes in the form of:

1 Practice allowances (fixed sum payments and fees based on type or place of practice);
2 Capitation fees (based on number of patients);
3 Item-of-service payments (based on services provided);
4 Fees based on qualifications;
5 Reimbursements and grants.

Table 1.6 summarises the main allowances and reimbursements of this complex remunerative system in which GPs enjoy the status of independent contractors.

A Government White Paper has recently provided the alternative choice of becoming salaried. Tables 1.6 and 7.2 summarise the status quo, but a mixed system of remuneration seems certain to develop in time. Possible implications are discussed in Section 1.7 (p. 66).

Table 1.6 Income from the NHS.

Category of fee	Red Book reference (para.)	Qualifications
Practice allowances		
1 Basic practice allowance	12.1	Paid to each principal with more than 1200 NHS patients on his list who fulfils the availability requirement of his terms of service (see Table 7.2) In a partnership the average must exceed 1200; for doctors with fewer patients pro rata payments are made
2 Designated area allowance	14.1	Paid to encourage doctors to practise in an under-doctored area. Two scales of payment, depending on the average number of patients on the doctor's NHS list. (Very few designated areas now exist)
3 Initial practice allowance (types 1 and 2)	41.1	Paid to doctors setting up practice or joining a partnership in a designated area for an initial period of up to 4 years
4 Inducement allowance	45.1	Paid to doctors practising in sparsely populated areas as a remuneration to offset losses due to their small list size. GPs in England and Wales must have fewer than 1200 patients. They will also receive full seniority and locum sickness allowances
5 Rural practice payments	43.1	Paid to doctors in rural areas where ≥20% of patients live ≥3 miles from the main surgery. Units are credited, not just on the basis of numbers, but also distance and difficulty of access. (Rural practice units are therefore subdivided into distance units, blocked route units, special district units and difficult walking units!)
6 Assistant's allowance	18.1	Paid to GPs employing assistants when their list size exceeds certain limits (for a full-rate allowance 3000 for a single-hander, or in a partnership 3000 patients for the first doctor and 2500 on average for the rest). Assistants must spend at least 25% of their time on NHS work
7 Associate's allowance	19.1	A scheme allowing two or sometimes three single-handed GPs to employ a doctor between them to allow time off for training. GPs must receive rural practice payments, receive an inducement payment or live >10 miles from the nearest surgery or district general hospital, and not employ assistants

Continued

Table 1.6 *Continued*

Category of fee	Red Book reference (para.)	Qualifications
8 Absence allowances	47.1–50.1	Allowances are available to cover locum costs during: • illness (single-handed GPs and partnerships with large lists) • confinement (up to a maximum of 13 weeks) • prolonged study leave (at least 10 weeks) • attendance at a PGEA-approved course (single-handed GPs)
Capitation fees		
1 Basic capitation fees	21.1	The basic fee that each patient on a doctor's list attracts in terms of income. Counted quarterly and paid on three scales depending on age: under 65s; 65–74; 75 and over (ages are those at the end of the preceding quarter)
2 Temporary resident's fee (form GMS3)	32.1	Paid for treatment or advice given to visitors to the practice area seeking medical assistance and staying more than 24 h but less than 3 months. Two scales—one for up to 15 days and a higher one for more than 15 days. (Temporary residents requiring a night visit attract two fees; those requiring only an item-of-service attract only the item-of-service fee)
3 Deprivation payments	20.1	Additional capitation fees for those patients living in areas of deprivation as identified by the Secretary of State (see Table 5.4—the Jarman Index)
4 Child health surveillance fee	22.1	Paid to GPs on the HA (or health board) child health surveillance list for each under-5 receiving a locally agreed programme of surveillance
5 Registration fee (form GMS4)	23.1	Paid to GPs carrying out the scheduled registration medical (see Table 8.2) within 3 months of a patient joining the list. No fee if: • the patient is under 5; • the patient was on a partner's list and had a similar medical in the last 12 months
Item-of-service payments		
1 Emergency treatment form GMS3)	33.1	For people in the practice area for less than 24 h (i.e. not eligible to register as temporary residents) and in need of immediate and necessary treatment. (Attracts a higher fee than the temporary resident fee)
2 Immediately necessary treatment (form GMS3)	36.1	Immediately necessary treatment or advice given to a patient permanently residing in the practice area whom the GP is unwilling to accept as a list patient or temporary resident (and who stays in the area too long to qualify for the emergency treatment fee)
3 Anaesthetic fee (form GMS4)	34.1	Paid when the administration of an anaesthetic requires the services of two practitioners
4 Dental haemorrhage fee (form GMS4)	35.1	For the arrest of a dental haemorrhage or the provision of aftercare
5 Night visit payments (form GMS4)	24.1	An annual payment to all partners *and* a consultation fee for each consultation requested and completed between 10 pm and 8 am with a list patient or temporary resident. The patient may be seen at home, or if appropriate, in the surgery or elsewhere in the practice area. The fee is paid whether the visit is made by the GP, his deputy, rota colleague, assistant, trainee, associate or locum

Continued on p. 58

Table 1.6 *Continued*

Category of fee	Red Book reference (para.)	Qualifications
6 Cervical cytology fee	28.1	Payable on two scales: • for full target payment, 80% of eligible women aged 25–64 (or in Scotland 21–60) must have had an adequate smear in the last $5\frac{1}{2}$ years; • for the lower payment, 50% (the time scale of $5\frac{1}{2}$ years is to allow for a 6-month call and recall delay). *Notes* **1** Women with hysterectomies involving complete removal of the cervix are exempt front the target group **2** Work can be delegated to attached staff **3** Where smears are taken by other GPs they count towards the target of the woman's registered doctor **4** The sum actually paid will be adjusted to account for the number of eligible women on the practice list as compared with the average anticipated nationally (430) and the number of adequate smears taken by GPs (rather than by others outside general practice)
7 Contraceptive fees (forms GMS4 and GMS3)	29.1	An annual fee (paid quarterly) for women on the doctor's NHS contraceptive list. Two scales are payable—for contraceptive advice and pill prescribing; and for the fitting of an intrauterine device and follow-up. Temporary residents may also receive advice or treatment (N.B.: The ordinary fee is payable for advice alone, even if the advice is a sheath or sterilisation; however, it is only payable in respect of the woman—to claim, the couple or woman alone must be counselled, not the man alone)
8 Maternity fees (forms FP 24/24A)	31.1	Maternity fees are paid on a dual-scale basis—one set for GPs not on the HA's obstetric list, and another (more than 70% higher) for those who are. 'Complete' services include care before, during and after delivery, but partial payments are possible, as described below
(a) antenatal care		Paid on three scales depending on the date in pregnancy on which the patient signs up for maternity services: • Scale 1—within the first 16 weeks; • Scale 2—between 17th and 30th weeks (a lesser sum); • Scale 3—on or after the 31st week (lower again)
(b) miscarriage		If the patient miscarries before 8 weeks and has not signed up for maternity care, no fee is payable. Otherwise (up to 24 weeks) a miscarriage fee can be claimed
(c) abortions		Termination arrangements are generally excluded unless the patient has previously signed up for maternity services
(d) confinement		Paid for intra-partum responsibility. Also fee payable if a doctor is called to a patient who is in labour but not booked under his own care. (In the case of premature confinements, if a live birth occurs after 28 weeks, the fee is paid as if the delivery were at full term)
(e) postnatal care		The full fee applies to services to mother and child over the first 14 postnatal days, plus a full postnatal examination between 6 and 12 weeks (the patient must leave hospital within 48 h of delivery). Partial fees are paid per visit (maximum five) and for the full postnatal examination

Continued

Table 1.6 *Continued*

Category of fee	Red Book reference (para.)	Qualifications
		(A GP can still claim the postnatal examination fee if he has made reasonable efforts to offer an appointment and the patient has not attended)
9 Minor surgery (form GMS4)	42.1	Paid to GPs on a minor surgery list for sessions consisting of at least five procedures per quarter from those activities itemised in Para. 42/Schedule 1 (Table 1.7) A maximum of three claims per quarter or an average of three per GP per quarter in group practices
10 Health Promotion Fees (form FP/HPP/1)	30.1	Paid annually to GPs and practices who conduct a programme of health promotion activities approved by a Health Promotion Committee. To be suitable, programmes must meet local and national priorities, and be in keeping with current medical opinion
11 Immunisations (a) children aged <2 (form FP/TC1)	25.1	Divided into four groups: • diphtheria, pertussis, tetanus (DPT; all three doses); • polio (three doses); • Hib (three doses or the over-13 months single dose); • measles or measles, mumps and rubella (MMR; one dose) Two payment scales—the higher if 90% of the appropriate children have been fully immunised on the first day of the quarter, and a lesser sum if only 70%. *Notes* **1** The actual sum is adjusted according to the number of courses done by GPs (as distinct from those given outside general practice), and the number of children on the list compared with the average nationally expected (which is 22) **2** Courses given by other GPs count towards those of the claiming GP **3** The GP who gives the final immunisation of a course will be credited with giving the full course (even if earlier doses were given by other doctors)
(b) Pre-school boosters (form FP/TPB)	26.1	To achieve the full payment, 90% of the list 5-year-olds must have received a reinforcing dose of DPT; 70% for the lower target. The actual sum paid will be derived in the manner described above
(c) Other domestic vaccinations	27.1	Payments can be claimed when vaccinations are approved according to the schedule set out in Para. 27/Schedule 1. In summary: *Diphtheria, tetanus, MMR, measles, polio*—to children aged ⩾6 who have not had a primary course; *Tetanus boosters*—to those leaving school and every 5 years thereafter; *Polio*—to school-leavers, as a booster for those under 40 or those whose children are being vaccinated; *Rubella*—to children aged 10–14 with no previous MMR; seronegative women of childbearing age; seronegative men in antenatal clinics; *Vaccinations for special-risk groups*—potentially exposed to polio, diphtheria, anthrax, typhoid, rabies or infectious hepatitis; *Emergency vaccination programmes*—as recommended by the community physician to contain local disease outbreaks

Continued on p. 60

Table 1.6 *Continued*

Category of fee	Red Book reference (para.)	Qualifications
(d) Foreign travel vaccinations		Approved vaccinations depend on the area to be visited: *Canada, USA, Australia, New Zealand, N. Europe*—no special recommendations (keep domestic vaccinations up to date); *Other places*—polio; *Known pockets of infection*—the appropriate vaccine (also when a vaccination certificate is a condition of entry); *Overland in areas of poor sanitation*—infectious hepatitis. Note that vaccines can be given separately or in combination—a fee is payable for each operation, not for each vaccine. In a course separate fees are paid for each stage. Vaccinations outside the schedule do not qualify for a fee, though you can ask for one from the patient

Fees based on qualifications

Category of fee	Red Book reference (para.)	Qualifications
1 Seniority allowance	16.1	Paid in three stages, depending on the length of time the doctor's name has appeared in the medical register, and the length of time with the NHS as a GP principal (Scale 1—registered 11 years and principal for 7; Scale 2—registered 18 years and principal for 14; Scale 3—registered 25 years and principal for 21) For the full allowance GPs must qualify for a full basic practice allowance
2 Postgraduate education allowance	37.1	An annual payment to GPs completing 25 days of accredited postgraduate education over the previous 5 years. Courses must include at least two from the three subject areas of: • health promotion and prevention of illness; • disease management; • service management Reduced payments are available pro rata for fewer days of accredited education

Reimbursements

Category of fee	Red Book reference (para.)	Qualifications
1 Dispensing fees	44.1	Paid to doctors who 'supply and personally administer' injections, vaccines, diagnostic reagents, suture and bandage material; and to doctors who qualify for a dispensing list (who receive the drug tariff cost of the prescription, less a discount, but with certain additions—on-cost allowance, VAT and container allowances, and the dispenser's fee—see p. 53
2 Practice staff scheme	52.1	Reimbursable costs include staff wages; employer's NI and pension scheme contributions; costs of providing training; redundancy payments. All GPs are eligible. HAs have the discretion to decide: • the percentage of costs to be reimbursed; • the date from which reimbursements will be made; • the minimum qualifications and experience of staff will need to be recognised These decisions, made in the light of local need, budget and priorities, can be reviewed at 3-yearly intervals. There are transitional arrangements for staff in post on 1 April 1990 (see Section 1.2 (p. 6)) Reimbursements may also be available for relief cover during holidays of reasonable length, sickness or maternity leave and training

Continued

Table 1.6 *Continued*

Category of fee	Red Book reference (para.)	Qualifications
3 Reimbursement of rent, rates and sewerage charges	51.1	Paid by the HA quarterly in arrears. The exact arrangement depends on the ownership of the premises: • in Health Centres the HA directly reimburses the HA and the doctors only pay a separate consolidated service charge; • in approved privately owned or leased premises rent reimbursement is 100% of the district valuer's 'fair rent' assessment (see Section 1.1 (p. 1))
4 Payments for computer systems	58.1	HAs have discretion to reimburse costs of computer equipment. The Dept of Health has suggested as a target: • 50% of capital and maintenance costs; • up to 70% of initial staff costs
5 Out of hours development scheme	59.1	A discretionary reimbursement of expenses incurred developing more efficient out of hours services. Includes reimbursement for: • communication equipment (mobile phones, pagers, etc.) • the non-doctor costs of a GP rota or deputising service (e.g. premises, computers, non-medical staff) • locum costs for isolated rural GPs All GPs are eligible, including restricted principals. HAs must be satisfied that the costs relate directly to providing a service; and that they represent good value for money.
6 Doctors' retainer scheme	39.1	Paid to the employing GP (up to half a day per week), provided that the scheme has regional PGEA approval
Grants		
1 Improvement grants	56.1	A grant of one- to two-thirds of the cost of improvements to surgery accommodation, but there are several qualifications on standards, project limits, use of the grant etc. (see Section 1.1 Improvement grants (p. 3))
2 Training grants	38.1	Paid to approved doctors who employ and supervise a trainee GP under the auspices of a training scheme. It comprises: • the trainer's grant; • the salary to be reimbursed to the trainee; • the employer's NI and superannuation contributions for the trainee; • an additional car allowance (to reimburse the trainee's travel expenses) • miscellaneous trainee expenses (phone extensions, defence union payments, removal costs)

The average GP's annual income is roughly made up as follows:

Capitation fees	60%
Allowances	17%
Items of service	15%
Health promotion clinics	4%
Minor surgery	2%
Target-based payments (smears and immunisations)	2%

However, these average figures disguise wide variations. Practices also vary widely in respect of their non-NHS income.

Outgoings

There are two broad categories of expense:
1   Running costs.
2   Capital expenses.

Running costs

The major running costs are as follows:
1   Cost of premises (including rent, rate, repairs, insurance).
2   Staff costs (including wages, NI contributions and pension payments).
3   Service costs (including heat and lighting, stationery and postage, telephones).
4   Professional fees (including accountancy, subscriptions, bank charges, personal health and professional insurance).
5   Travel expenses (including petrol, road tax and depreciation).

1 and 2 are discussed in more detail in the sections devoted to reimbursements (see Sections 1.1 and 1.2 and Table 1.6). Suffice to say they are to a large extent reimbursable, while 3 and 4 leave only a limited scope for economy. The running costs associated with a car (5) include such items as: petrol, oil and antifreeze; road fund licence and car insurance; servicing, MOT and replacement parts (e.g. tyres); AA/RAC membership; cleaning, etc. These items are tax-deductible but only for the proportion attributable to practice use. A percentage (negotiable with the Inland Revenue) is not allowable, representing private use. Commonly 90% of expenses are allowable for a first car and 50% on a second 'back-up' car. (In addition the Inland Revenue allows GPs an allowance that qualifies for tax relief on the *capital* expense (see below) of their vehicle—25% of the 'written down' value of the car annually, subject to a maximum allowance of £2000, and with a reduced allowance for a second car.)

Capital expenses

Non-recurring expenditure on buying (or building) something new is classified as capital expense. Replacement items are included, but repairs are treated as running costs. Examples of capital expenses include a new computer or an ECG machine. For tax purposes 25% of the 'written down' value is allowable annually in the same manner as for GPs' cars.

Doctors' pensions

GPs pay 6% of their gross remuneration (less practice expenses) into the NHS superannuation scheme. Benefits from this include:
1   a pension (1.4% of the aggregate, over the whole service period, of gross remuneration less practice expenses—corrected to take account of inflation);
2   a retirement lump sum (three times the pension);

3   a widow's pension;
4   an incapacity pension;
5   a death gratuity.

Tax allowances
All running expenses legitimately and wholly incurred in the running
of the practice are tax-deductible. The special concessions related to
car use and the tax position on capital expenditure have been
described above. GPs also benefit from two other sources in addition
to the usual practice-based expenses:

1   *Wives as employees.* Most male GPs pay their wife as a receptionist,
and claim from the Inland Revenue an annual expense just short of the
amount at which NI contributions are required and well short of
the wife's earned income allowance (after which income tax is paid).
The validity of this claim has been queried by the Inland Revenue,
and some authorities recommend that wives perform measurable
book-keeping and secretarial duties at home, and that the transaction
is sealed by the transfer of funds by cheque, preferably paid through
the practice account. Participation in a co-operative may limit the
scope to claim tax relief, although periods of home telephone cover do
often still arise.

2   *Use of the home for consulting.* Providing a substantial number of
patients are seen at home, the GP can claim tax relief on:
    (a) his mortgage interest payments (over and above the MIRAS
    allowance);
    (b) his rates and water rates;
    (c) maintenance, lighting and heating costs.

Normally a proportion of the total expenses (say 20%) is deemed
tax-deductible and for business use, and the rest is not deductible,
representing private use. The exact proportion is negotiable with the
Inland Revenue.

Concern has been expressed that GPs selling their home may then
be liable to capital gains tax (CGT) on the part claimed as business
property but, providing no particular area of the house has been designated for exclusive use in this way, and the doctor merely changes
his primary residence, this attracts 'roll-over relief', and CGT is not
payable.

1.7 THE DEVELOPMENT OF GENERAL PRACTICE

The 1966 General Practice Charter represented in its time something
of a watershed in the development of modern general practice. Until
the middle of the 20th century it was normal for GPs to be single-
handed, to work from their own homes, employing their wives as secretaries, and with a minimum of supporting staff; premises were often

substandard, gloomy places; and there were no financial incentives for change. Lack of a clear postgraduate training structure and lack of academic prestige also left GPs the poor relations of their hospital colleagues in the glamour specialties, and recruitment to general practice was a problem. The Charter of 1966 made a great impact on this situation. Its principal ingredients were better pay, seniority, group practice and designated area allowances, financial recognition of out-of-hours services, and the reimbursement schemes for staff salaries.

In 1967 the GPFC was founded as a source of loans, and hand in hand with these two changes there emerged an improvement in staffing, premises and general practice recruitment.

Several further developments helped to boost professional status:

1 Granting of the Royal status to the College of General Practitioners (1967).

2 The recommendation of a 3-year Vocational Training Scheme by the Royal College on Medical Education (1968), later to become compulsory.

3 Direct access to laboratory facilities, helped by the Report on Organisation of Group Practices (1971).

4 The emergence of general practice as a specialty capable of original research and publication.

5 The building of multidisciplinary Health Centres by HAs.

Table 1.7 Minor surgery procedures eligible for a fee.

Injections	Intra-articular
	Periarticular
	Varicose veins
	Haemorrhoids
Aspirations	Joints
	Cysts
	Bursae
	Hydroceles
Incisions	Abscesses
	Cysts
	Thrombosed piles
Excisions	Sebaceous cysts
	Lipomas
	Skin lesions (for histology)
	Intradermal naevi, papilloma, dermatofibroma and similar conditions
	Warts
	Removal of the toe nails (partial and complete)
Curette cautery and cryocautery	Warts and verrucae
	Other skin lesions (e.g. molluscum contagiosum)
Other	Removal of foreign bodies
	Nasal cautery

Such was the impact of these changes (and the lack of a satisfactory career structure in hospital medicine) that general practice became oversubscribed, with a glut of eager well qualified trainees chasing a shortage of principal vacancies!

Surprisingly, however, over the period 1964–1977, when Cartwright and Anderson conducted two major general practice surveys, the patients became more critical of the service, although the overall level of satisfaction was high in both studies. Some significant changes in attitude and service were highlighted, for example:

1   A dramatic swing towards appointment systems.
2   Improved access to hospital facilities.
3   Fewer frustrations concerning lack of leisure and poor pay amongst practitioners.
4   A slight increase in the percentage of practitioners expressing satisfaction with their careers, and a slight decrease in the number reporting frustration with unreasonable patients and trivial consultations.
5   A four-fold increase in the criticisms that patients made concerning doctors' availability to visit.

The rising tide of consumerism which characterised the 1980s, ballooning health service costs and reported inconsistencies in the standard and delivery of family services led to another major landmark in the development of general practice, presaged by the Government's White Paper *Working for Patients* and crystallised in the NHS Community Care Act 1990 and revised terms of service for GPs.

The key changes of the 1990 contract included:

1   An increase in the proportion of income derived from patient numbers as compared with automatic fixed-item allowances.
2   The setting of strict performance targets.
3   New separate payments to encourage minor surgery, child health surveillance and health promotion, as well as to encourage doctors practising in deprived areas.

In addition the Government sought to encourage:

1   Greater accountability for the spending of public funds, e.g. stricter availability requirements; medical and financial audit; indicative prescribing budgets; the fundholding scheme; compulsory practice reports.
2   More patient choice:
    (a) practice information leaflets and a local directory of family doctors;
    (b) an easier system for changing doctors;
    (c) a revised complaints system.
3   Greater HA autonomy (e.g. to set performance standards and to determine staff reimbursement levels).
4   Cost-consciousness and downward pressure on HA budgets.
5   The wider use of modern information technology (computers).

A reader approaching this account afresh may wonder why these proposals met with such a hostile reception. Some changes were felt to be regressive, some financially or politically motivated, some of unproven medical value. Concerns were expressed that patient care would suffer; that bureaucracy would increase; that many of the details were ill conceived and impractical.

What happened is now history. In a national ballot GPs decisively rejected the new terms of service, but the Health Secretary imposed them amidst calls for legal or industrial action, even resignation. The popularity of general practice slumped in the aftermath, and serious recruitment shortages emerged. Ballooning workloads further contributed to the discontent, and to the GMSC stance on 'core pay' for 'core duties'.

Big bang?

Further radical change is in prospect following a recent Government Bill. As discussed on p. 51 (big bang pilot schemes) new legislation has provided GPs with a choice of employment terms over and above the time-honoured model of self-employed contractor. It is now possible to be salaried, working for an NHS trust, a partnership or another body within the 'NHS family'; to hold a local, rather than a national employment contract; and to contract independently for non-core services. GPs may also run more extensive services, at least on a pilot basis, and there has been talk about GPs taking control of cottage hospitals, employing hospital consultants or other GPs on a sessional basis and even founding 'primary care trusts'. There may be less palatable outcomes too. Until now decisions on manpower provision in general practice have been made by the Medical Practices Committee (MPC), who assess the local need for doctors and regulate the supply to prevent areas becoming 'over-doctored'. However, under the new proposals the power to approve pilot scheme appointments passes to the Secretary of State. Supply may be allowed to exceed demand, forcing GPs to compete with one another in the struggle to retain patients. The scheme may introduce private capital and private enterprise into the primary care sector, and presage free market competition and the deregulation of primary care (the primary care 'big bang').

The place of delivery for primary care services will doubtless change under the new arrangements. Hospital trust–GP alliances, particularly inner-city ones, may offer primary care 'shops' on hospital premises; and the cost-rent scheme is being revamped in part because GPs will be working in bigger units. The merging of primary and secondary care budgets, will enable these larger units to offer secondary, as well as primary, care services.

The first wave of 'big bang pilots' (April 1998) could involve up to 2000 GPs. It is too early to say how this latest twist in the fortunes of the profession will develop. However, some practices have reacted to change with tremendous energy and vigour, and there is enough vitality and talent around to have confidence that general practice will emerge from this period of transition with its fundamental values unscathed.

2 The Consultation

According to Stott and Davis (1979) the potential exists within the consultation to address several issues:

1   The management of presenting problems.
2   The management of continuing problems.
3   The modification of health-seeking behaviour (education).
4   Opportunistic health promotion (education, screening and preventive activities).

Research into the consultation has examined the extent to which this potential is realised. Studies have attempted to define process (what the doctor and patient do) and its relationship to outcome (what happens to the patient afterwards). This chapter considers processes and outcomes, the methods used to examine them, the extent to which the consultation realises its potential, and how consultation techniques can be improved. The chapter concludes with sections on prescribing and the referral of patients for secondary care.

2.1 CONSULTING

Studying processes

Studies from other fields suggest that social skills and social competence have a great impact on overall effectiveness in dealing with people. Thus, Argyle (1972) found a variation up to 16-fold in absenteeism and labour turnover in industrial workforces led by supervisors with different styles. There is evidence that this competence consists of a repertoire of learned behaviours that may be identified and taught to less adept people. This approach has proved successful in training sales staff and American medical students, and has stimulated a great deal of interest in general practice processes and how to improve them.

The methods used to observe the consultation include:

* audiotaping;
* videotaping;
* the use of two-way mirrors;
* sitting in on colleagues' consultations;
* role-play.

No single method has proved entirely satisfactory: audiotapes miss important non-verbal information and contain uninterpretable pauses; role-play is to some extent artificial; and the presence of a video camera, or a second doctor, or the knowledge that there are eavesdroppers may modify the behaviour of doctor or patient or both. Despite these problems much useful descriptive information has been obtained. Taped consultations may be replayed and subjected to peer review and small group analysis, or dissected into their various social, linguistic and psychological components.

Analysis of this sort has led to several complex models of the doctor–patient relationship:

1 *The sociological model*—doctors and patients have beliefs based on the norms and values of their peers; their behaviour is consistent with the rules of these roles.

2 *The anthropological model* (e.g. Hellman 1981)—illness behaviour is promoted by the attempt to answer questions like 'What has happened?', 'Why now, and why to me?', 'What would happen if I did nothing?' Patients form a theory based on their experience, imagination and peer group views, to answer these questions, and this colours the consultation.

3 *The transactional model* (e.g. Berne 1964) — at any one point in time, three states of mind (ego states) operate in doctor and patient: parent, adult or child. Correct combinations communicate in transactions occurring in a predictable way and leading to a predictable outcome (rituals). Sometimes transactions are *crossed* (when, for example, the doctor talks like a parent and the patient adopts the role of subservient child), or *oblique* (when an ulterior message is aimed at another ego state in the recipient). A familiar example is the 'Why don't you? — Yes but . . .' ritual in which the doctor plays the parent ('I can make you grateful for my help, whether you want it or not') and the patient plays the child who always wins ('You go ahead and try . . .').

4 *The psychological model* (e.g. Rosenstock 1966) — patients vary in their health motivation, perceived vulnerability, the perceived seriousness of a problem, and the perceived costs and benefits; they behave rationally and consistently in the light of their own beliefs, which are fostered by a variety of cues, and modified by different outcomes.

One variation of this model (Rotter 1966) proposes that patients can be subdivided into those who explain what happens to them in terms of their own actions (i.e. have an internal locus of control) and those who explain everything as if they have little control (i.e. have an external locus of control). This aspect of the patient's psychological make-up influences outcome — thus, internal controllers are more likely to accept advice, keep appointments and take their prescriptions.

5 *The verbal model*—doctors develop a style, vocabulary, fluency and familiarity that control the relationship and structure it predictably. Byrne and Long (1976) analysed 2500 audiotaped consultations and defined various characteristic phases (phase 1 — relationship established by doctor; phase 2 — reason for consultation established by doctor; phase 3—examination conducted by doctor, etc.); about 75% of the medical content of the consultation was doctor-initiated. Workers have observed that doctors develop a style and vocabulary early in their careers that subsequently varies little from one consultation to another.

6 *The non-verbal model*—more information is conveyed by non-verbal cues than by speech; doctors and patients read one another's non-verbal messages and sometimes acknowledge and act on them, but non-verbal messages that are inconsistent with spoken ones hinder communication.

7 *The Balint model*—Balint (1957) pioneered a school of thinking altogether more sensitive to the nuances of the consultation. The main themes of his philosophy were:

(a) that patients' problems cannot be divided into physical and psychological categories: the two always coexist to a greater or lesser extent. Psychological problems often manifest physically, and physical diseases usually have psychological sequelae;

(b) that doctors have feelings and these have a function in the consultation;

(c) that doctors vary in their awareness of (a) and (b), but they can be trained to improve their awareness level.

Valuable though these models are, they often suffer the shortcoming of failing to relate process to outcome.

Studying outcomes

Measures of outcome are imperfect. It is extremely difficult, for example, to measure the average health, medical knowledge or prognosis of a doctor's list and to relate it to variations in his consultative approach. Three important outcomes that can be counted are patient satisfaction, patient recollection and patient compliance. When the consultation is judged according to these criteria it is clear that its potential is often not fully realised.

Are patients satisfied?

Communication is an aspect of care in which patients are most dissatisfied.

1 In one hospital study (McGhee 1961):

(a) less than 40% were dissatisfied with medical care, food, amenities; but

(b) 65% were dissatisfied with communication and 21% satisfied only with reservations.

2 In general practice surveys (e.g. Kincey *et al.* 1975) only about 50% expressed complete satisfaction with communications.

3 In outpatient surveys (e.g. Reader *et al.* 1957):

(a) 67% of patients wanted more information;

(b) 75% wanted to know 'as much as possible';

(c) 40% wanted the results and implications of all tests conducted.

What do patients remember?

1 Numerous studies suggest that more than 50% of information has
been forgotten when patients are interviewed within a few minutes of
leaving the surgery.

2 The characteristics of *memorable* information are that:
  (a) the patient believes it to be important (often diagnosis rather
  than treatment);
  (b) the patient understands it;
  (c) the information is given early in the consultation;
  (d) not too much is given at once.

How good is patient compliance?
Compliance is assessed in a variety of ways (by biological methods,
subjective ratings, self-report, pill counts and direct observation).
Whatever the method of evaluation, non-compliance rates are high—
varying from 12 to 70% (e.g. Davis, 1968)—and it seems likely that 50%
or so of medical advice is not taken. Richard Podell (1975) proposed
the 'rule of threes':
• one-third follow advice closely enough to make it effective;
• one-third follow *some* advice, though *not* closely enough to make it
effective;
• one-third do not accept or follow advice at all.

Other studies on outcome
Two other types of outcome sometimes studied are patient well-being
and the ability of doctors to make true and accurate diagnoses.
1 Egbert *et al.* (1964) demonstrated that patients counselled prior to
surgery on the likely postoperative course experienced less pain and
required less analgesia postoperatively than others who were unpre-
pared. This is an example of the beneficial effect that process can have
on the outcome of well-being.
2 Shepherd *et al.* (1966) reported wide variations between London
GPs in the level of psychiatric illness they detected—from 38 per 1000
up to 323 per 1000, which is a nine-fold discrepancy. Goldberg (1981)
has identified certain patterns of behaviour practised by GPs adept at
identifying mental ill-health:
  (a) empathy;
  (b) early eye contact;
  (c) directive rather than closed questioning;
  (d) clarification of the complaint at an early stage.

Improving consultation techniques
Consultation analysis has suggested various explanations for the relative failure in communication observed in doctor–patient studies:
1 *Patient factors*:
  (a) limited knowledge of illness (many misconceptions and folk-
  models of illness);

(b) diffidence in asking for clarification. This is class-related. Only 45% of hospital patients obtain the information they want by asking, but 65% of class 1 ask, while only 40% of class 5 do (Cartwright 1964);

(c) the negative effect of anxiety;

(d) the 'hidden agenda' — patients often legitimise their desire to consult over one matter by presenting with another one that they think is a more respectable reason in the eyes of their doctor. If their complaint is taken at face value, the 'hidden agenda' may remain hidden and the patient leaves the room dissatisfied.

2 *Doctor factors*:

(a) professional and personal attitudes. Doctors vary at the extremes from autocratic, high-status information-withholders to egalitarian sharers of information who place emphasis on the patient's role;

(b) medical uncertainty and doubt — which doctors prefer to hide;

(c) inappropriately technical language;

(d) too much information too quickly;

(e) failure to establish what concerns the patient;

(f) non-verbal cues of uncertainty or doubt, at variance with what is said.

3 *Doctor–patient relationship factors*:

(a) communication and compliance are better if there is doctor–patient rapport (usually a doctor who is perceived to be empathetic and a patient who conforms to the doctor's idea of a model patient!);

(b) class differences between doctor and patient are important. There appear to be linguistic and other social factors that produce better communication if doctor and patient come from a similar background. Thus, Cartwright and O'Brien (1976) found that middle-class patients, on average, spend longer in consultation, raise more questions and cover more problems with their doctor than working-class patients do.

Consideration of these factors suggests that various techniques can be employed to improve such outcomes as diagnostic accuracy, patient satisfaction, communication and compliance. Thus, Ley *et al.* (1976) and others have stressed the need for:

• a good relationship (caring and confiding; Korsch & Negrete 1972);

• establishing and giving due weight to the patient's concerns, beliefs and expectations;

• giving information early in a consultation;

• keeping the message simple and clear (and not imparting too much in one session);

• repeating the message and stressing its importance;

• providing specific information and concrete examples;

- giving written instructions as a reminder.

In addition:

- according to Bertakis (1977), recall and satisfaction are both enhanced when patients are asked to repeat and give feedback on the instructions they are given;
- Francis *et al.* (1969) have shown that compliance and satisfaction are enhanced when explanations are spontaneously volunteered by the physician;
- outcome is improved by the correct use of non-verbal cues (e.g. body posture can communicate concern; several studies have shown that good communicators smile more, look at the interlocutor more and have a different intonation when compared with less successful colleagues);
- patient-centred behaviour (seeing illness through the patient's eyes and with his expectations) has been linked with higher patient satisfaction, better compliance with treatment, better treatment of chronic health problems, and better recovery from ill-defined illnesses;
- Law *et al.* (1995) report from videotape analysis that women doctors tend to be more patient-centred than men; also that the highest 'patient-centredness' scores are achieved between women doctors and women patients—the lowest being between male doctors and female patients;
- the structure of the consulting environment affects the amount of information exchanged (e.g. seating arrangements can reduce or enhance exchanges by a factor of six; Pietroni 1976).

One interesting paper has looked at the doctor himself as a therapeutic instrument in the consultation, and the extent to which this is enhanced by a positive, assertive approach. Thomas (1987) found that in the 40–60% of consultations where no firm diagnosis can be made, patients feel better in the hands of a positive physician.

The difficult patient

In the MRCGP exam (and in real life), there is a special interest in how to handle the difficult patient, the non-compliant 'troublemaker', the addict who will not relinquish his tranquilliser, the liberated rebel giving birth in an unheated caravan, contraceptive and ethical conundrums, problem families and so on. Such characters feature prominently in Paper 1 of the exam (see Section 10.4, p. 278), and are thick on the ground in the viva too!

At the simplest level the courses of action open, given a contentious request are: to agree, to disagree, or to refer/bargain/educate/counsel—and each will have predictable implications.

At a slightly more sophisticated level, there have been several attempts to classify the so-called 'heart-sink' patient (Cohen 1986).

Groves (1951) has defined four categories of difficult patient (Table 2.1).

Table 2.1 Types of 'difficult' patient.

Class	Features
1 The dependent clinger	Expresses excessive gratitude for doctor's, actions, but seeks regular reassurance over minor problems
2 The entitled demander	Frequently complains about imagined shortcomings in the service received
3 The manipulative help-rejecter	Presents a series of symptoms the doctor is powerless to improve
4 The self-destructive denier	The patient who refuses to accept his behaviour affects his disease and will not modify self-harming habits

Gerrard and Ridded (1988) define 10 categories of patient, from 'black holes' to 'secrets'. Others have found heart-sink patients to be a disparate group of individuals, defying obvious classification and sharing in common only the ability to 'exasperate, defeat and over-whelm' (O'Dowd 1988).

The common response to such patients is unnecessary investigation or inappropriate referral, arising from a need to escape for a time from contact with the patient.

Coping strategies include:

1 Recognition by the doctor of his true feelings.

2 Help from counsellors and psychologists (for the patient, or doctor, or both!).

3 Alternative sources of therapy — the extended family network, religious organisations, self-help groups.

4 The work of Balint groups.

5 Peer group meetings — for support, information-sharing and to formulate multidisciplinary management plans.

6 Challenging (with tact and sympathy) inappropriate patient demands; and if necessary making a pact with him, e.g. the 'allowed' frequency of attendance; or a hierarchical problem list, so that one query is handled at a time.

Problem patients will occupy a disproportionate amount of our time, both within exams and outside them, and this is an area worthy of special preparation.

The consultation is *the* central process in the practice of medicine. It is not surprising therefore that attempts at raising standards have placed such an emphasis on consultation techniques. This chapter is a simple résumé of a large and complex body of literature. For a more comprehensive review the interested reader is referred to *Doctor–Patient Communication* by Pendleton and Hasler (see Further Reading).

Is it all necessary?

At least 50% of all consultations end with a prescription being written, amounting to 13 000 scripts per GP per year. The cost is considerable: the number of prescriptions dispensed in the UK almost doubled from 240 million to 500 million between 1964 and 1996; £4 billion was spent, amounting to £120 000 per annum per GP, and an average of seven prescriptions per head of the population.

Though large in absolute terms, these figures stand up well to international comparison (Tables 2.2 and 2.3). Yet we are all familiar with examples of unnecessary prescribing; for example, when:

- diagnosis is still in doubt;
- ingredients are probably ineffective;
- combinations and formulations are irrational;
- the value of treatment is debatable (in obviously self-limiting illness).

The variation in prescribing habits between doctors is often high-lighted. In prescribing surveys net ingredient cost per item may vary more than threefold and prescribing rates from 24.5 to 160.9 items per 1000 patients per month within a local area (Troup 1989). But can this amount of variation be satisfactorily explained? In one study of 90 Health Authorities (HAs) 81% of the variation was explained in terms of demand variables like age and mortality risk (Morton-Jones *et al.* (1993).

In general there is a lack of hard data relating prescribing practices to outcome, and without this it is difficult to judge performance and cost-effectiveness. However, the 1994 Audit Commission report, *A Prescription for Improvement*, criticised GP prescribing, and a public enquiry by Sainsbury (1967) into more than 2200 prescribed drugs concluded:

1 50% were effective;
2 8% were rational combinations;
3 35% were undesirable (obsolete, ineffective or irrational).

Table 2.2 International comparison of prescribing rates.

Country	Scripts/patient/year
USA	16.6
Italy	11.3
West Germany	11.2
France	10.1
Spain	9.6
New Zealand	8.5
Australia	7.7
UK	7.0
Sweden	4.7

Table 2.3 Health care spending—international comparisons.

	Health care and drug spending as a percentage of GDP (1995)	Spending per head on health care (£)
Switzerland	9.1	2176
France	9.2	1435
Germany	8.5	1677
UK	**6.8**	**814**

This raises important issues, such as:

1 Why are these drugs made?
2 Why are they allowed?
3 Why are they prescribed?

The first two questions are really political and economic: drug companies, operating within legal guidelines and the international codes of pharmaceutical practice, produce drugs for which they claim there is a market (proven by doctors' willingness to prescribe them and patients' willingness to take them). They make profits, some of which are ploughed back into research and development, they pay a large amount in taxes, and their employment record is good. A lot of money is spent on drug promotion and on political lobbying, but some drugs are of undisputed importance.

The Government seeks to maintain a delicate balance: it must appear a neutral watchdog and must keep faith with doctors and drug companies, but it also has to control its own budget. To curb drug company profits on non-essential drugs might affect research into future winners; to regulate too strictly could alienate drug companies and doctors alike and produce adverse political propaganda. Earlier Government strategies focused on education:

1 Free prescribing information for doctors (the *British National Formulary*, *Prescriber's Journal*, *Drugs and Therapeutic Bulletin*).
2 Feedback from the Prescription Pricing Authority, and visits from the Regional Medical Officer (to doctors who deviated markedly from the norm in their prescribing habits).
3 Attempts to control costs by negotiating with drug companies to limit prices and profits (various voluntary price-regulation schemes have been tried).
4 Voluntary initiatives have also been encouraged — many on an intraprofessional basis with the Royal College and leading academic practices taking a prominent role. However, beginning with the Limited List (1985), the Government sought a more direct control over prescribing costs.
5 The Limited List scheme was based on successful precedents in NHS hospitals and in other countries like Norway and New Zealand, and saved the NHS £75 million in its first full year of operation.

6 Fundholding (see p. 46) represented another Government plan to make doctors more aware of the costs of their prescribing, and to involve them in managing and moderating it.

Two other initiatives are noteworthy:

7 The Prescribing Analysis and Cost (PACT) package.

8 Prescribing allocations and the prescribing incentive scheme.

The PACT scheme

The PACT scheme comprises a series of quarterly prescribing reports for GPs in England (in Wales and Scotland there are parallel systems). Prescribing and dispensing reports relate to principals and partnerships and information is fed back at three possible levels (Table 2.4).

PACT analyses are based on the *prescription item*, a measure which has been shown to vary in quantity as well as cost (Bogle *et al.* 1994). Average cost per item may reflect unfairly on GPs who prescribe larger quantities per script to patients who have to pay prescription charges. Furthermore, the results, like other counting exercises which deal in quantity but not in quality, need to be related to outcome.

Prescribing allocations and the prescribing incentive scheme

At present there are two schemes for setting a practice's drug budget. *Fundholding practices* manage their own monies, but their HA recommends an annual level (called a prescribing allocation). In the case of *non-fundholding practices* the annual prescribing allocation set by the HA's Prescribing Medical Adviser imposes on them an effective drug budget. In each case the amount recommended (or set) is determined individually, based on:

• historic prescribing patterns;
• average prescribing costs locally;

Table 2.4 The PACT scheme.

PACT level	Format	Availability
1	The simplest level. A four-page report with basic information: • quarterly prescribing costs; • average costs per item; • relationship to list size; • subdivision by therapeutic group; • comparison with practice, local and national averages	All GPs receive this overview
2	More detailed information with special emphasis on the most expensive sections	On request. Also sent automatically to high-cost practices*
3	Full reports running to more than 100 pages with an index and technical guide	Only on request

*Practices whose total costs exceed HA averages by at least 25% or where costs in one of the six major therapeutic categories is at least 75% above average.

- list size and age profile (a key determinant);
- special factors not previously recognised but identified by the practice;
- with time and experience, special factors identified by 'improved NHS management systems'.

In both cases practices are expected to regularly monitor their prescribing profiles throughout the financial year to ensure that the year-end target is met. They are assisted by:

- quarterly PACT reports;
- an indicative prescribing statement and monthly budget information (including a year-end projection);
- an annual summary return;
- more detailed breakdowns from the Prescription Pricing Authority on request.

A number of bodies and posts exist to assist the effort (Table 2.5).

From April 1999 when fundholding is abolished, there will be one method of budgetary allocation for GPs in England and Wales: indicative prescribing budgets will be set by PCGs and their HAs. The basis of allocation, and the monitoring and feedback requirements have not yet been spelled out fully, but probably will be based on existing mechanisms.

At present a system of sanctions exists to penalise profligate prescribers (fundholders may have their budget privileges withdrawn, or may have to pay back an overspend later, or the HA may discuss with a practice ways of containing its costs); some sanctions procedure is likely to continue in future where there is clear evidence of overspending.

Incentives exist as well as sanctions. Fundholding practices may channel part of any savings they make back into approved patient services. Similarly, in non-fundholding practices local voluntary incentive schemes enable HAs and Local Medical Councils to plan a target saving, part of which can be ploughed back into agreed projects. In

Table 2.5 Bodies and posts designed to improve prescribing practices.

The National Medicines Resource Centre	Centrally funded. Located in the Merseyside Regional Health Authority. Staffed by drug information pharmacists. Produces a monthly bulletin
Prescribing Unit, Department of General Practice, Leeds University	To investigate the range of normal prescribing and to assist research
Medical prescribing advisers	Doctors appointed at HA level to establish, monitor and advise on indicative prescribing
Medical Audit Advisory Groups	Established at local level to assist GPs' efforts at audit
The Prescribing Allocation Group	Advises the NHS Executive on methods of allocating drug budgets to regions and practices

future PCGs will be able to offer incentives in a similar fashion. Recently a quarter of 450 non-fundholding practices in the Northern region hit their savings target, demonstrating that the incentive approach can be successful (Bateman *et al.* 1996).

Clearly all medical practitioners are under pressure to consider the cost of their prescribing policies, and need tight management controls that identify exceptional costs as they arise. The practice formulary is likely to be one of the essential administrative tools in cost containment.

What is rational prescribing?

Though it is relatively simple to collect prescribing statistics, it is not simple to interpret them. For example, it has been pointed out (Stott 1989) that doctors with above-average prescribing costs may:
- have expensive patients (for example, those on growth hormone, or domiciliary oxygen, or fertility treatment);
- do more good (be more aware of the therapeutic possibilities; keep patients out of expensive hospital beds; keep them productive and at work, etc.);
- be more efficient in screening for (and then treating) latent problems like hypertension or hyperlipidaemia.

The implicit assumption that above-average prescribing is 'bad medicine' and below-average is 'good medicine' has been challenged, since process has not been related to outcome.

The Government has made HAs responsible for both hospital and family practitioner services, and hopes thereby to compare the relative costs of alternative approaches, but information is not presently available at this level of sophistication. How then are we to define rational prescribing?

One serviceable definition would be that prescribing conforms to consensus opinion of the best current practice.

How to prescribe rationally

The choice of a drug is influenced by several considerations:
1 Is the diagnosis known?
2 Is a drug required?
3 Will it work?
4 Will it harm?
5 How much will it cost?
6 Have all the alternatives been considered?
7 Is the likely benefit : risk ratio acceptable?

What to look for in a prescriber

The responsible prescriber has several duties:
1 To ensure the diagnosis is right.
2 To make a positive and correct decision that a drug is needed.
3 To choose a drug appropriate to the patient's needs.
4 To consult the patient, and to ensure there is informed consent.

5   To explain the patient's role and to secure his co-operation.
6   To keep accurate prescribing records.
7   To oversee the course of treatment.
8   To terminate it when it is no longer needed.

Social reasons for prescribing

However, doctors often prescribe without proof efficacy. Why should this be? Contributing factors include:

1   True variations in medical opinion (in Germany in 1974 doctors issued 154 000 hypertensive scripts per million populus; in the UK the figure was 200 per million).
2   The pressure of pharmaceutical advertising.
3   Habit, peer group recommendation and ignorance.
4   Patients' demands (there is evidence that this is overestimated and that a larger percentage leave a consultation with a prescription than those expecting one beforehand. Indeed, up to 20% of patients do not even have their scripts dispensed!).
5   Attempts at placebo prescribing (see below).
6   A variety of social reasons:
    (a) to play for time until the true picture becomes clearer or natural recovery occurs;
    (b) to cover uncertainty, rather than admit it;
    (c) because of medico-legal worries;
    (d) to keep faith with patients, to justify their efforts and to demonstrate concern;
    (e) to hasten the conclusion of a consultation;
    (f) to avoid confrontation;
    (g) to keep faith with their partners (hence the 'Friday afternoon antibiotic');
    (h) personal experience: we like to think we are scientific, but often base our prescribing on limited and subjective experiences with our own small patient samples.

Many patients are adept at securing social prescriptions, and use well recognised ploys to obtain what they want (e.g. insistence, flattery, bargaining, comparison with other doctors).

Placebo prescribing

The response rate to placebos is high, of the order of 30–40%. According to some sources there are particular personality traits (e.g. extroversion, sociability, neuroticism, awareness of autonomic function) that identify the placebo responder. However, other studies suggest no clear correlation and show that most people can respond given the correct situation.

Many conditions can be helped (Table 2.6). Note that the response is not entirely psychological: physiological changes have been observed, suggesting a 'real' effect, e.g. placebos have:
• reversed the motility effects of ipecacuanha;

Table 2.6 Some conditions susceptible to the placebo response.

Angina	Enuresis	Insomnia
Anxiety and depression	Hayfever	Peptic ulcer
Arthritis	Headaches	Postoperative pain
Asthma	Hyperglycaemia	Premenstrual tension
Blood pressure	Hyperlipidaemia	Social problems

- lowered blood sugars;
- lowered blood pressure;
- reduced cholesterol (and mortality from ischaemic heart disease according to one study).

The time–response of placebo treatment also mimics the pharmacokinetics of active drugs.

Up to 40% of patients experience placebo side-effects including: headache; anorexia; diarrhoea; nausea and vomiting; dry mouth; vertigo; lassitude; palpitations; dermatitis; even addiction!

Factors affecting the placebo response include:

1 Pain levels—the more severe, the more likely is a placebo response.
2 Anxiety levels.
3 Tablet size, appearance and formulation. To be effective tablets should be:
   (a) very small or very large;
   (b) unlike an everyday medicine in appearance;
   (c) capsules or injections rather than tablets;
   (d) bitter to taste.
   Colour is also important (Table 2.7).
4 Patient expectation.
5 High technology: attendance at outpatient clinics, X-rays, and especially invasive investigations have a therapeutic effect.

The conviction of the prescriber, his charisma and the doctor–patient relationship probably also contribute. Male patients tend to respond more frequently than females, and higher social classes are especially prone.

Ethical problems
Proponents of the placebo argue that:
1 It is effective (what does the mechanism matter if the result is satisfactory?).

Table 2.7 The effect of tablet colour on placebo response.

Colour	Best response in:
Blue or green	Creams/ointments
Green	Anxiety
Red	Analgesia
Red or brown	Elixirs
Yellow	Depression

2 It is reassuring, and helps morale in chronic/incurable disease.
3 It fulfils patient expectations.
4 There is no significant toxicity.
5 There is evidence of an underlying physical basis (e.g. naloxone has been shown to reverse placebo pain relief suggesting a possible endorphin-based mechanism).

Those against placebo prescribing argue that:
1 It is deception and an abuse of a relationship of mutual trust.
2 It may generate hurt and ill-feeling if the deception is uncovered.
3 It delays true diagnosis.
4 It reinforces the sick role.

Whatever the rights and wrongs, placebo prescribing is widely practised, and (if we admit it to ourselves) so is the habit of prescribing for largely social reasons.

Generic vs. branded prescribing

Prescriptions are still commonly written by brand name, although health officials have counselled the use of generic alternatives, and suggested that the taxpayer should not pay for expensive brands when there are cheaper alternatives. The two sides of the argument have been well expressed by Collier (1988) and Cruickshank (1988). Table 2.8 illustrates that the matter is not as clear cut as might be supposed.

Self-medication

The last decade has seen a world-wide move to increase the number and range of medicines available over the counter. Drugs may be reclassified from prescription-only to over-the-counter (OTC) provided that they are safe, of low toxicity in overdose, and used only for 'minor' self-limiting conditions.

Doctors and patients may perceive some advantages:
• an opportunity for patients to take more responsibility for their own health;
• an opportunity to save the cost, inconvenience and time involved in obtaining a prescription;
• to ease the pressures on surgery appointments.

In addition, a shift in the costs of purchasing minor ailments medicines from NHS to patients should preserve tax-payers' funds to meet more urgent needs.

However, there are some potential disadvantages and concerns:
1 an increased risk of drug interaction with prescription medicines;
2 an increased risk of self-medication side-effects;
3 the risk of inappropriate self medication—for example:
   (a) self medicating for a serious illness whose presentation is thereby masked or delayed;
   (b) taking the wrong preparation or wrong formulation;

Table 2.8 Generic versus named-brand prescribing.

Supporting more generic prescribing (Collier 1988)	Defending brand prescribing (Cruickshank 1988)
1 There are fewer generic names, making learning and teaching simpler	1 There are more than 40 generic versions of propranolol alone: changes in tablet size, colour and taste confuse patients and may prejudice compliance
2 Generic names are international and used routinely in scientific publications: this allows clear exchange of information. Generic names convey an indication of chemical class, facilitating an understanding of their uses	2 Generic names are often long and confusing. Brand names are shorter, simpler and more memorable
3 Stocking a smaller line of drugs would be simpler and more efficient for the chemist, who could achieve savings through bulk purchase	3 Chemists, reimbursed on a fixed price basis, have an incentive to purchase only the cheaper generics; in the case of overseas sources quality may be suspect
4 The NHS drug bill may be reduced by up to 100 million pounds per annum	4 Relatively small savings to the NHS (in percentage terms) represent punitive losses to research drug houses who need reserves to develop new drugs
5 Under the Medicines Act the licensing authority and its inspectorate guarantee comparability of quality between like products	5(a) There have been examples of clinical inequivalence between generic versions in some studies; (b) therapeutic data are not always required by the authorities and no data on efficacy/side-effects; (c) ingredients other than the active agent (up to 95% of the tablet) can differ from the original product; (d) ultimately, if the manufacturer of a generic cannot be identified, product liability may fall on the supplier (doctor or pharmacist)

(c) taking the wrong dose (or the correct dose for too short or too long a period);

4   a risk that a 'pills for all ills' culture will become fostered in consumers;

5   less feedback on adverse drug reactions;

6   less chance to offer opportunistic health promotion activities.

Bradley *et al.* (1995) have pointed out that the trend to self-medicate has practical implications for GPs, who will need to:

• ask routinely about patients' use of non-prescription medicines;

• consider these, and the potential for drug interactions and side-effects;

• educate patients on responsible and safe use of OTC preparations;

• forge better links with local pharmacists, who will increasingly be offering advice to their patients.

Practice formularies

Every doctor, consciously or unconsciously, uses a personal drug formulary for his routine prescribing needs—often on the basis of familiarity, previous training, habit, the preference of colleagues or local consultants, and so on. However, many authors argue that this piecemeal approach is no longer sustainable — legally, administratively, contractually or ethically. The Government has strongly advocated the development of local prescribing formularies. Others too have made the case.

Advantages

1 In writing practice formularies doctors are forced to look critically at their personal prescribing habits, and to make choices which are hopefully safer, better, cheaper, more rational and more cost-effective. The process is very educational.

2 There has been a four-fold increase in the number of available medicines over the last 30 years, producing a mountain of product information too large for anyone to assimilate. If prescribers are to keep abreast of current knowledge they must by necessity read and choose selectively.

3 Drug formularies can reduce practice prescribing costs (Beardon *et al.* 1987). Doctors with formularies can justify their spending, and their efforts are more accessible to audit. It also makes it easier for fundholders to balance their budgets.

Home-produced vs. standard formularies

Several excellent formularies already exist, including a respected version by the Royal College of General Practitioners' Northern Ireland Faculty. There are advantages to adopting one of these standard formularies:

- the hard work of preparation has already been done;
- such sources will be periodically updated;
- they provide an accepted standard of excellence.

Alternatively doctors can produce their own practice formulary. This has the advantage that they will learn a lot of therapeutics and pharmacology along the way, and can adapt to local needs and hospital colleagues' known preferences.

Disadvantages include:

- the considerable effort required;
- the need for regular updating;
- possible medico-legal problems arising from errors and omissions.

In writing a practice formulary, several practical steps need to be taken:

1 Secure the agreement and involvement of all the partners.

2 Divide the work up between them (different doctors may choose different therapeutic groups).

3   Get each person to research his topic, and then select and justify an appropriate list of drugs.

4   Meet and agree a first-draft formulary. If necessary seek arbitration (e.g. from the head of the local drug information service).

5   Agree circumstances under which deviation from the formulary is permissible.

6   Check and counter-check all prescribing information before producing a final version, which should include information on side-effects and drug interactions.

7   Agree policies for:
    (a) initiating drug treatment;
    (b) drug treatment started by hospital colleagues and other GPs;
    (c) reviewing maintenance therapy.

8   Review in the light of new developments and information.

Local prescribing groups may make lighter work of the task. The Audit Commission has recommended closer co-ordination between GPs and hospital prescribers, and this has led to joint local prescribing committees and formularies agreed between GPs and consultants.

2.3 REFERRING

Questions have arisen recently concerning the general practice referral system — its effectiveness, strengths and weaknesses; consumer choice and the equitable rationing of health care services; how to refer rationally and how to identify rational referrals.

The rationale for the present system

The present referral system from generalist to specialist arose historically from mid 19th-century demarcation disputes between apothecaries, physicians and surgeons. Although this restrictive practice was intended to protect the livelihood of doctors, it has since been justified as a rational and effective basis for allocating health care resources.

Patients can only bypass the gatekeeper system in the case of urgent personal need (casualty), or public interest (sexually transmitted disease services). It is argued that the generalist can, from this position:
• ration access according to need;
• target care more specifically;
• protect against over-investigation and over-medicalisation;
• prevent the misuse of expensive high-technology facilities, and needless trafficking between specialisms.

The GP is also best placed to appreciate the whole picture, and the patient benefits from two complementary views — personal and technical.

Criticisms of the present system

Although there are obvious arguments in favour of this approach, critics have pointed out that:

- GPs exercise a virtual monopoly in their control of access to secondary care in the UK;
- other countries' health care systems function without such a restriction of choice;
- there is unacceptable variation in the performance standards of the gatekeepers, with expensive and potentially unfair consequences.

To what extent are these criticisms justified?

A restrictive practice?

The referral system was granted special dispensation from the Restrictive Practices Act 1976 because of its perceived advantages to the public. However, this is a topic on which the Monopolies and Mergers Commission has been seeking a review, and doctors cannot assume that the status quo will remain unchallenged. Marinker (1988) considers that doctors will need to take active steps to fight their corner.

Quality and quantity of GP referrals

Descriptive studies have established a variation in referral and investigation rates not accounted for by characteristics of the population studied. At extremes they varied from 2.9 per 100 consultations to 11.8 per 100 consultations in one study (Wilkin & Smith 1987); and in another study from 5 per 1000 per month to 115 per 1000 per month (Last 1967). A 20-fold variation in referral rates seems stunning. Is it an indictment of standards within the profession?

Variations can arise through errors of counting, random fluctuation of demand, true differences in demand or different referral thresholds between physicians. There is some evidence that a combination of these factors contributes. Thus:

1 There is scope for error in:

(a) not counting private referrals (in some practices a substantial percentage of the total);

(b) relating referral rates to personal list size rather than workload and consultation rates in practices with shared-list systems.

2 There is also doubt as to which denominator (list size, episodes of illness, number of consultations, category of disease) best measures the rate in question.

3 Using too short a study time may lead to random peaks and troughs in demand. Moore and Roland (1989) point to the many factors influencing referral rates and suggest that a significant part of the variation may be due to the fairly small number of referrals in most studies and the effect of chance. They conclude, however, that 'there remains a substantial part of the variation that cannot be accounted for'.

Two points are worth noting:

1 Variations in referral rates do not seem to correlate with the age of doctors, their use of investigations, postgraduate qualifications or experience in a specialty (which actually increases referrals to that specialty; Morrell *et al.* 1971).

2 High referrers are not necessarily profligate or inadequate: they may be more aware of the diagnostic and therapeutic possibilities and offer a better service. It requires a better measurement of outcome to make this judgement.

Referral thresholds

Nevertheless, there are a number of criteria — not all medical — that doctors apply by common agreement in making their referral decisions, and other circumstances that doubtless sway them (Table 2.9). Differences in subjective judgement inevitably arise.

One study has focused on doctors' capacity to cope with uncertainty, comparing the referral thresholds of Dutch, Belgian and British GPs (Grol *et al.* 1990). There was a marked difference in their comfort with a wait-and-see policy: all doctors dislike uncertainty but some can live with it better than others.

In principle, risk-taking can be quantified through a closer understanding of the sensitivity, specificity and positive predictive value of clinical symptoms and signs in the community: doctors with desk-top computers should 'learn the language of probability' and its application in improving the assessment of referral need, according to a leading editorial (Lancet 1990). Perhaps this day will come.

Emergency admission trends

Emergency hospital admissions have been rising in the UK over the past four decades, to the point whereby bed shortage 'crises' have become commonplace. But, with the exceptions of childhood asthma and self-poisoning, little evidence exists that disease has become genuinely more common.

Part of the blame has been laid on modern primary care services. It has been suggested, for example, that GP deputies are less inclined to fulfil the gatekeeper role; that GPs have been browbeaten by rising

Table 2.9 Factors influencing referral decisions.

1 Distance from local hospitals
2 Availability of public transport
3 Family and social expectations
4 Community support services
5 Quality and quantity of available hospital services
6 Variations in morbidity, age–sex structure and other environmental factors within the population
7 The training, interests and experience of the GP
8 The GP's ability to abide uncertainty

patient demands and expectations, as well as fear of litigation; and that the problem has not been helped recently by a fundholding scheme that charged practice budgets for elective, but not for emergency services.

Certainly the rise in admissions has mirrored an increase in surgery attendances and out-of-hours calls. But a recent review has highlighted the likely multifactorial nature of the situation (Capewell 1996). Other factors may contribute that lie outside the hands of GPs, such as:

- population ageing;
- premature hospital discharges, leading to 'revolving door' readmissions;
- social change, e.g. decreased support for the elderly, increased social deprivation;
- consumer demand, heightened by Patient Charter initiatives and media scare stories;
- new hospital-based emergency interventions (e.g. thrombolysis for myocardial infarctions);
- (paradoxically) increased capacity. According to Roemer's Law admissions rise to fill the available beds, just as new roads attract new traffic jams!

Whatever the explanation, a bed crisis in the hospital sector has serious repercussions for GPs too: they experience difficulties in securing urgent admissions, and in coping with the extra workload arising from patients discharged earlier in their convalescence. A variety of solutions have been proffered, such as open-access outpatient clinics, and the staffing of accident and emergency departments by experienced GPs and practice nurses; but a more basic understanding of the underlying causes of the phenomenon will be required before it can be adequately tackled.

3 Prevention and Screening

3.1 PRINCIPLES

Definitions

There is some confusion over the use of the terms primary, secondary and tertiary prevention. One school of thought defines the three degrees of prevention as follows:

1 *(primary) prevention*: removing the causal agent, e.g. sanitation measures of the 19th century;

2 *(secondary) prevention*: identifying presymptomatic disease (or disease risk factors) before significant damage is done, e.g. screening for hypertension;

3 *(tertiary) prevention*: limiting complications/disability in patients with established disease by regular surveillance, e.g. trying to prevent diabetic problems by good control, regular fundoscopy, foot care, etc.

According to this definition *screening* is a form of secondary prevention. It can be defined as the application of sorting procedures to populations by doctor initiative with the aim of identifying asymptomatic disease or people at particular risk from it.

Others have taken primary prevention to mean measures taken *before* an event (e.g. in trying to prevent a myocardial infarction), and secondary prevention to mean those measures taken *after* an event to limit damage or prevent recurrence.

Anticipatory care

Anticipatory care is an approach to medicine that concentrates attention on anticipating and precluding problems. It is in fact an effort to offer all appropriate forms of prevention (however defined) within the consultation and the organisational framework of primary care.

Methods of screening

Methods of screening follow two broad lines:

1 *Case finding (opportunistic or anticipatory care)* — this means taking the opportunity when the patient attends on another matter to screen him for the desired characteristic. This method is simple, involves no extra administration or expense and reaches 75% of the practice population in 1 year and 90% in 5 years.

2 *True screening* — the active pursuit of cases by questionnaire, letter, home visit, purpose-designed clinic, etc. This involves more administrative work and the expense (partly offset by item-of-service payments where applicable) is borne by the GP.

The major disadvantage is that patients do not always share their doctor's passion for screening and there is often a significant non-

Table 3.1 Pros and cons of opportunistic versus formal screening.

	Pros	Cons
Opportunistic screening	Simple, cheap to administer Does not depend on patient compliance Reaches a section of the public who will not attend for preventive advice alone Can be made relevant to the circumstances of attendance	Requires organisation, time and commitment Does not offer 100% coverage to the target group The time used is not 'protected': more urgent demands may take precedence Patients seen when ill may be less receptive to health education
Formal screening approaches	'Protected' time for discussion Purpose of attendance understood by all parties Attendees are (by definition) motivated and more receptive to advice they have personally solicited Comprehensive coverage of related health areas can be planned Financial incentives now favour the formal health promotion clinic	Requires organisation, time and commitment Important non-attendance problem, wasting health care resources Users are often those least in need of the service Administrative obstacles are considerable

attendance rate. The advantages and disadvantages of these two approaches are compared in Table 3.1.

Requirements of a screening programme

Wilson (1966) proposed these criteria:

1 The condition must be:
   (a) common;
   (b) important;
   (c) diagnosable by acceptable methods.

2 There must be a latent interval in which effective interventional treatment is possible.

3 Screening must be:
   (a) simple and cheap, if possible, and in any case cost-effective;
   (b) continuous;
   (c) on a group agreed by policy to be at high risk.

To this we can add the requirements that the disease is readily treatable and that screening tests are highly sensitive (few false negatives), highly specific (few false positives), safe, non-invasive, acceptable to the patient and easy to interpret. If used in mass screening programmes a test should have a high positive predictive value (Table 3.2).

Relatively few conditions exist for which all criteria could be said

Table 3.2 Sensitivity, specificity and positive predictive value of screening tests.

1 In order to assess a new screening test, comparison is made with a reference method (which is the best currently available)
2 Cases and non-cases are identified by applying both tests and a 2 × 2 contingency table constructed:

	Reference method		Totals
	+ve	−ve	
New screening test			
+ve	a	b	$a + b$
−ve	c	d	$c + d$
Totals	$a + c$	$b + d$	$a + b + c + d$

3 If it is assumed that the reference test is always correct,
- a cases are true positives
- d cases are true negatives
- c cases are classified falsely negative
- b cases are classified falsely positive

4 The *sensitivity* of a test is the proportion of true positives detected as positive by the test, i.e.:

$$\text{sensitivity} = (a/(a + c)) \times 100\ (\%)$$

In a highly sensitive test c is very low, i.e. there are few false negatives
5 The *specificity* of a test is the proportion of true negatives detected as negative by the test, i.e.:

$$\text{specificity} = (d/(d + b)) \times 100\ (\%)$$

In a highly specific test b is very low, i.e. there are few false positives.
6 The *positive predictive value* of a test is the proportion of those detected as positive by the test who truly *are* positive, i.e.:

$$\text{positive predictive value} = (a/(a + b)) \times 100\ (\%)$$

More simply, it is the likelihood that the test is right in an individual whom the test declares positive

to be met. It is certainly true, since screening is doctor-initiated, that benefits should outweigh costs.

Weighing costs and benefits
Several theoretical and practical considerations have a bearing on the cost–benefit equation:
1 There is always a trade-off between sensitivity and specificity in a screening test, i.e. the looser the definition of a case, the fewer the number of borderline cases missed, but the larger the number of false positives.
2 Even tests of high specificity and sensitivity may have a low predictive value in populations where the prevalence of a condition is low (odd but true).
3 Screening tests often unearth disease at an earlier stage in its genesis; this may lead to the spurious belief that survival has been

| Clinical case: | A | ━━━━━━━━━━━━━━▶ B ━━━━━━━━━━━━━━━━━━━━▶ C |
| Screened case: | A | ━━━━▶ B ━━━━━━━━━━━━━━━━━━━━━━━━━━━━━━━━━▶ C |

A = Start of the disease process
B = Point of awareness (presentation as a case or detected during screening)
C = Death

In this case the time course of the disease (A–C) has not changed, although earlier detection has created the impression that survival time (B–C) has improved.

Figure 3.1 Spurious effects on survival produced by an earlier diagnosis (lead-time bias).

prolonged, when in truth treatment has been ineffective and the true time course is unaltered (Fig. 3.1).

4   Decisions about the target population (e.g. age group) and recall frequency are often arbitrary and based on imperfect ideas of natural history.
    Costs and benefits are not easy to establish.

Benefits
1   Improvement in mortality and morbidity needs, if possible, to be confirmed by randomised trials.
2   The possible economic saving on future treatment is particularly hard to quantify.

Costs
1   Costs to patients:
    (a) unnecessary anxiety or even psychological harm;
    (b) false reassurance (some of the time);
    (c) economic costs (e.g. time off work).
2   Costs to doctors: time and resource costs (test and follow-up).
3   Costs to the NHS:
    (a) costs of the test (direct and indirect);
    (b) costs of follow-up, further investigation or treatment.
    Financial cost-benefit assessments have been attempted, as shown below, but these estimates remain tentative.
1   Cervical cytology—40 000 smears, 200 excision biopsies and up to £300 000 per life saved.
2   Mammography—£3000–5000 per quality-adjusted life year saved.
3   Hypertension—£1700 per quality-adjusted life year saved.
    Psychological costs are well described:
1   Telling patients they have hypertension has led to absenteeism, lower self-esteem and poor marital relationships (Haynes *et al.* 1978).
2   Unfortunately, the damage once done is not easily undone:
    (a) Bloom and Monterossa (1981) followed up people who had been told they were hypertensive, and who were later assured it was a false alarm: they had more depression and a lower state of general health than matched controls initially told they were normotensive;

(b) other studies confirm that once the seeds of doubt have been sown by a false-positive result, people suffer lasting unease.

3   There are also concerns that the communication of a negative result may be harmful. It may, for example, reinforce an unhealthy lifestyle or make participants less likely to return for repeat tests.

Marteau (1989) suggests that sensitive pre-test counselling is necessary in anticipation of these problems, and that the long-term behavioural outcomes of widespread screening initiatives need to be fully assessed. Others too see this as an ethical imperative, as in many instances the efficacy of intervention and cost-effectiveness of screening initiatives can be questioned.

Health promotion activities and targets

Many types of screening and health promotion activity have been advocated as appropriate to primary care, despite the failure in some cases to demonstrate objective benefit (Table 3.3). Amendments to GPs' contractual terms now allow them to be remunerated for self-fashioned health promotion programmes, provided that these have been approved by a Health Promotion Committee (HPC). The HPC, which includes members of the Health Authority (HA), LMC and MAAG, considers submissions annually in the light of:

- modern authoritative medical opinion;
- patient needs;
- local health priorities; and
- national strategies.

The idea is to allow GPs and HAs to produce programmes which are sound and appropriate. In contrast to two unhappy earlier

Table 3.3 Possible preventive activities.

Screening
Hypertension screening, detection and follow-up
Cervical cytology
Developmental surveillance
Well-woman and well-man clinics
Visiting the elderly at home
Mammography
Blood fat estimation
Faecal occult bloods
Screening for psychiatric illness/alcohol abuse
Well-person periodic medicals

Preventive interventions
Immunisations/vaccinations
? Post-menopausal hormone replacement
? Lifestyle counselling
Advice on smoking
Keep-fit and aerobic programmes
Weight-watching

attempts, the new package is meant to be flexible: clinic-based and opportunistic screening, and chronic disease management pro-grammes may all qualify.

The current focus is most likely to reflect the Government's declared *Health of the Nation* priorities and the five key preventive areas subject to explicit targets (Table 3.4). It may also be influenced by the Department of Health's newly established National Screening Committee, which has compiled a 'national screening inventory' of screening measures, divided into those that should be available nationally, those that are still at the research stage, and those that the Committee feels the NHS should not support.

Table 3.4 Governmental *Health of the Nation* targets for England.*

Key areas	Principal targets†	Some suggested interventions‡
Coronary heart disease and stroke	• Reduce mortality in under 65s by 40% • Reduce mortality in 65–75s by 30% (MIs)—40% (CVAs)	• Reduce smoking prevalence to ≤20% (by year 2000) • Reduce food energy from saturated fats by 35% and total fat by 12% • Reduce frequency of obesity (BMI 30+) by 25% in men and 33% in women • Reduce mean systolic blood pressure in adults by 5 mmHg • Reduce frequency of men drinking ≥21 units of alcohol per week to 18%, and women drinking ≥14 units/week to 7% • Encourage more exercise (no explicit target)
Cancer	• Reduce mortality rate from lung cancer in under 75s by 15–30% (by year 2010) • Reduce mortality rate from breast cancer in women invited for screening by 25% • Reduce incidence of invasive cervical cancer by at least 20% • Halt the year-on-year increase of skin cancer (by year 2005)	• Reduce smoking prevalence (see above) • Encourage women aged 50–69 to accept invitations for breast screening • Ensure all women aged 20–64 who have not had a smear in the last 5 years receive one • Educate patients on avoidance, particularly those who burn easily or have a family history of melanoma
Mental illness	• Reduce suicide rate by 15% overall, and by 35% in those with severe mental illness • Significantly improve the social function of mentally ill people	• Closer enquiry, especially in high risk groups • Maintain at risk register for attempted suicides • More attention to diagnosis • More thorough treatment (e.g. full drug doses)

Table 3.4 *Continued*

Key areas	Principal targets†	Some suggested interventions‡
HIV/AIDS and sexual health	• Reduce rate of conception in girls under 16 by 50% • Reduce proportion of injecting drug misusers sharing syringes/needles by 75% • (No specific target for HIV/AIDS)	• Better information about contraceptive services, including the Family Planning Association's Helpline • Better education on HIV risk factors and drug abuse, with sustained attempts to change behaviour
Accidents	• Reduce mortality rate from accidents by 33% in under 15s, by 25% in 15–24 year-olds and by 33% in the over 65s (by 2005)	• Education—on wearing seatbelts; not drinking and driving; keeping medicines locked away • In the elderly: checks of household safety and lighting, eyesight checks and encouragement of daily exercise

*Similar national initiatives have been launched in Scotland, Wales and Northern Ireland.
†By year 2000 unless otherwise stated CVA, cerebrovascular accident; MI, myocardial infarction.
‡By year 2005 unless otherwise stated.
CVA, cerebrovascular accident; MI, myocardial infarction.

Obstacles to prevention
An effective programme will take account of some of the barriers to success.

Patient-related obstacles
Patients weigh costs against benefits and often perceive costs to be high. Taking smoking as an example, the costs of giving up include:
1 Sacrifice of physical pleasure — the anxiolytic pharmacological action of cigarettes.
2 Sacrifice of the psychological and social benefits—smoking is:
   (a) a social activity that binds groups;
   (b) a relaxation ritual;
   (c) a conversation filler;
   (d) a risk-taking, and hence exciting, exploit;
   (e) in adolescence, a form of rebellion.
   Hence people rationalise or ignore:
• 'It won't happen to me' (the ostrich approach).
• 'I don't believe they know the true facts' (the sceptic's approach).
• 'You go when it's your turn and you can't change that' (the fatalist's approach).
   Sometimes people are genuinely ignorant of relative risks ('Life's a risk—you're just as likely to be knocked over crossing the road. . . .').

Doctor-related obstacles

Costs to the doctor include:

1   Time and resources.
2   Frustration (if returns are low).

There are also barriers of organisation and enthusiasm, problems with effective, clear communication (see Section 2.1) and in some areas medical debate and uncertainty that make advice-giving harder. In group practices commitment to preventive activities often varies between the partners, and this produces a source of potential friction and a check on the effectiveness of the service.

Overcoming patient-related obstacles

Fowler, Gray and others have suggested the following plan:

1   Point out the debits (seriousness and magnitude of risk).
2   Point out the benefits (social and financial as well as physical; positive as well as negative).
3   Anticipate and be prepared to discuss difficulties.
4   Suggest coping strategies.
5   Give simple advice and supplement it with written information.

The application of this approach to smoking is discussed in Section 6.1 and the subject of improving patient compliance is discussed in Section 2.1.

Setting up a screening programme

Zander (1982) has pointed out the major differences between preventive and routine care:

Routine care	*Preventive care*
Patient-initiated, i.e. demand is unpredictable	Doctor-initiated, i.e. the demand should be predictable
Immediate-type demand	Non-urgent
Usually involving the doctor	Easily delegated to other primary health care team members
Focused on individuals	Focused on high-risk groups
Good records are a help but audit is difficult	Good records are essential; audit is usually straightforward

In general terms the stages involved in setting up a screening programme are:

1   Identifying a problem which meets the Wilson criteria and which the practice agrees is a priority.
2   Auditing the records to establish the baseline performance of the practice, and then deciding whether to proceed.
3   Counting numbers — how big is the undertaking? Do you know the names of the high-risk group? (Age–sex register is obviously important here.)

4   Defining *objectives* (e.g. to measure the blood pressure of all males over 40 years old).

5   Defining *methods*:
   (a) Opportunistic?
   (b) By patient invitation?
   (c) By patient visiting?

6   Defining the *participants* (e.g. practice nurse in hypertension screening and well-woman clinics; geriatric health visitor in over 75s home surveillance).

7   Participants may need training and/or equipment and need to have a protocol. They also need time to do the job.

8   Review after a trial period. Has the performance improved? Are objectives being met? Are teething problems disturbing the balance and effectiveness of the practice in other respects? Then decide whether to continue and what refinements are needed.

These are the principles involved, but the MRCGP candidate might well be expected to discuss screening with reference to specific examples as they exist (or might exist) in his own practice. The remainder of this chapter is therefore devoted to some topical examples of how screening services could be organised. The principles involved are really the same in each case, but they are described in full so that each topic can be read on its own if required. (Note that the methods suggested are not the only way to deliver the service but merely examples of the type of approach commonly employed.)

3.2 CERVICAL SCREENING

Background and rationale
A total of 2.5–3.0 million smears are performed annually. Despite this:
- deaths occur each year in the UK;
- the death rate is rising amongst young women;
- 16% of women aged 20–64 have not had a smear in the last $5\frac{1}{2}$ years.

Cervical screening has been shown to be effective in the Nordic countries and the US. High coverage of the target populations has been followed by sharp declines in mortality.

The current campaign is based on evidence that the natural history of cervical cancer involves several pre-malignant stages (grades of dysplasia and carcinoma *in situ*) detectable by regular cervical screening several years in advance of frank carcinoma.

Certain *high-risk* groups have been described:
- low socio-economic class;
- early age of first sexual intercourse;
- early age of first pregnancy;
- multiple sexual partners;

- frequent pregnancies;
- venereal disease.

Smoking probably doubles the risk of cervical cancer.

Limitations to cervical cytology

1 A false-negative rate of about 10% for carcinoma *in situ* (even necrotic tumours can give a negative result).

2 A false-positive rate of about 5% (smears showing mild dysplasias).

3 Sampling problems: the squamocolumnar junction is not always accessible.

4 Other technical problems which upset interpretation (e.g. delayed application of fixative, menstruation, pregnancy, the contraceptive pill, intrauterine devices and polyps).

5 Limitations of the *cervical smear campaign*:

(a) Guidelines have been complex, inconsistent and often lagging behind current research;

(b) the number of smears taken has probably been inadequate;

(c) the right women have probably not been screened, in particular the high-risk groups from low social classes use the service least but need it most (the inverse care principle);

(d) organisation has often been inadequate:

- in some inner-city studies nearly 70% of invitation letters were inaccurately or inappropriately addressed (Beardow *et al.* 1989);
- a study by Elwood *et al.* in Nottingham (1984) found that only 59% of positive smears were properly followed up;
- Ellman and Chamberlain (1984) reviewing 100 cervical cancer deaths in Sutton found that:

68 had never been screened;

10 had negative smears, but over 5 years previously;

13 suspicious smears were not followed up.

The old DHSS recall system was disbanded in 1988. Instead an HA call–recall system and an NHS cervical screening programme national co-ordination network were established to bring more coherence to bear. The recent target-based system of fees has also encouraged GPs to organise themselves more efficiently. This has been reflected in improved coverage of the target population (up from 61% in 1989–90 to 83% in 1992–3; Austoker 1994).

How to set up a cervical screening and recall system

The steps involved (which will become familiar by the end of this chapter!) are as follows:

1 Define *objectives and priorities*, e.g.:

(a) decide whether you want to screen every 3 years or every 5;

(b) should you screen every sexually active woman or just the over 25s and antenatal patients?

(c) consider your priorities (older women are least likely to have had a smear, so some practices start with them first; others have a policy for high-risk groups and make extra efforts here).

2 *Count numbers and obtain names.* Identify the desired population using the age–sex register.

3 Define *methods*, e.g.:

(a) a cervical smear/well-woman clinic;

(b) opportunistic smears;

(c) a combined approach (trials suggest that call–recall systems are usually better than opportunism alone, but those who do not respond to a clinic invitation may respond to opportunistic counselling).

participants, e.g.:

(a) all the partners;

(b) family planning trained nurse or health visitor;

(c) clerk to operate the recall system;

resources, e.g. allocate consulting time.

4 *Establish a recall system:*

(a) practice computers now enable the target population to be readily identified and their current smear status ascertained (provided the data has been input to begin with);

(b) the chosen recall criteria can be selected, and women's records ordered according to their next due date;

(c) this information can be used to generate a clinic invitation around the due date, offered in the form of a word-processed letter of invitation; a reminder letter to non-attendees; and an opportunistic prompt, e.g. when the patient next makes an appointment, or the doctor accesses the computer-held record;

(d) the recall list can be ordered according to defined priorities such as extent of overdueness, risk grouping or significant previous findings.

(Formerly this was done by setting up a manual card index system with patients' cards filed in order of recall, and such a system would still be required in practices without a computer system).

5 *Implement the screening*, e.g.:

(a) draw up a list of immediately due smears;

(b) devise a plan to clear the backlog (e.g. temporary extra clinics);

(c) if an opportunistic approach is favoured, mark the notes as a reminder or organise a computer-generated prompt ('smear due next time'); otherwise draft carefully worded letters of invitation and offer smear appointments.

Invitations that offer the choice of a female doctor or nurse are generally thought to improve uptake. An opportunistic approach will often be required to improve uptake in reluctant attendees.

6 *Review.* Periodically count numbers:

(a) What percentage of the target group is having smears taken?

(b) What is the success rate of an opportunistic approach?

(c) What is the take-up rate if appointments are offered?

(d) Can the figures be improved (e.g. by offering smears with the nurse, smears at more flexible times or educational information)?

A computer-held database is easier to interrogate, and of great value in monitoring progress towards planned targets.

Dealing with smear results

It is important to establish a secure system that ensures patients know their smear result. Patient initiative may not be sufficient (as a tragic case in Oxfordshire has made clear) and various approaches have been adopted: at one extreme there are doctors who take the view that the patient should have responsibility for her own health and should therefore make her own arrangements to contact the surgery; at the other extreme there are doctors who adopt the practice (expensive in time and administration) of writing to every patient. The middle-ground approach concentrates on positive smear results: some doctors write to all of these patients, others keep ledgers or leave the result out, and contact patients who do not enquire after a defined interval. A computer prompt offers a further back-up option. The important point is that there is a system that is fail-safe and subject to regular review.

3.3 WELL-PERSON ASSESSMENTS

The well-woman clinic

The well-woman clinic has its origin in the old cervical cytology clinics run through local authority services, where it became recognised that women in need of cervical smears also appreciated the opportunity to discuss other problems in a setting specifically tailored for them. The potential to offer health education to women who are in a receptive frame of mind is considerable, and these clinics have therefore become popular.

Advantages

1   These clinics may attract women who might not otherwise come to the surgery, who are inhibited about seeing a doctor and using up his time unless ill.

2   Patients attending such clinics are in a health-conscious and receptive frame of mind.

3   It is often possible to offer more time and a more informal atmosphere.

4   There is greater scope in this elective setting to offer the woman a doctor of the sex she prefers than in the higher-pressure, immediate-demand setting of routine surgeries.

5   A separate clinic also avoids the real pitfall of opportunistic

screening, that it is often inconvenient (the surgery is running late; the patient is having a period, etc.).

6 Separate clinics are often more convenient if different members of the team (e.g. doctor, health visitor and nurse) all wish to attend: they can arrange their timetables to suit.

7 There is a large potential for health promotion and educating towards self-help for common, minor problems (perhaps reducing demand on consulting time in the long run, and helping to relieve health-related anxieties in those with neurotic illness).

8 Income may be boosted (e.g. increased item-of-service work, higher list sizes because a well received competitive range of services is on offer).

9 Greater satisfaction for the patient and doctor, and an extended (more satisfying) role for the practice nurse.

Disadvantages
1 The obvious costs of:
    (a) time and energy;
    (b) administrative effort and overheads.
2 These clinics may still reach the *most* motivated people, when the need is to reach the *least*.
3 There are dangers that:
    (a) it will degenerate into a sick-woman clinic through patient misuse;
    (b) a poor uptake will affect morale and enthusiasm and more-over, unaccepted invitations will squander consulting time. At the very least, demand may be unpredictable.

How to set up a well-woman clinic
1 *Define objectives and priorities*, e.g.:
    (a) to screen for cervical cancer;
    (b) to screen for breast cancer;
    (c) to screen for hypertension;
    (d) to screen for gynaecological problems;
    (e) to promote family planning;
    (f) to give pre-conceptual counselling;
    (g) to teach self-examination of the breasts;
    (h) to give health education and advice (self-help for thrush and cystitis; facts about premenstrual syndrome; psycho-sexual counselling; encouragement to lose weight, stop smoking, eat a healthier diet, etc.);
    (i) to develop self-help groups (weight-watchers, toddler groups, etc.).
2 *Count numbers and obtain names*—using the age–sex register.
3 Define *methods*, e.g.:
    (a) is the format of the clinic to be by letter invitation, or open access or a mixture of the two?

(b) will there be a follow-up for non-attendees?

(c) what is the recall frequency?

(d) should invitations be issued according to priority?

participants, e.g.:

(a) interested female partner (taken on for this purpose?);

(b) health visitor;

(c) practice nurse;

resources, e.g.:

(a) a slot in the timetable; training of staff as required;

(b) letters of invitation and posters advertising the service.

4 *Establish a recall system*. Practice computers lend themselves to defining subsets of patients for call–recall, and generating prompts or letters of invitation at specified intervals; and help in monitoring patient contacts and outcomes.

5 *Ensure the protocol is approved for HA remuneration.*

6 *Review*. Periodically consider:

(a) how many attendees (and defaulters) there are;

(b) how many new cervical smears have been done;

(c) whether patients are satisfied;

(d) whether it has affected the pattern of normal surgeries.

Demand can be measured readily, but satisfaction and understanding are harder to quantify.

Well-man clinics

Less common, but growing in popularity, are the well-man clinics, aimed in particular at the overweight and overstressed businessman, and the male smoker from the lower social classes.

Aims may include:

- screening for hypertension and alcohol abuse;
- advice on weight reduction, safe levels of drinking, giving up smoking, a more healthy diet, exercise and fitness;
- optional activities like urinalysis and lipid estimations.

Costs and benefits of well-person screening

GPs' Terms of Service require well-person health assessments on those registering with their practice for the first time. The content of this medical assessment is detailed in Table 8.2 (p. 242). It includes some measures whose strict scientific value have been questioned, in particular:

1 There is no evidence that the routine measurement of height and weight is of benefit.

2 Non-selective routine urinalysis has a low yield.

The cost-effectiveness of inviting infrequent attendees to attend for a periodic health check has likewise been challenged—Thompson (1990) scrutinised 1488 records: out of 114 patients who had not attended in the last 3 years, 17 were eventually persuaded to attend. Thirteen needed anti-tetanus injections but five refused and five failed to return for immunisation; three needed a repeat smear, but all failed to return for it, and one case of mild hypertension was discovered at an estimated cost of 28 h of staff time and 15 h of doctor time.

Multi-phasic screening of asymptomatic patients has been a notable disappointment (Oboler & LaForce 1989; South-East London Screening Study Group 1977).

These arguments led to the abandonment of the former requirement for a 3-yearly medical, but the requirement to collect baseline information at initial registration has so far been retained.

3.4 DIABETIC CARE

The problem
The prevalence of diabetes in the population is about 1–2%. The incidence is about 1–2 new cases per GP per year. On average each GP has about 30–40 diabetic patients: three-quarters of these are non-insulin-dependent, leaving about 8–10 insulin-dependent diabetics. However, 'the rule of halves' is thought to apply, i.e.:
- half of a practice's diabetics are unknown;
- half of the known diabetics are not followed up;
- leaving one-quarter of the total followed up (often haphazardly).

There are two important aspects to diabetic care:
1 *Case finding* or screening.
2 The *follow-up* of known diabetics.

These will be considered separately.

Screening for new diabetics
Since the prevalence is 1–2%, routine urinalysis as a screening procedure would have a small but definite yield. This could be improved by considering the at-risk factors, and therefore screening high-risk groups, e.g.:
- the obese;
- those with a family history of diabetes;
- those with big babies (birth weight 10 lb or 4.5 kg);
- those with a history of gestational diabetes (the risk of full diabetes is about 20% at 5 years).

Follow-up care
Should GPs run separate diabetic clinics?

Potential *advantages*:
1 It avoids the drawbacks of hospital clinics, namely that they are:
  (a) overcrowded;
  (b) impersonal;
  (c) staffed by a succession of changing junior doctors;
  (d) subject to care which is more haphazard and more restricted in access than in a well run surgery clinic.

2 Patients prefer the convenience of a trip to their own surgery and the security of seeing a familiar doctor who knows their personal problems.

3 There is also an opportunity to improve doctor–patient rapport.

4 More time can be offered for counselling and advice than at busy hospital clinics.

5 It is more convenient for the GP, e.g.:

(a) time has been calculated and set aside to do the job properly (this cannot be guaranteed in the unpredictable hurly burly of the routine surgery);

(b) the relevant staff and equipment are to hand;

(c) delegation is then possible;

(d) with only one subject to concentrate on, a more systematic and thorough approach is possible.

6 If diabetic patients are followed up methodically rather than haphazardly, there should be better control, which may mean:

(a) fewer complications;

(b) earlier referrals;

(c) fewer out-of-hours calls.

7 There is greater professional satisfaction if the primary health care team can offer a good service to a group of its own patients with a common chronic condition.

8 Although strictly speaking a tertiary prevention activity (some would say a treatment service), supervision of diabetics qualifies for the health promotion fee if organised into a recognisable clinic.

Potential *disadvantages*:

1 The extra time and effort involved.

2 Administrative costs—now offset in part by the health promotion fee.

3 It needs interest, enthusiasm and commitment to the subject (not always heart-felt!). There is, for example, an onus to keep abreast of current thinking on the subject and, as with all preventive exercises, enthusiasm may need to be maintained in the face of an apathetic and frustrating response.

4 Doctors may feel underqualified and that patients would do better under the care of a specialist (although evidence exists that this is not the case).

Shared care or full care?

Assuming a practice wishes to provide a diabetic clinic, two further questions arise:

1 Which patients are suitable?

2 Should practices operate a shared-care or full-care system?

Diabetics suitable for exclusively practice-based care would probably include:

• stable, complication-free diabetics treated by diet, tablets or insulin (perhaps 75% of the total);

Specialist input (shared care) is almost certainly required in the case of:

- children;
- pregnant women;
- patients with known complications;
- the unstable insulin-dependent diabetic.

Increasingly practices operate shared-care liaison schemes with local specialists. These may include:

- a co-operation card;
- consultant visits at the surgery;
- a visiting dietician, chiropodist and/or diabetic liaison sister;
- extra laboratory facilities.

There are clear advantages to this system:

- high patient convenience;
- a specialist input which benefits patients and educates GPs;
- extra services on tap;
- a lower running cost as compared with the hospital outpatient setting.

How to set up a diabetic clinic

1 Define *objectives and priorities*, e.g.:

(a) decide on baseline observations (e.g. blood sugar, glycosylated haemoglobin, blood pressure, lipids, urinalysis, full history and examination);

(b) decide on the follow-up parameters and recall frequency (e.g. a 6-monthly check on weight, blood sugar, glycosylated haemoglobin, fundi, feet and pulses, visual acuity, etc.);

(c) decide on the desired level of control;

(d) decide on an advice package (advice on monitoring, hypos, foot care, smoking, etc.).

2 *Count numbers and obtain names.* If the practice has a morbidity index, the job is done. If not, produce one using:

(a) the memories of partners and reception staff;

(b) repeat prescription records;

(c) hospital correspondence;

(d) opportunistic or systematic review of patient records.

3 Define *methods*, e.g.:

(a) the format of the invitation;

(b) the format of the clinic;

(c) whether shared care or full care;

(d) how the protocol can be streamlined and administered (would a flow chart in the notes or a patient education leaflet speed things along? Would a computer pro-forma ensure more thorough coverage?);

participants, e.g.:

(a) interested partner(s);

(b) practice nurse;

(c) clerk operating the recall system;

(d) empathetic local consultant;

resources, e.g.:

(a) a slot in the timetable; training of staff as required;

(b) a practice glucometer;

(c) sound out the local physician on available back-up (visiting dietician, chiropodist, diabetic liaison sister, etc.);

(d) a practice brochure and display posters to advertise the service.

4   *Establish a recall system*, e.g.:

(a) produce a full index of known diabetics, tag their notes and establish when desired checks are next due. It is commonplace now to log such information on the practice computer, enabling call and recall programmes, letters of invitation and target monitoring as an integrated package;

(b) issue an appointment, and after attendance update the record and choose the desired recall interval;

(c) send reminders to clinic non-attendees; and catch them opportunistically using the computer or tagged patient record as a prompt;

(d) have a system for adding new names as newly diagnosed diabetics appear.

5   *Ensure HA approval of the protocol*—to qualify for payment.

6   *Implement the system*: should extra clinics be laid on temporarily to clear the backlog of patients whose check-ups are urgently overdue?

7   *Review*, e.g.:

(a) what is the attendance/default rate?

(b) has diabetic control improved?

(c) what percentage of diabetics are now seen on a regular basis?

(d) have emergency out-of-hours calls from diabetics become less frequent?

3.5 HYPERTENSION SCREENING AND FOLLOW-UP

The problem

Dilemmas in the diagnosis and management of hypertension are fully discussed in Section 4.1. To summarise briefly, problems have been caused by:

• the arbitrary nature of treatment values;

• the validity of measuring techniques;

• doubts regarding natural history, especially in relation to the elderly;

• the size, cost and logistic (organisational) problems of the undertaking;

• conflicting trial results and differing opinions on cost vs. benefit.

If the active treatment of mild hypertension is pursued, this could involve 15–20% of the population.

Despite these problems hypertension is perceived to be *par excellence* a condition that should be managed in general practice. According to a survey by Fulton *et al.* (1979), two-thirds of GPs feel general practice is the ideal place for blood pressure screening. However, embarrassing gaps have been described between expectations and performance, e.g.:

- in one central London general practice survey only 24% of the population had their blood pressure recorded in the last 5 years, and only 39% of hypertensives so found were followed up (Fulton *et al.* 1979);
- apparently hospitals are no better—in one study only 32% of new outpatients had their blood pressure recorded, and only 38% of hypertensives so detected were followed up.

The 'rule of halves' has long been described:

- half the hypertensives are unknown;
- half the known ones are not treated; and
- half those that receive treatment are not controlled.

In 1990 a Scottish study reaffirmed this unhappy 'rule' (Smith *et al.* 1990).

Is screening feasible?

D'Souza *et al.* (1976) found that 93% of patients with a diastolic blood pressure above 95 mmHg visited their GP in a 5-year period. A strong case can therefore be made that opportunistic screening is entirely feasible and has a high yield. Fowler estimates that for a 5-yearly blood pressure check on all the patients of an average list, only 1–2 extra measurements would be required each day (and, of course, there is no need for the doctor to do this task personally — it can easily be delegated).

How to set up a screening and treatment service

1 *Define objectives and priorities*, e.g.:

   (a) the age group to be screened (e.g. over 20s or over 40s?; all women on the contraceptive pill);

   (b) the frequency of screening (e.g. 5-yearly);

   (c) devise a protocol which standardises recording methods, treatment values, baseline investigations, recall frequency, drug policy, etc.;

   (d) fix a target blood pressure so that quality of control can be assessed;

   (e) compile a morbidity index and tag the records in every case.

2 Define *methods*, e.g. opportunistic screening or a separate clinic (hypertension, well-woman or well-man clinics), or a walk-in service operated by the nurse;

participants, e.g.:

(a) all the partners;

(b) the practice nurse;

(c) the clerk who maintains the recall system;

resources, e.g.:

(a) a flow diagram sheet for the notes;

(b) prominent posters advertising the service.

3 *Establish a recall system*, e.g.:

(a) identify all known hypertensives (from memory, repeat pre-scription cards, correspondence, summary notes and surveying the records) then compile a morbidity index; tag the notes and computer-held patient record;

(b) use the practice computer (or a manual card index system) to generate letters of invitation at specified intervals; reminders to non-attendees; and opportunistic prompts to ensure blood pressure measurement is not overlooked at the next patient contact;

(c) some practices categorise patients according to the so-called 'three box' method—that is to say into three groups on the basis of their blood pressure:

- a treatment group;
- a borderline group;
- 'normals'.

The name derives from the era of manual recall systems when patient names were written down on cards and filed in three separate box indexes subject to a different recall frequency:

- the treatment group may need to be seen (say) every 4 months;
- the borderline group annually; and
- the majority with normal blood pressure only 5-yearly.

Although the same result is now more easily accomplished by practice computer software, the basic approach remains valid.

For a list of 2000 patients there will be roughly 55 hypertensives under treatment, and up to 120–160 'mild' hypertensives needing annual monitoring.

4 *Review*, e.g.:

(a) What is the percentage of the target population being screened?

(b) What percentage of the known hypertensives has been seen in the last 6 months?

(c) Have the chosen investigations produced a reasonable yield? (If not, the protocol could be simplified.)

3.6 GERIATRIC SCREENING

At present 15–17% of the population are over 65 years old, but the proportion of the elderly is increasing, and the proportion of the very elderly is increasing even more. By the year 2000 the ranks of the over-75s may have swelled by 20–35%, and the over-85s by 45%.

Fifty per cent of all non-psychiatric NHS beds are already occupied by the over-65s, and concern has been expressed that hospital services will not be able to cope. The solution to this dilemma may lie in better prevention and in identifying disability before it becomes severe. Better prevention could also raise the quality of life in old age.

Preventive measures

Preventive measures that may help include advice on:

- the avoidance of smoking and obesity;
- increasing dietary fibre;
- winter 'flu vaccinations;
- keep-fit activities (and vigorous rehabilitation after acute illness);
- mental recreation;
- avoiding the typical negative attitudes associated with ageing.

Regular attention from the chiropodist, optician and dentist may be beneficial.

Is screening worthwhile?

Screening studies on the elderly show a high prevalence of unreported problems, so it might be supposed that they would benefit from the regular attention of a screening physician. In fact, only a minority of practices displayed an interest in geriatric screening before it became a condition of service. This is explained in part by doubts repeatedly cast on its feasibility and effectiveness, e.g.:

- Wallis and Barber (1982) estimated that to screen all patients over 75 years of age in their Glasgow practice needed 18 h of health visitor time per week for the first year, and 11 h per week in subsequent years;
- Tulloch and Moore (1979) found that screening produced an increased use of health care and social *facilities*, but not a great change in *health*;
- Hendriksen *et al.* (1984) found a reduction in hospital admissions but no reduction in the number of nursing home admissions;
- Coleman (1989) identified in a practice list of 11 000 patients 132 elderly people who had not been seen in the last 2 years: 22% could not be contacted, 51% did not welcome the approach, and in the 36 who were finally seen eight remediable but minor problems were detected at a direct cost of £3400 and at a time cost of 425 h (only 5%, spent with patients);
- Epstein *et al.* (1990) conducted a large-scale US study in which patients were randomly allocated between usual and intensive specialist care (geriatrician, geriatric nurse, geriatric social worker): at 3 and 12 months the health differences between the groups were marginal.

It has been argued by some that most newly diagnosed problems in the elderly are trivial or irreversible, so health spin-offs are small.

Advantages of screening

Proponents of geriatric surveillance point out:

1 that some spin-offs (morale, self-esteem and satisfaction) are immeasurable and come forth when it is shown that someone cares;

2 that today's trivial problem (e.g. uncorrected presbycusis or loose doormat) is tomorrow's major one (e.g. fractured neck of femur);

3 that some worthwhile diagnoses *can* be made (up to one in five over 75s are said to suffer some degree of depression; 6–12% have some degree of dementia, with carers stressed and unsupported);

4 that some worthwhile interventions can also be made, e.g. influenza vaccinations reduce mortality from 'flu by 70% in the over 65s, and halve the rate of serious associated complications and hospital admission.

It has also been suggested:

1 that an opportunistic approach is feasible, since 90% of the over-75s see the primary health care team anyway over a 1-year period;

2 that *selective* screening of high-risk patients (e.g. the very old, the recently bereaved, the socially isolated, the immobile, the recently discharged) is a more realistic proposition with a higher yield in prospect.

One study on selective screening showed that out of every 12 screened patients:

- three could be helped;
- four needed no help;
- five had irremediable problems.

Other studies have also raised question marks over the discriminating power of the commonly suggested high-risk criteria.

Although lingering doubts remain regarding the cost-effectiveness of screening, this is now a condition of service and doctors have been forced to face head-on the logistic problems entailed.

How to set up a geriatric screening service

1 *Define objectives and priorities*, e.g.:

(a) who to screen (everyone over 75; perhaps high-risk groups over 65);

(b) what to screen for (the minimum standard is determined by Schedule—see Table 8.2 (p. 242)).

2 Define *methods*, e.g.:

(a) opportunistic?

(b) home visiting? (must be offered annually to the over-75s)

(c) a combination of these?

(d) a questionnaire pro-forma (locally or nationally agreed? HA-approved?)

participants, e.g.:

(a) district nurse;

(b) health visitor;

(c) doctor;

(d) volunteer (e.g. local Age Concern group);

(The obligation to screen can be delegated within the primary care team.)

resources, e.g. equip and train the screening personnel.

3 *Identify the patients at risk*, e.g.:

(a) using the records and age–sex register;

(b) construct an at-risk register.

4 *Implement the screen* — after first making contact with the elderly person to establish his interest.

5 *Review*:

(a) feedback on problems discovered;

(b) deal with them;

(c) review the progress (and benefits of screening);

(d) ensure proper records are kept to demonstrate compliance with Terms of Service.

3.7 IMPROVING IMMUNISATION RATES

Immunisation rates are clearly affected by media publicity (as indicated by the fluctuation in pertussis vaccination rates after various media scares), but within this variation some practices achieve rates worse than average and some achieve rates of nearly 100%.

Recall schemes run by HAs and those offered through the school health system have ensured a reasonable level of coverage, but there exist some shortcomings that primary care can address.

Ultimately the success of immunisation programmes depends on the compliance and commitment of parents and the efficient organisation of the vaccinating service. A characteristic of practices with high vaccination rates appears to be a clear predetermined practice policy, discussed, agreed and understood by all health care team workers. Particular attention to methods of recall, screening and advertising is needed. A plan might include:

1 Discussion with parents at all available opportunities (for example, in the antenatal period, again at birth, when the health visitor calls, and at the 6-week postnatal check — the times when mothers are likely to be receptive).

2 Further education of parents by means of surgery posters and notices, a lending library of tapes or review articles (especially on the controversial vaccines).

3 A reminder to doctors in the form of:

(a) immunisation record cards;

(b) a box on the antenatal/postnatal record card (to be completed when immunisation advice is given);

(c) the tagging of records when vaccinations are completed.

4 A computer-generated recall system run based on age–sex and vaccination summary data, especially to recall:

(a) girls for rubella vaccination (some practices send a reminder in the form of a 10th birthday card);

(b) teenagers (15–19 years old) for tetanus and polio.

5 Opportunistic approaches:

(a) checking tetanus status every time a patient attends with minor trauma;

(b) the routine generation of overdue prompts upon patient contact, e.g. linked in with the computerised appointment and repeat prescription system;

(c) offering polio boosters to parents, when their children are vaccinated;

(d) checking rubella antibodies when women are first offered contraceptive care and tagging the record to indicate a satisfactory result.

6 A practice immunisation protocol (updated so everyone knows the latest recommendations and gives the same advice).

High immunisation rates have virtually eradicated serious infective illnesses like diphtheria, polio, tetanus and measles. In addition to improving the well-being of the population, immunisations generate income in the form of item-of-service payments and these payments are contingent on meeting taxing coverage targets.

3.8 PAEDIATRIC SURVEILLANCE

Infant mortality rates have been dropping in all countries, but not as fast in England as some others, notably Japan and France. This has led to the critical examination of the preventive services for children. Developmental surveillance has been practised in some form for at least 50 years. Until quite recently one out of every 10 GPs participated in this process with much regional variation. Amendments to the remunerative system may in future encourage many more family doctors to participate. However, doubts still exist about its value and about how, where and by whom it should be done.

Is it worthwhile?

The early detection of remediable conditions, notably congenital dislocation of the hip, squint and undescended testes, is the main value of the exercise.

1 In one study in 1978 it was found that 232 children out of 2157 needed specialist agency referral.

2 In Glasgow problems requiring treatment or follow-up were encountered in 23% of pre-school children, and 15% had a previously unrecognised physical abnormality.

3 Another London study involving pre-school children followed for the first 5 years of life found a significant health problem in 20% at each age.

Other apparent benefits include a better relationship with children and their parents, opportunity to educate and to offer self-help advice, and perhaps better compliance. However, as Bain (1989) points out, there are costs:

- time and resources are limited;
- non-attendance figures at clinics may be as high as 40%, especially amongst low socio-economic groups with the greatest need;
- the number of major abnormalities detected will be relatively small in relation to the effort and expense.

Several screening programmes have been evaluated. On average 5–10%, of those screened are referred for assessment, but more severe abnormalities freshly detected by this route amount to less than 1% of all those seen. Large-scale studies in Sweden have found only a marginal direct impact on health, while the British Paediatric Association has cautioned that a number of routine tests are unreliable, invalid or poorly performed. So, there is uncertainty over the value of routine mass screening.

Should it be scheduled or opportunistic?

Houston and Davis (1985) and others have suggested that children attend sufficiently often to adopt an opportunistic approach to screening. This has the advantage of simplicity and convenience and does not depend on patient response. However, Walker (1986) has highlighted some of the pitfalls in this approach:

1 Attendance for medical care falls off sharply after the first year of life.

2 If visits are not planned, children may appear at times that are inappropriate for the assessment of key milestones.

3 Interpretation of screening efforts would be difficult because of background illness.

4 Communities that habitually bypass general practice services might never be included.

The positive benefits of a separate clinic have also been stressed. Thus:

1 Time is specifically allocated for that purpose and the relevant personnel and equipment are to hand. It is easy to see how the best intentions of opportunists may be spoiled by the pressures of a busy surgery.

2 There is a value to meeting children when they are well.

3 A clearly defined service is appreciated by parents and has benefits for the doctor–patient relationship.

4 The item-of-service payment scheme encourages GPs to organise their child health work into identifiable clinics.

Who should do the work?
It has been argued that it is artificial and unsatisfactory to divide the responsibilities for surveillance and care in illness, and that general practice is the natural setting for screening. Movements to promote its wider practice by GPs include:

1 The Sheldon (1967) and Court (1976) reports.
2 The Conference of Local Medical Councils (1977).
3 The publication of the Royal College of General Practitioners' Working Party *Healthier Children—Thinking Prevention* (1982).
4 Its subsequent joint publication with the GMSC, *Handbook of Preventive Care for Pre-school Children* (1984).
5 Remuneration in the form of the child health surveillance fee.

Traditionally most of the work has been done by clinical medical officers and health visitors who have been adequately trained and have the necessary time and experience. Now GPs are showing a greater interest, but several possible question marks hang over GPs as an alternative or supplement to this service.

Do they have the experience?
Court (1976) argued that GPs need a specialist skill, and should spend up to 70% of their time working with children and train formally as GP paediatricians. The proposal of specialists within primary care was rejected by the GMSC and by GPs who felt the necessary skills were already present. In 1982 the Royal College proposed compulsory paediatric training for new GPs or the creation of a Paediatric List, reluctantly echoing the two-tier proposal of Court. In effect this proposal has now been adopted: to be paid for developmental screening, doctors must be registered on their HA's approved list and must be appropriately qualified. The issue of experience remains controversial, as the required standard has not been centrally defined, leaving HAs to formulate their own criteria under the influence of the various interested pressure groups. Common criteria for acceptance include substantial prior experience in such clinics or in hospital paediatrics, specific training on an approved course, or a relevant qualification (DCH, DCCH or MRCP (Paeds)).

Do they have the time?
The Royal College has calculated on the basis of five recommended examinations over a 5-year period that the average GP would see 7–8 extra children per week, so the time involved would be roughly equivalent to a weekly session of 2 h.

Do they have the incentive?
Until 1989 no form of extra remuneration was provided to doctors undertaking this work. Those who adopted it as a matter of good practice were, in fact, penalised by higher overheads. A paediatric surveillance fee was introduced to rectify this position and to encourage

more participants. The fee for this work is comparatively modest, but the uptake has been strong. Some doctors find their clinics useful lossleaders in the push to achieve lucrative child immunisation targets; others never viewed the clinics in financial terms anyway, believing in their implicit value to patients, and for them some element of recognition has been welcome.

Screening schedules

In its 1982 report the Royal College of General Practitioners confined its recommendations to feasible, simple, well validated procedures that did not require elaborate equipment (Table 3.5). Research suggests that screening often throws up false positives, so rather fewer procedures are currently recommended than in the past. The Hall Working Party, whose membership is drawn from the British Paediatric Association and BMA, as well as the Royal College of General Practitioners, proposes six examination schedules:

1 At birth (hospital staff, GP or midwife).
2 At 6–8 weeks (usually GP).
3 At 6–9 months (GP and health visitor).
4 At 2 years (health visitor).
5 At 3 years (simple review by primary care member).
6 At 5 years (usually school medical service).

The content and significant findings at the various stages are summarised in Table 3.6 and important developmental milestones in Table 8.1 (pp. 240–241).

Setting up a screening clinic

The principles follow the usual five-point plan suggested throughout this chapter.

1 *Define objectives and priorities*, e.g. aim to complete the schedules in the 1984 GMSC and Royal College of General Practitioners handbook or those of the Hall report for all the practice's pre-school children. Make sure your programme is recognised by the HA for remuneration.

Table 3.5 Screening objectives recommended in the Royal College of General Practitioners report (1982).

Adults	New-born	Pre-school children
Contraception	Chemical screening (e.g.	Immunisation (polio, tetanus,
Prenatal and antenatal care	phenylketonuria,	diphtheria, pertussis,
Promotion of breast feeding	hypothyroidism)	measles)
Anti-smoking education	Testes (for descent)	Hearing
	Hips (to exclude congenital	Visual acuity
	dislocation)	Squints
		Colour vision

Table 3.6 Recommended schedule and some significant findings in child health surveillance (adapted from *Health for all Children* 1996 (3rd edn) Hall D.M.B. (ed), OUP, Oxford; and *Handbook of Preventive Care for Pre-school Children*, GMSC & RCGP 1984).

Schedule	Examination check	Findings
Birth	Weight, head circumference	Unusually small or large head
	External inspection	Congenital abnormality (e.g. cataract, coloboma, cleft lip/imperforate anus, etc.
	Listen to heart and check colour	Murmurs
	Eescent of testes	Undescended testes
	Hips	Congenital dislocation of the hips
	Tests for phenylketonuria or hypothyroidism	Chemical evidence of these disorders
6–8 weeks	Weight, head circumference	Unusually small or large head
	Hips	Restricted hip abduction (refer urgently)
	Descent of testes	Undescended testes (refer)
	Listen to heart and check colour	Murmur, cyanosis
	Inspect eyes	Cataract, absent visual response
	Enquire about vision and hearing	Parental concern
6–9 months	Weight or length (if required)	Failure to thrive
	Hips	Restricted hip abduction
	Inspect eyes	Squint, nystagmus, failure to fixate
	Distraction test of hearing	Failure of the test
2 years	Enquire about behaviour, vision and hearing	Major maternal anxiety
	Check walking	Abnormal gait
	Height (if required)	Crossing the centile lines on growth chart
3½ years	Enquire about behaviour, vision, hearing and language acquisition	Major maternal anxiety, evidence of clumsiness, visual problems (?refer to orthoptist), hearing problems (?refer for testing) or behavioural problems
	Height (if required)	Crossing the centile lines on growth chart
5 years	Height	Crossing the centile lines on growth chart
	Vision (Snellen chart)	Evidence of myopia
	Hearing ('sweep' test)	20–30 dB loss at one or more frequencies on repeat testing

2   *Count numbers and obtain names*—using the age–sex register, health visitor's records or computer.

3   Define *methods*:

(a) opportunistic or separate scheduled clinics?

(b) recall frequency and approach to the follow-up of non-attendees;

(c) liaison with health visitors;

participants, e.g.:

(a) health visitor;

(b) interested GPs;

resources, e.g.:

(a) a slot in the timetable;

(b) separate record cards for the notes, mother or both;

(c) simple screening equipment.

4 *Establish a recall system*, e.g.:

(a) a computer-generated call–recall system, including letters of invitation and reminder, and opportunistic prompts for non-responders;

(b) update the system when an examination has been completed.

5 *Review*, e.g.:

(a) How much time is involved?

(b) What is the yield?

(c) What is the uptake?

(d) Should the service be advertised by booklet or poster?

3.9 SCREENING FOR BREAST CANCER

The size of the problem

1 Breast cancer is *the* major form of cancer among women in the UK. It accounts for:

(a) over 12 500 deaths per annum;

(b) 20% of all female cancer deaths. It is the most common cause of death in women aged 35–54.

2 The UK has a high breast cancer mortality rate compared with other developed countries.

Risk factors

1 Factors known to increase the risk of breast cancer include:

(a) increasing age;

(b) late childbearing (first child after the age of 30);

(c) nulliparity;

(d) early menarche;

(e) late menopause;

(f) family history (first-degree relative);

(g) obesity;

(h) ionising radiation.

2 Other factors (e.g. high-fat diets, hormone therapy and the contraceptive pill) are still being evaluated.

Prognosis

On average two-thirds of all women with breast cancer are alive 5 years after diagnosis. However, those with early local disease fare better than those with metastatic spread (Table 3.7).

Screening by mammography

1 Mammography involves low-level X-ray exposure on one or two planes. The amount of radiation involved is small (1 rad).

Table 3.7 Survival rate at 5 years according to stage of breast cancer.

Stage	Features at diagnosis	5-year survival rate (%)
I	Small mobile tumour confined to the breast; no nodes	84
II	As for stage I plus nodes	71
III	Locally advanced tumour attached to chest musculature	48
IV	Distant metastases	18

2 The tissue of young women's breasts is dense, resulting in practical difficulties in interpretation. Perimenopausal thinning makes the task easier, so screening is easier in older (50+) women.

3 The sensitivity of modern mammography is about 80%, and the specificity is 95%. (Clinical examination picks up 50–60% of abnormalities.)

4 Estimates of positive predictive value vary from 9 to 60%, with the Forrest report (1987) suggesting a 2:1 ratio of benign to malignant biopsies.

5 A programme of screening by mammography is necessarily complex, requiring:

(a) a sophisticated call–recall system;
(b) a relatively expensive test;
(c) interpretation by a trained radiologist;
(d) (in suspect cases) biopsy by a skilled surgeon;
(e) interpretation of biopsies by a skilled histopathologist;
(f) treatment where cancer is found.

There are potential pitfalls at every stage—failure of uptake, loss to follow-up, technical problems, errors of interpretation, treatment failures.

Benefits

It might be supposed, these problems not withstanding, that mammography is bound to be of benefit: after all, it detects breast lumps too small to be palpated, and 5-year survival figures are better for early disease. In fact, as Fig. 3.1 illustrates, earlier diagnosis can result in longer survival times from diagnosis without altering the time-course of a disease at all.

Several major trials have considered whether there is a true benefit (Table 3.8). Early results appeared to show an improvement in mortality, although estimates of the benefit differed. Nystrom *et al.* (1993) in an overview of five Swedish studies (altogether 283 000 women followed over 5–13 years) reported a 24% fall in breast cancer mortality overall, comprising a 29% benefit in women aged 50–69; a 13% fall in those aged 40–49; and a marginal effect only in women aged 70 and over.

Table 3.8 Some important trials of breast cancer screening.

Study	Design	Screening method	Age group studied (years)	Screening interval (years)	Reduction in mortality (%)	Comments*
Shapiro et al. (1982) Health Insurance Plan, New York	Randomised control trial	Clinical examination + two-view mammography	40–60	1	30	$P < 0.05$
Tabar et al. (1985) Sweden	Randomised control trial	One-view mammography	40–74	2–3	31	$P = 0.013$ High compliance (up to 90%) Reliable population lists from tax office
Andersson et al. (1988) Malmo, Sweden	Randomised control trial	Two-view mammography	>45	1.5–2	No significant difference between screened and control groups overall	In over-55s a 20% reduction in mortality Relative risk 0.79 Confidence intervals 0.51–1.24 74% response rate
Verbeck et al. (1984) Nijmegen	Case control trial	One-view mammography	≥35	2	52	Odds ratio, screened vs. unscreened = 0.48, but wide 95% confidence intervals (0.23–1.00) compatible with 'no effect' Low attendance rates in older groups
Roberts et al. (1990)	Controlled trial	Two-view mammography + clinical examination	45–64	1–2	17% (at 7-year follow-up)	Odds ratio = 0.83, but wide 95% confidence intervals (0.58–1.18) compatible with no effect Low attendance rates
UK Trial of Early Detection of Breast Cancer Group (1988)	Controlled trial (eight locations in the UK)	Two centres: clinical + two-view mammography (46 000 women) Two centres: breast self-examination (64 000 women) Four centres: controls (127 000 women)	45–64	1–2	14%	Odds ratio = 0.86, but wide confidence intervals (0.69–1.08) compatible with 'no effect'

*The interpretation of P values, relative risk, odds ratios and confidence intervals is explained more fully in Chapter 11.

Costs

1 A typical mammography screening unit comprises a radiologist, radiographer, histopathologist, surgeon, receptionist, nurse and administrator. The capital cost of equipment is high, as is the replacement and maintenance bill. The Forrest report (1987) estimated the financial cost to be £3000 pounds per life-year saved, but other estimates place it much higher.

2 There is also an opportunity cost, as skilled personnel and capital funds could be deployed elsewhere.

3 A low positive predictive value implies over-diagnosis, over-investigation and over-treatment of some false positives, with all the heartache this entails.

4 All women experience anxiety awaiting and undergoing tests, and awaiting results; some experience indignity; some may become phobic.

The UK National Breast Screening Programme

In 1988 health authorities began phasing in a programme of screening recommended by the Forrest report. The target population is currently defined as all women aged 50–69 years (although it has been suggested the programme may be extended to women under 50). A single oblique mammogram is offered at 3-yearly intervals. The call and recall procedure is organised as follows:

1 The screening office identifies groups of eligible women.

2 The HA produces a 'prior notification' list for each GP.

3 GPs amend the list (correcting errors) and then return it.

4 Women are invited and attend for mammography.

5 The results are conveyed to women and their doctors, and follow-up arranged where appropriate.

6 A recall procedure is established.

A 70+% uptake is being achieved. Of those screened:

- 5.5% are recalled for investigation;
- 0.75% have a biopsy;
- 0.6% have confirmed cancer.

The benefit of the scheme has been hotly disputed. Mortality from breast cancer in the UK has been falling since 1985. Proponents of the screening programme have hailed some of the decline as evidence of success; whereas Baum (1995) points out that a scheme that did not become fully operational until 1990 could not be expected to have an impact before the next millennium, and that the fall must have another explanation. Other points of contention include the cost per life saved; and the relative cost-effectiveness of money spent in screening and in breast cancer research.

The role of the GP

Austoker (1990) suggests that GPs can make an important practical contribution to the campaign, improving uptake and acceptability by:

- checking prior notification lists to ensure data are accurate;
- allaying fears;
- providing information and counselling;
- following up the non-attenders.

Breast self-examination (BSE)

There is a long-held view that BSE is a worthwhile preventive exercise, to be taught at every available opportunity. However, the evidence for this view is shaky. Hill *et al.* (1988) reviewed 12 trials: six of them purported to show some benefit as judged by the stage of disease at diagnosis. However, as already discussed, earlier diagnosis does not necessarily confer benefit.

In the UK Trial of Early Detection of Breast Cancer those invited to classes to learn BSE (after 400 000 women-years of observation) actually had a higher death rate than women in control districts!

The *disadvantages* of BSE include inconvenience, embarrassment, anxiety and the risk of false positive cases. Furthermore guilt may be engendered in those patients with cancer who did not self-examine before diagnosis.

Some doctors have suggested that it is unethical to offer a test that may harm without clearer evidence of benefit. It is not surprising, given the debate concerning mammography, that a less sensitive screening test should be challenged in this way.

3.10 LIPID SCREENING

Who should be screened?

The case for measuring serum cholesterol is built on several tiers of evidence:

1 Substantial epidemiological data that raised serum cholesterol concentrations are associated with more coronary heart disease.

2 Experiments in animals showing that dietary manipulations that alter serum cholesterol can accelerate or retard atherosclerosis.

3 Evidence from human primary and secondary intervention studies that those who lower their cholesterol level suffer fewer coronary heart disease events.

In the US in 1985 a consensus of experts agreed that all American adults should have their cholesterol measured at least once; similar views have been expressed by the European Atherosclerosis Society and the American National Heart, Lung and Blood Institute. However, many others take a contrary view on who should be screened, and as Leitch (1989) points out, there is no consensus expert opinion on which GPs can advise and act. Recommendations range from no screening at all to screening everyone before the age of 30 years (Tables 3.9 and 3.10); while a survey of UK HAs and Health Boards revealed that only 70 have formulated a screening policy, with

Table 3.9 Recommendations on who should have their serum cholesterol concentration measured.

Source	Main recommendations
Working group on cardiovascular disease of the Faculty of Community Medicine, 1989	Screening of the population not recommended
Study group of the European Atherosclerosis Society, 1987	General screening to be carried out only if provisions have been made for treatment and follow-up by medical practitioners; screening of specified high-risk groups; screening of patients opportune during routine medical contact (examples given)
British Heart Foundation, 1987	Screening of people with a family history of coronary heart disease
Coronary Prevention Group, 1987	Screening of specified high-risk groups*
Journal of the Royal College of General Practitioners (editorial), 1986	Screening of specified high-risk groups*
Journal of the Royal College of General Practitioners (editorial), 1988	Screening of specified high-risk groups* if screening all adults not practical
Royal College of General Practitioners, 1988	Ideally screening of all adults aged 20–70 or, if this is not possible, of specified high-risk groups*
Drugs and Therapeutics Bulletin, 1987	Ideally screening of all adults or, if this is not possible, of specified high-risk groups*
British Hyperlipidaemia Association 1987	Screening of all adults, preferably before age 30

*See Table 3.10. Adapted from Leitch (1989) with permission.

much divergence of opinion. It is instructive to consider how such a situation has arisen.

Do lipid-lowering interventions prolong life?

At least 10 large cohort studies, three international studies and 25 randomised controlled trials have confirmed the relation between cholesterol levels and coronary heart disease events. A 10% reduction in cholesterol has been associated with a 27% difference in coronary heart disease (Law *et al.* 1994), but low cholesterol levels have regularly been linked with deaths from other causes, and it has been suggested that too low a cholesterol can similarly cause harm. Thus, Isles *et al.* (1989) identified in men a strong correlation between low cholesterol and lung cancer, and a U-shaped association with colorectal cancer, also true for women. There are 21 reports, of which 13 identified a link with cancer and low cholesterol, and eight showed no relationship. An increased incidence of cholelithiasis has also been reported, as well as a number of other effects, including a puzzling increase in deaths from violence and suicide.

These associations may arise by chance, or because disease causes a low cholesterol (rather than the other way around), or because of

Table 3.10 Advice on screening high-risk groups (adapted from Leitch (1989) with permission).

Source	High-risk groups								
	A	B	C	D	E	F	G	H	I
Study group of the European Atherosclerosis Society, 1987	Yes, especially if history is in relative <50	Yes	—	Yes (specified)	Yes	Yes	Yes	Yes	Yes
Coronary Prevention Group, 1987	Yes (age unspecified)	Yes	Yes	Yes (specified)	Yes	Yes	—	—	—
Journal of the Royal College of General Practitioners (editorial), 1986	Yes, if patient is <60	—	Yes	—	Yes	Yes	—	—	Possibly
Journal of the Royal College of General Practitioners (editorial) 1988	Yes (age unspecified)	—	Yes	Yes (specified)	—	Yes	Yes (gross)	—	—
Royal College of General Practitioners, 1988	Yes, if history is in relative <60	Yes	Yes	Yes (specified)	Yes	Yes	—	—	—
Drugs and Therapeutics Bulletin 1987	Yes, especially if history is in relative <50	Yes	—	Yes (specified)	Yes	Yes	Yes	—	—

A, people with family history of coronary heart disease; B, people with family history of hyperlidaemia; C, people with personal history of coronary heart disease; D, people with physical signs of hyperlidaemia, for example, arcus xanthoma, xanthelasma; E, people with hypertension; F, diabetics; G, obese people; H, people with a history of gout; I, smokers

some specific side-effect of drug treatment or diet on behaviour. One interesting report links the natural post-partum decline in serum cholesterol with post-natal depression, providing tentative evidence of a biological mechanism in suicide cases (Ploeckinger *et al.* 1996), but controversy still abounds.

The practical problems
1   *The cholesterol screening test.* Several practical considerations apply:
   (a) the test is not perfect—it has a sensitivity of 38% and a specificity of 75%;

(b) serum cholesterol is not static, it varies up to 20% in the course of a day, and rises with age until the fifth or sixth decades;

(c) the range of values is a continuum without a sharp cut-off point between health and disease for most of the population;

(d) high cholesterol is not in itself a diagnosis: it may be primary or secondary, and if primary, one of a complex group of disorders.

This leads to a situation that has an analogy in the problems of defining hypertension:

(a) strictly speaking we should take the mean of several readings before confirming an abnormality;

(b) then proceed to a range of supplementary tests;

(c) then take an arbitrary decision, based on actuarial risk, as to who should be treated.

2 *The size of the problem.* The mean cholesterol level in the UK is 6.3 mmol/l. Many authorities believe dietary advice, further investigations and individual intervention become appropriate at or around this value—that is to say, for nearly half the population!

(a) An American study has estimated (after assuming a 10% decline in serum cholesterol with appropriate dieting) that 7% of men and 4% of women would need drug treatment, 41% lipoprotein analysis, and 84 million people would need interventionist treatment costing several billion dollars (Sempos *et al.* 1989; Wilson *et al.* 1989);

(b) A British study estimated that even more people would need drug treatment. Assuming 100% compliance and no harmful effects from this, over 4000 people would have to be treated to save one life every 5 years. Twice the number of coronary events might be saved by devoting the effort instead to reducing the mean population cholesterol by 0.5 mmol/l by public health measures;

(c) Pharoah *et al.* (1996) estimate that drug treatment of middle-aged men with a cholesterol >6.5 mmol/l and no prior history of coronary disease will cost £136 000 per life saved—a cost that could not be met from current NHS resources.

3 *The compliance problem.* It has been pointed out that:

(a) only a proportion of those screened and found to be at increased risk will return for follow-up counselling;

(b) only some of these will receive and remember accurate dietary advice;

(c) only some of those remembering advice will take it;

(d) only some of those will comply enough to influence their serum cholesterol.

Even if compliance at each step is reasonable, the cumulative effect of drop-outs over the various stages will considerably detract from the potential benefit inherent in the initial screening (Table 3.11).

4 *The negative effect of a normal cholesterol level.* Communication of a normal result could engender unwarranted complacency in the

Table 3.11 Compliance at each stage of a high-risk strategy cholesterol screening campaign.

Study	% of those with high cholesterol returning to their doctor	% of those returning who report receiving dietary advice
Kinlay and Heller (1990), Australia*	82	82
Heart health programme (1988), Minnesota	58 (>6.9 mmol/l)	73
Wynder *et al.* (1986), New York	33 (>5.7 mmol/l)	36

*In Kinlay and Heller's study, three-quarters of those who reported receiving dietary advice acted on it. However, this represented only $0.82 \times 0.82 \times 0.75 - 50\%$ of those found in screening to be at greater risk.

recipient. Indeed, there is some evidence on re-testing that serum cholesterols are higher the second time around!

Furthermore, the Multiple Risk Factor Intervention Cohort Study (of 300 000 men over a 6-year follow-up) found that 30% of deaths occurred in those with cholesterols <5.2 mmol/l, and 60% in those with cholesterols <6.5 mmol/l. These are people who might well assume, on the basis of their blood test, that their diet was satisfactory. It is important not to obscure the community message — that we should all consume less fat.

Selective versus general screening

Many authorities argue that selective testing is more cost-effective than whole-population screening. The pragmatists identify the foregoing problems, which are considerable; the theorists invoke the findings of the Multiple Risk Factors Intervention Trial, in which subjects were grouped according to age, sex and smoking habits, and banded into fifths according to blood pressure and serum cholesterol. It was possible to calculate, by subtraction between groups, the maximum theoretical benefit on mortality when moving from the top fifth to the bottom fifth of the population's cholesterol league-table, for any given combination of other risk factors. This so-called cholesterol-attributive risk was found to vary enormously depending on the size of other risk factors: in men aged 35–45 who had a normal blood pressure and did not smoke, the extra risk from a high cholesterol was minute, whereas in the presence of other risk factors the risk was multiplied manyfold. Isles *et al.* (1996) also report wide differences in cholesterol-attributive risk, such that women with cholesterol levels >7.2 mmol/l are at less risk than men with values <5 mmol/l.

All authorities agree that assessment of coronary heart disease risk must be multifactorial: some have argued on the basis of these findings that cholesterol screening can be reserved selectively for those in whom other significant risk factors have been identified.

3.11 SCREENING FOR BOWEL CANCER

In the UK there are about 30000 new cases of colorectal cancer and 20000 deaths each year. Increasingly enthusiasts advocate screening for bowel cancer using faecal occult blood-testing kits.

The *advantages* are obvious. The technique is:

- non-invasive;
- cheap;
- simple to administer.
  Disadvantages include:
- inconvenience;
- relative insensitivity (occult blood is not uniformly distributed in faeces, and some lesions bleed intermittently);
- relative non-specificity (lesions other than cancer can generate positive tests);
- poor compliance (around 50–70% with wide variation);
- technical interference (from red meat and vegetables rich in peroxidase).

How good is the test in practice?

1 If asymptomatic individuals are screened, about 2% come out positive.

2 If the test is positive there is a 1 in 10 chance of cancer and a 1 in 3 chance of an adenoma; over half of the detected tumours are Duke A at presentation (5 times more than in the unscreened group).

3 If the test is negative there is still a 1 in 200 chance of a cancer and a 1 in 50 chance of an adenoma in the next 4 years.

4 Overall, 3–20 malignancies are detected per 10000 screened, but faecal occult bloods are only positive in 50–60% of cases.

5 Bleeding tends to occur relatively late in the tumour's natural history.

A randomised trial of faecal occult blood testing in Minnesota reported a 33% decline in mortality from colorectal cancer with annual screening, but no benefit from a biannual programme. The false positive rate was high (38%) and a large number of colonoscopies were performed, making it difficult to ascribe the benefit wholly to occult blood testing. However, other randomised trials in Denmark and Nottingham have reported a 15–18% decline in mortality (in cohorts only 4% of whom underwent colonoscopy).

In the Nottingham study (Hardcastle *et al.* 1996), which followed more than 150000 people over a 14-year period, 60% of those randomised to testing completed at least one screening, and 38% completed all tests (3–6), suggesting reasonable acceptance of the procedure. There are now calls for a national screening programme (Lieberman & Sleisenger 1996). The bulk of the cost in such a programme would lie in investigating the false positives.

Do realistic alternatives exist?

Alternative screening strategies (endoscopy, radiology) are expensive and invasive. Flexible sigmoidoscopy would miss one-third of significant lesions; even total colonoscopy is not 100% effective and carries a distinct morbidity (1/1000 perforate); and resources are not adequate to cope with mass screening. However, it has been estimated that a single screening by flexible sigmoidoscopy around the age of 60 could prevent 3500 deaths each year (Atkin *et al.* 1993).

Some authors advocate endoscopic screening of high-risk groups (e.g. those with a personal or family history of bowel cancer or polyp), but even here the recall interval remains undefined. Further progress in the field may depend on the new developing generation of circulating tumour markers and gene probes.

3.12 PREVENTING OSTEOPOROSIS

The size of the problem

Around 45000 people in England and Wales suffer a fractured neck of femur annually. Two-thirds are elderly women.

Treatment costs run into hundreds of millions of pounds a year. The major contributory factor is osteoporosis — one-tenth of women in their 60s and one-half in their 70s suffer an osteoporosis-related fracture.

Preventive strategies

In the first 20–25 years of life bone mineral density (which correlates highly with bone strength) increases with age to reach a peak; it then remains constant in women until the menopause when it falls sharply for 5–10 years (oestrogen withdrawal bone loss); and more slowly thereafter (age-related bone loss). Preventive strategies focus on encouraging new bone formation, discouraging bone resorption and achieving a higher bone mineral density at peak. Several initiatives may confer benefit:

1 *Regular exercise* — highly effective in preventing bone loss. (Ideally exercise should start well before and continue through middle age.)

2 *An adequate diet* — there is debate concerning the role of dietary calcium, but it would be prudent to ensure an intake of 1400 mg per day. The effect probably depends on age. Prospective cohort studies are currently examining whether calcium supplements can help achieve a higher peak bone mineral density in young adults (many adolescent girls probably risk a suboptimal intake).

3 *Enough sunlight* — 15 min per day may be enough to allow skin synthesis of vitamin D.

4 *Hormone therapy* — oestrogen is effective in reducing bone loss, and hormone replacement therapy can halve the risk of a fracture if given

perimenopausally. Treatment should probably be long-term (more than 10 years) with a mixed oestrogen/progestogen regimen for those who have not had a hysterectomy. (This mitigates against the risk of endometrial cancer. The risk of breast cancer is probably slightly higher, but that of coronary heart disease is substantially reduced by oestrogen, implying a strong net beneficial effect.) Compliance tends to be poor because of side-effects and the recurrence of withdrawal bleeds, but tissue-specific oestrogens may soon provide a more acceptable alternative.

5   *Giving up smoking*—smoking lowers circulating oestrogen levels.

6   *Bisphosphonates* — evidence is emerging that these drugs may be effective inhibitors of bone resorption. Several are now licensed for the treatment of osteoporosis.

7   *Calcitonin*—increases bone mineral density and probably reduces fracture rate, but has to be given by injection. Alternative routes of administration (nasal and rectal) have not so far proved so effective.

Osteoporosis is a common and important condition, deserving closer attention that it presently receives from GPs. It is perhaps one of the areas where well-woman advice may reap dividends in years to come.

3.13 DISEASE MANAGEMENT PACKAGES

This US concept involves a long-term relationship between commercial (usually drug) companies and a health care provider — in which the doctor agrees to offer an agreed disease treatment or tertiary prevention package in return for cheap or free drugs, staff or other benefits. Formerly such alliances were banned by the Department of Health, but now there is active discussion about a framework that would enable partnership.

The scheme offers obvious advantages. An opportunity exists at little or no extra cost to provide new dedicated services (e.g. asthma, diabetes or hypertension nursing clinics) to better manage chronic health problems.

However, a number of potential concerns have been raised too:
- a risk that confidentiality may be breached if drug companies gain access to the prescribing data;
- likely delay in the introduction of new drugs to the market;
- curtailment of GPs' clinical freedom, and their ability to make holistic and individual judgements;
- public unease that doctors' behaviour will be determined by commercial, rather than clinical considerations;
- concern that drug companies may selectively target high prescribers, leading to a two-tier provision.

The Royal College of General Practitioners has expressed reservations about the concept. However, its financial attractions are considerable. If the more serious clinical and political concerns can be addressed, and the necessary quality thresholds can be met, packaged disease management programmes may become a feature of primary care.

4 Clinical Dilemmas

Few topics in general practice (as in medicine as a whole) are straight-forward. Usually there is room for debate — definite clinical uncertainty. Sometimes the areas of clinical debate are shared throughout medicine (does strict control of diabetes prevent complications? when to treat hypertension?) and sometimes there is an important or unique general practice bias — the management of the sore throat, earache or backache; home care for coronaries or maternity cases.

Of course the debate in general practice does not stop with purely clinical issues; it encompasses the fields of administration, legal and ethical dilemmas, finance and priority allocation. The remit is wide: how to run a business; how to maximise resources; how to handle sensitive issues; how to manage tonsillitis; how best to do X, Y or Z.

A large part of this book is devoted to the non-clinical issues: appointment system; deputising services; computers; personal lists. This chapter reviews some of the clinical dilemmas and is meant to illustrate how debatable most of our actions are.

Note that in many cases totally opposite points of view are defensible or at least merit consideration. This is important in an examination like the MRCGP where you are expected to be sensitive to the debate, to be aware of the breadth of opinion, to avoid dogmatism and admit contrary possibilities.

For the examination you are expected to marshal facts into an argument, so some facts are marshalled into arguments in this chapter, but remember that as the debate unfolds these 'facts' may change, so keep up to date! Try to supplement this chapter with a list of your own topics because the arena of debate in general practice is now very wide. This is important exam preparation which should pay off in the examination.

4.1 WHEN TO TREAT HYPERTENSION?

The treatment of hypertension is an area that can be broken down into a series of dilemmas.

The dilemma of definition
1 Systolic and diastolic blood pressures (BPs) are continuous variables with a 'normal' distribution in the population and no clear cut-off point between disease and health.
2 Actuarial tables (produced for insurance purposes) show a direct relationship between height of BP and longevity for all values, so everything is relative: all other things being equal a person with a BP of 135/90mmHg will not live as long as another with a BP of

120/80 mmHg. Clearly the cut-off point for treatment is *arbitrary* and depends on views about costs and benefits.

The dilemma of measurement

1 Everyone's BP *fluctuates* (e.g. with posture, level of arousal). Replicate measurement of BP is required to confirm a diagnosis of hypertension, but a Dutch survey has revealed that even four measurements may be insufficient for the purpose (Brueren *et al.* 1996). If due account is not taken of within-person variations, hypertension will be over-diagnosed in borderline cases. The recent development of non-invasive techniques for constant measurement of BP has allowed ambulatory BPs to be compared with the traditional cuff method in the surgery: they are often lower.

(a) Pickering *et al.* (1988) described so-called 'white-coat hypertension' in 22% of 292 patients with borderline high BPs.

(b) In a retrospective study of 638 patients with hypertension in a cardiology unit, 89% satisfied the World Health Organization hypertension criteria on resting measurements, but only half that number were judged hypertensive on ambulatory monitoring (Kenny *et al.* 1987).

2 Other sources of variation include:

(a) measuring technique (size of cuff; observer bias; inaccurate machines);

(b) different end-points (phase V in most trials but phase IV in most surgeries). Which measurements are representative of true health risk?

We should remember that traditional guidelines (e.g. three readings on separate occasions) are arbitrary. A solitary raised reading from the actuarial point of view means a shorter life on average.

The dilemma of natural history

In Fry's (1979) untreated group of 1000 hypertensives over a 15-year period:

- diastolic BP decreased spontaneously in 30%;
- diastolic BP remained unchanged in 20%;
- diastolic BP increased in 50%.

It appears there is almost a one in three chance that diastolic BP will fall spontaneously in follow-up.

There is also a dilemma of *heterogeneity*: hypertensives are not a uniform group; they vary in their associated cardiovascular risk factors and hence in the likely natural history. Treating these different groups at the same BP level is an oversimplification.

Dilemmas in the elderly

1 In Fry's study of untreated hypertensives the standardised mortality ratio falls with age and after 60 years is not more than expected.

2   In another study, death rate clearly increased with systolic BP below age 70 years but there was no correlation above this.

Recent trials have confirmed the benefit of lowering blood pressure in the over 60s (see Sanderson 1996), although the risks of iatrogenic illness (e.g. postural hypotension) are higher. Paradoxically the British Hypertension Society Working Party recommends treating the elderly at a lower diastolic blood pressure than younger adults, although the evidence suggests that GPs adopt the opposite policy (Dickerson *et al.* 1995).

Logistic dilemmas

As Fry has observed, there are 5–7 million hypertensives in the UK (85% of these classified as mild). This is prevalence of 10–15%. If they are all seen 2–4 times per year and given a script worth about £10 each time, the drug bill alone could cost £150 million, and added to this is the use of the resources and time of doctors and nurses on a large scale. This is a sizeable and costly undertaking. As described in Section 3.5 general practice has so far failed to organise itself to meet this challenge; perhaps only one-eighth of all hypertensives are currently well controlled.

The cost–benefit dilemma

Benefits

The benefit of treating severe hypertension is generally undisputed and so is the effect on longevity of untreated mild/moderate hypertension; the problem arises in demonstrating a benefit from treatment in the milder groups. Several expensive large-scale trials have examined this (Table 4.1) but unfortunately this brings us on to *the dilemma of the muddling trial results*. Contradictory methods and recommendations have left the clinician in a confused position (Fahey & Peters 1996).

Even where there is agreement that treatment is needed the target BP is in doubt. The traditional counsel has been to lower raised BPs to as near normal as possible, but some authorities have recently argued that the relationship between mortality from coronary heart disease and BP achieved after treatment is J-shaped—in other words, lowering BP too far may actually *cause* extra deaths!

Costs

The costs are more readily counted:

1   The *labour* cost (considerable administrative problems; doctors' time, allocated in the face of competing priorities).

2   The *financial* cost (in drug bills and the salaries of medical and paramedical staff).

3   The *iatrogenic* cost (claudication, complete heart block, heart failure, impotence, fatigue, drug interactions, etc.). This aspect may be underestimated: according to the Stroke Association almost one-third

Table 4.1 Some important hypertension trials.

Trial	Groups examined and methods	Results	Possible criticisms
Veterans Administration Co-operative Study, USA (*Journal of the American Medical Association* 1970; **213**, 1143)	380 male 'veterans', average age 50 years, with diastolic BPs averaging 90–115 mmHg. Double-blind randomisation between placebo and active treatment	Risk of developing a morbid event over 5 years was 18% in the treated group and 55% in the controls, most impact being in the higher BP patients and for cardiac failure and strokes, rather than coronary artery disease	Veterans were highly selected for their adherence to a drug regimen and the persistence of their hypertension
Hypertension Detection and Follow-up Program, USA (*Journal of the American Medical Association* 1979; **242**, 2562)	Patients with diastolic BPs in the 90–105 mmHg range. Hospital stepped care was compared with referral back to GP. (Stepped care included systematic follow-up, education and financial assistance)	Deaths from cardiovascular disease were reduced. BP control was better in the stepped-care group	1 There were no controls 2 The stepped-care group also showed a fall in non-cardiovascular deaths (cumulative 5-year mortality 5.9/100 compared with 7.4/100) suggesting better overall care in this group
Australian National Board Hypertension Study, Australia (*Lancet* 1980; **i**, 1261)	3427 men and women aged 36–69 years with a diastolic BP in the range 95–110 mmHg, randomised in a single-blind fashion between placebo and active drugs. There were 14 000 patient-years of observation	1 A two-thirds reduction in cardiovascular deaths 2 A fall in overall mortality 3 Most effect was seen when diastolic BP was greater than 100 mmHg	1 The trial stopped prematurely because of the results, at a time when they were just marginally significant 2 About one-third of patients prematurely stopped the regimen to which they had been randomised
Multiple Risk Factor Intervention Trial (*Journal of the American Medical Association* 1982; **248**, 1465–77)	8000 men aged 35–57 with diastolic BPs of 90–114 mmHg randomised between an intensive heart disease prevention programme (addressing diet, smoking habits, hyperlipidaemia and hypertension) and 'usual care'	No reduction in CVAs observed in the treated hypertensive subgroup	The incidence of CVAs in the control group was unusually low, suggesting a high standard of 'usual care' in the control group
MRC mild hypertension trial, UK (*British Medical Journal* 1985; **291**, 97)	A 15-year trial costing £4 million. 85 570 patient-years of observation by 176 GP groups: 500 000 people screened; 50 000	Deaths per thousand *Treated* *Untreated* CVAs 1.4 2.6 MIs 5.2 5.4 Overall 5.8 5.9	1 30–40% withdrew from the treated group because of side-effects 2 Bendrofluazide was used in doses we now

Continued on p. 134

Table 4.1 *Continued*

Trial	Groups examined and methods	Results	Possible criticisms
	were eligible but only 17 000 joined the trial. 35- to 64 year-old age group with diastolic BPs of 90–109 mmHg. Single-blind randomisation between bendrofluazide, propranolol and placebo	i.e.: **1** A reduction in CVA rate **2** No reduction in MIs or overall mortality **3** One CVA saved per 850 patient–years of treatment	fear may exacerbate other cardiovascular risk factors (raising glucose, uric acid and lipids without additional hypotensive benefit)
European Working Party on Hypertension in the Elderly (*Lancet* 1985; **i**, 1349)	Patients over 60 years. Double-blind randomisation between placebo, hydrochlorothiazide and triamterene (with or without methyldopa). Conducted in 18 European collaboration centres over 12 years	**1** Deaths reduced from MIs **2** Deaths from CVA *not* reduced **3** Overall mortality *not* reduced	**1** Only 840 patients were recruited (on average 4 per centre per year) **2** The trial was so long that only one-third of patients were still in the double-blind part at the end
MRC trial of treatment of hypertension in older adults (*British Medical Journal*; **304**, 405–12)	Randomised placebo controlled single blind trial. 4396 patients aged 65–74 with mean systolic BPs of 109–160 mmHg and mean diastolic BPs < 115 mmHg randomised between diuretic, beta-blocker or placebo	**1** Actively treated subjects had a 25% reduction in CVAs and a 19% reduction in coronary events **2** The reduction arose in those treated with diuretics, but not beta-blockers **3** All-cause mortality was similar in treated and placebo groups	The study, in common with others of similar size, did not have sufficient power to detect small effects of treatment on all-cause mortality

CVA, cerebrovascular accident; MI, myocardial infarction.

of hypertensives who stop their treatment are reluctant to tell their doctor.

4 The *psychological* cost (the illness label which some previously asymptomatic individuals wear around their necks!).

Studies suggest that many vague and non-specific side-effects (headaches, tiredness, light-headed feelings, lack of well-being) are no more common in treated than untreated groups, but some real costs, like impotence in thiazide-treated hypertensives, may go unrecognised for some time, and the unexpected complications of practolol therapy have made people rightly critical in appraising the need for long-term drug treatment.

Conclusions

The British Hypertension Society Working Party recognised the need

Table 4.2 The British Hypertension Society Working Party's recommendations (1993) for drug intervention in hypertension.

Diastolic BP*
Treat if:
- ≥110 mmHg (several measurements closely spaced)
- ≥100–109 mmHg if there is (a) evidence of end-organ damage or (b) persistence
- 90–99 mmHg if (a) persistent or (b) coexisting with other risk factors (e.g. smoking, hyperlipidaemia, strong family history) or (c) elderly

Systolic BP*
Treat if:
- ≥200 mmHg; or 160–199 mmHg with dBP > 95 mmHg
- ≥160–199 mmHg and (a) persistent or (b) evidence of end-organ damage

Other points
- Advise weight reduction in obese patients
- Warn all patients against smoking and heavy alcohol intake

*Several readings, generally spaced over a few months. The full report (*Br Med J* 1993; **309**, 983–7) contains more details.

for some sort of consensus conclusion, and produced a set of recommendations (Table 4.2). However, these answers to the cost–benefit dilemma are not definitive, so the clinician faced with real patients will have some hard decisions to make. The element of uncertainty in these decisions should be recognised, as well as possible implications.

4.2 IS STRICT CONTROL OF DIABETES WORTHWHILE?

Some element of control is indisputably important in diabetes; for example, hypoglycaemic coma is potentially fatal; prior to the development of insulin, diabetes was a rapidly fatal disorder and pregnancy was very dangerous. But good control is bought at a cost, be it the risk of more hypoglycaemic episodes or the disruption of a person's lifestyle. Does strict control prevent complications? Does strict control benefit those who already have complications? And does the benefit outweigh possible risks and costs?

The relationship between diabetic control and vascular complications
Most studies on the relationship between diabetic control and vascular complications founder because of:
1 Problems in accurately assessing control;
2 Other confounding risk factors (e.g. smoking and hypertension) not considered.
   Knowles (1970) reviewed 300 studies:
- only 85 had no major design errors;

- 50 of these found a positive correlation between poor control and vascular complications;
- a further 25 found no correlation;
- the remaining 10 were undecided.

Three studies in favour of a correlation are listed in Table 4.3. The dilemma could best be resolved by a prospective study in which newly diagnosed patients were randomly allocated into well and poorly controlled groups, but this approach would take many years to provide an answer and is, of course, unethical.

The relationship between existing complications and strict control

This is also unclear:

1   *Retinopathy* — initial studies involving sudden normalisation of blood sugar levels in patients with existing retinopathy actually provoked deterioration, even progression to a proliferative form. More recent studies suggest this is a transient effect. The situation is now being studied using continuous subcutaneous insulin infusions (CSII) to perfect control:

> (a) in the Oslo study (1986) patients did better on CSII—there was no regression of vascular damage, but the rate of deterioration was slowed;
>
> (b) in the Stena study (1983) the most marked deterioration in retinal function was seen in those with the worst and best degree of control. This suggests there is an optimal range of glycaemia, and that being too strict may be as harmful as being too lax.

2   *Nephropathy* — A small number of studies have demonstrated a regression in the basement membrane changes of kidneys showing diabetic nephropathy when transplanted into non-diabetic patients.

More recently in a comparative study of 1400 patients, those receiving intensive therapy were 75% less likely to suffer progressive retinopathy and 39% less likely to develop microalbuminemia.

The hazards of stricter control

The most obvious risk of stricter control is hypoglycaemia (in fact

Table 4.3 Studies supporting an association between diabetic control and vascular complications.

Study	Conclusion
The Bedford study	Retinopathy only develops in patients whose blood glucose exceeds 11.1 mmol/l at 2 h in a glucose tolerance test (GTT)
Epidemiological studies of the Pima Indians of Arizona (50% of whom are diabetic)	Retinopathy and nephropathy were confined to those with fasting sugars over 8 mmol/l or 2-h GTT sugars over 13 mmol/l
Chemical pancreatectomy studies in dogs and rats	High blood sugar levels damage eyes and kidneys in this experimental model of human diabetes. Sugar itself appears to be the toxic agent when present in excess

many patients sabotage their control to avoid it). Hypoglycaemia seems to be very common: for example, in a 1-year Nottingham study at least 9% of the insulin-dependent clinic population received hospital treatment for hypoglycaemia. Despite the high frequency, death and measurable brain damage seem rare. Also it is by no means clear that hypoglycaemia is more common in those who strive for stricter control: many authorities believe it is more common in the 'casual' diabetic.

For whom is strict control not suitable?

This is contentious. The decision may be swayed by such factors as:

- the presence of complications;
- the age of the patient;
- the competence of the patient;
- the degree of psychological and social interference, stricter control causes.

4.3 ANTIBIOTICS FOR SORE THROATS?

On average the practitioner sees about 600 upper respiratory tract infections including 100–150 sore throats each year. Despite the frequency of this condition there is no universally accepted management policy.

Although the presence of palatal petechiae and vesicles is suggestive of viral inflection, and tonsillar exudate in patients under 15 years of age is more likely to be streptococcal, while in those over 15 it is more likely to be glandular fever, it is generally felt that the aetiology cannot be predicted from appearance with any degree of certainty.

When a throat swab is taken from an acute throat the following results are obtained:

- 40% yield no growth;
- 30% grow a beta-haemolytic *Streptococcus*;
- 20% grow a virus;
- other less common growths are *Haemophilus*, *Candida*, *Pneumococcus* and the organism of Vincent's angina.

However, anti-streptolysin titres (ASOT) titres can rise without symptoms and beta-haemolytic *Streptococcus* can be grown from asymptomatic throats without any rise in ASOT titre (Haverkorn *et al.* 1971).

Hence, the correlation of symptoms, throat appearance and even throat swab growth with infection is imperfect. Prescribing habits, not surprisingly, vary between the extreme views of 'antibiotics for all' and 'no antibiotics at all' with many GPs occupying the middle ground and prescribing for various indications of their own choosing (e.g. fever, malaise) which again correlate poorly.

Benefits?

1 *Complications.* Although the incidence of rheumatic fever and post-streptococcal glomerulonephritis has fallen dramatically, the evidence suggests this has more to do with improved living standards than the widespread prescription of penicillin (the fall started early in the 20th century, pre-dating the introduction of antibiotics).

2 *Duration of illness.* Several studies suggest that this is not much affected, e.g. Whitfield and Hughes (1981) found that illness was not shortened at all, irrespective of whether there was fever, purulent tonsils or lymphadenitis; Brumfitt and Slater (1957) felt that duration was shortened by about 24 h.

3 Doctors, however, perceive a pressure to prescribe, which provides several *social* benefits (see also Section 2.2):

(a) it demonstrates concern;

(b) it lets the patient down gently, justifying the efforts made to attend;

(c) it represents an attempt to do something, which patients appreciate and expect;

(d) it is a quick way to conclude a consultation;

(e) the precedent of other doctors' prescriptions often makes it hard not to prescribe.

In fact doctors perceive more pressure than really exists. According to Cartwright and Anderson (1981), 41% of patients entering consultations expect a prescription but 67% leave with one!

Problems?

1 There is a very small risk of anaphylaxis but a much greater risk of nuisance side-effects (e.g. gastrointestinal upset, vaginal candidiasis).

2 Although penicillin is a cheap drug, the cost to the NHS when prescribed on a huge scale is considerable.

3 Widespread antibiotic prescribing encourages drug resistance.

4 Prescribing fosters a patient's dependence and reinforces the sick role, teaching him that he needs medical attention with his next illness episode. Apparently patients only take a sore throat to their doctor on 1 in 18 occasions (Banks *et al.* 1975), which is fortunate as the system might well be overwhelmed otherwise! It is possible that ready prescribing saves time in the short term but generates more work in the long term.

4.4 MIDDLE EAR PROBLEMS IN CHILDHOOD

Acute otitis media is predominantly a disease of the first 10 years of life, especially the pre-school years, and is very common. Thus:

1 The attack rate has been estimated to be between 10 and 15% in the under 10-year-olds.

2 One in four children is affected at some time.

3 On average a GP expects to see about 100 cases per year.

139

Chapter 4
Clinical
Dilemmas
4 This amounts to about 1.5 million episodes annually in England and Wales.

Approximately 40% of children will suffer at least one recurrence in the following year and those with unresolved middle ear effusions from the original attack are particularly prone.

If the middle ear fluid is aspirated and cultured:

1 66% of cases grow bacterial pathogens, usually *Haemophilus influenzae* and *Streptococcus pneumoniae*;

2 25% of aspirates are sterile;

3 mycoplasma and anaerobes are sometimes grown, and Gram-negative organisms in 10–20% of neonatal cases;

4 viruses are isolated in 4% of cases (although viral titres are raised in 25%, suggesting that viral infection may precede bacterial infection).

Other predisposing factors include:

1 Persistent eustachian tube dysfunction. This may be:

(a) functional;

(b) due to large adenoids;

(c) due to allergy (there is an increased family history of allergy in recurrent sufferers).

2 Unresolved middle ear effusions (a high percentage of asymptomatic effusions grow bacteria).

The debate

Major issues include:

1 The role of antibiotics in management.

2 The role of alternative treatments in the acute stage and in recurrent disease.

3 The management of the middle ear effusion.

These will be considered briefly in turn.

Antibiotics or not?

Proponents of antibiotic treatment argue that:

1 It is rational since a bacterial aetiology is likely in most cases (more so than the sore throat).

2 Antibiotics are cheap and generally very safe.

3 There has been a decline in the incidence of serious complications, especially chronic suppurative otitis media and mastoiditis since their widespread use.

4 Clinical experience suggests patients obtain quick pain relief after prescription.

5 Some trials support a prescribing policy, e.g. Laxdal *et al.* (1970) found in a non-double-blind study that children under 3 years of age did better on ampicillin than placebo.

The case against antibiotics runs as follows:

1 Several trials do not show an objective advantage for the majority

(Table 4.4) — spontaneous resolution occurs in up to 85% of cases without treatment.

2 There is a low frequency of serious complications. This may not be due to the widespread use of antibiotics but to a decline in the virulence of pathogens or improved herd immunity.

3 Antibiotics prescribed *en masse* cost the NHS a lot of money.

4 Widespread prescribing may discourage the development of natural immunity, or promote drug-resistant organisms.

5 Ready prescribing may promote dependence on doctors.

6 Up to 29% of treated cases report nuisance side-effects.

7 The rising incidence of glue ear is thought to be iatrogenic, with antibiotics as the culprit.

Alternative treatments?

1 *In acute attacks*:

(a) myringotomy has not been shown to be beneficial in routine cases;

(b) antihistamine decongestants are prescribed in 50% of cases but there is not much evidence that they affect the outcome.

2 *In prophylaxis*:

(a) antibiotics appear to reduce the recurrence rate in susceptible children;

(b) grommets in some studies reduce recurrence rate to an even greater extent than prophylactic ampicillin;

(c) adenoidectomy and/or tonsillectomy: this is controversial. Maw (1983) found adenoidectomy had a beneficial effect, not enhanced by tonsillectomy, for up to 12 months in 40% of chronic cases with effusion, but other studies have reached different conclusions.

The management of middle ear effusions

Persistent middle ear effusions are a common sequel to acute otitis media. In studies:

- approximately 40% have fluid at 3 months;

Table 4.4 Studies suggesting that antibiotics are not needed routinely in acute otitis media.

Study	Finding
Fry (1958): more than 500 cases	85% resolved completely without antibiotics. At follow-up the degree of hearing loss and frequency of recurrence were no different from the antibiotic group
Halstead *et al.* (1968): 89 cases randomised between antibiotic and placebo	No advantage found in the antibiotic group
Van Buchem *et al.* (1981): 240 cases of acute otitis media randomised between antibiotics, placebo and myringotomy	No significant difference found. Most placebo cases resolved after 24–48 h with analgesia alone

- 20% have hearing losses of 20 dB or more 6 months after treatment;
- 17% have hearing losses 5–10 years after an attack.

Referral policy is unclear, but some authorities suggest:

- sustained hearing loss of 30 dB on two or more frequencies or 20 dB throughout the normal frequency range.

The management of the overlapping disorder *glue ear* is also debatable. Here approximately one-third of all children are affected by the fifth year of life for reasons which are unclear, but suggested to be:

- viral or bacterial otitis media modified by immunological factors;
- otitis media modified by antibiotics;
- a catarrhal disorder with eustachian tube dysfunction;
- large adenoids;
- allergy;
- cigarette smoke (case control studies suggest up to one-third of cases may be due to passive smoking).

The natural history is *benign*:

- most children grow out of their catarrhal phase by 7–8 years old;
- no permanent deafness results;
- there is natural self-resolution over months to years (75% by 6 months).

Medical (drug) treatment includes antibiotics, antihistamines and decongestants. Efficacy is not proven.

Surgical treatment is by myringotomy and the insertion of a grommet which aerates the middle ear and corrects hearing loss. After eventual extrusion of the grommet 70% of children remain trouble-free, but the remainder have recurrence and a further grommet is often necessary; thus very young patients may be submitted to several procedures. Various concerns have been raised about this operation which has been performed with much greater frequency over the last decade:

1 It is used to treat a condition that is common and benign.

2 Although glue ear does not cause permanent deafness, an operative complication may do so.

3 Surgery can cause scarring of the drums, the long term effects of which are unclear.

4 Ninety-five per cent of ENT surgeons advise children with grommets not to swim.

5 Glue ear surgery costs the NHS around £30 million per year.

The serious complication rate is probably less than 2%, however, and the social and educative cost of even temporary hearing loss to the young child is difficult to determine and perhaps considerable.

4.5 THE MANAGEMENT OF BACKACHE

The scale of the problem

There are about 400 consultations per 1000 patients each year (i.e. 3–7 million GP consultations per year) and 50 million working days lost per year.

The natural history

- 50–80% recover completely in 4 weeks without treatment;
- in 80% of cases no specific diagnosis is made;
- however, nearly 70% of patients who ever experience an episode will suffer three or more recurrences.

Should cases be referred?

Of the 3–7 million people who consult with backache annually:

- 1.5 million (about one-third) are referred for an opinion;
- a similar number are X-rayed;
- 1 million attend NHS physiotherapy departments;
- 100000 people are admitted and 24000 undergo surgery (less than 1 in 200 of the original sufferers, and 1 in 60 of the referrals).

Many patients are referred for primarily social reasons: patient insistence on a second opinion; to reassure the patient that all possible avenues have been explored; to demonstrate continuing concern; or to reassure the doctor that no serious pathology has been missed. However, since relatively few cases are amenable to specialist help this represents a questionable use of orthopaedic resources.

The element of referral due to medical ignorance could be reduced by clear specialist guidelines such as those produced by the Clinical Standards Advisory Group on Back Pain (1995):

- Evidence of cauda equina syndrome or widespread neurological disorder (disturbed micturition/anal tone, saddle anaesthesia, widespread progressive motor weakness, gait problems) demand *emergency* referral;
- 'Red flag' signs (e.g. weight loss and malaise; history of cancer, steroid use, drug abuse or HIV; inflammatory features) require *urgent* referral (within a few weeks);
- Simple backache and non-progressive nerve root entrapment should *normally be managed within general practice*, but referred if prolonged (6 weeks or so) and unresolved.

The element of referral due to social factors is more difficult to tackle, although counselling may help once it is acknowledged for what it is.

Should X-rays be used?

The yield from lumbosacral X-rays is low. Thus:

- in one district general hospital where there were 3000 such X-rays per year, 30–40% were reported normal and about 40% showed degenerative changes only;
- many large studies have found a very poor correlation between degenerative changes and symptoms;
- Nachemson (1976) estimated that a routine lumbosacral X-ray in

the absence of suspicious features reveals unexpected disease on only one occasion in 2500.

Despite these drawbacks surveys indicate that a high percentage of backache sufferers eventually present to the X-ray department, e.g.:

• 20% of all American sufferers (according to the National Ambulatory Medical Care Survey 1980);

• in the UK there are half a million lumbar spine X-rays annually.

Why then are so many patients referred for X-rays at great cost in terms of personnel, money and convenience? In general many of the social reasons for referral are mirrored in the use of X-rays and other investigative procedures. Important factors include:

1   The insistence of poorly counselled or impatient patients.

2   Impatience or ignorance on the part of the doctor.

3   The fear that something important may be missed.

4   The psychological benefit that patients (and doctors) gain from a normal X-ray report.

What treatment should be given?

Mobilisation

The Clinical Standards Advisory Group recommends that bed rest should not normally exceed 1–3 days for simple acute backache, and 1–2 weeks for nerve root pain (for longer periods there is no evidence of benefit, but there are well documented disadvantages). Active exercise and rehabilitation often promote recovery: the particular type of exercise may be less important.

Manipulation

1   Some studies have found short-term benefits, not sustained at 3–7 days (e.g. Glover *et al.* 1974).

2   In one study Doran and Newell (1975) randomly allocated 450 patients between manipulation, physiotherapy, corset and rest/analgesia groups and found no difference in outcome.

3   A more recent study (Mead *et al.* 1991) has claimed significant benefit from chiropractor manipulation, but its methods and conclusions have been challenged.

4   The Clinical Standards Advisory Group say that short term symptomatic benefit may be expected in acute back conditions, but that in chronic low back pain the evidence of benefit is more limited.

5   Manipulation requires some expertise and is potentially harmful in the presence of neurological complications and certain pathological conditions (fractures, metastases, osteoporosis).

6   Some patients derive comfort from manipulation and believe in it.

A survey by Little *et al.* (1996) highlighted that GPs' management of back pain did not match up to the Standards Group guidelines. Doctors often failed to examine thoroughly and to advise on back exercises; and only 20% offered manipulation.

Is education helpful?

In cases and ex-cases

1   In one study patients attended four lectures on back anatomy and function, and received instruction in lifting and exercising. Recovery was hastened but no difference was observed in the likelihood of recurrence.

2   Another study prescribed regular exercise programmes but found no difference in the duration of recurrences (Berquist-Ullman & Larsen 1977).

3   However, in a randomised controlled trial used to evaluate an educational booklet in general practice, significantly fewer of the counselled group consulted with back pain in the following year; fewer were referred and admitted; but there was no significant change in certified absence from work with back problems (Roland & Dixon 1989).

In non-cases (primary prevention)

1   A number of studies in industry have shown initial benefits from lifting training programmes, but the benefit generally diminishes with time.

2   Routine radiographs have not proved effective in screening out workers who are at increased risk of back injury prior to employment in heavy industries (e.g. coal mining).

The economic consequences of backache

Each year about 50 million working days are lost because of backache. In 1993 this represented £480 million in direct costs to the NHS, but several billion pounds in indirect costs (lost economic activity, DSS payments, etc.). Some 80000 people are permanently crippled through chronic backache, many of whom are in receipt of welfare benefits. Lumbar spine X-rays form 4–5% of the average X-ray department's workload and about 20% of all new orthopaedic referrals are for backache. At least one out of every two people in western society suffers from back trouble at some time, and on a world scale the annual toll runs into many billions of pounds.

4.6 MATERNITY CARE

Obstetric standards have improved over the last few decades, e.g.:

1   There has been a fall in the perinatal mortality (PNM) rate (from 38 per 1000 total births in 1949 to 8.8 per 1000 in 1995).

2   A 10-fold decrease has occurred in maternal mortality (from more than 90 per 100000 in 1949 to 6 per 100000 births recently).

Several other trends have emerged over the same period:

1   The transfer of childbirth from home to hospital maternity units (66% of births were in hospital in 1960, but 98% in 1994).

2   A steady fall in maternity beds available to GPs as a percentage of the whole (now down to 18%).

3   A change in the disposition and deployment of maternity staff (more consultants and hospital midwives; fewer community midwives).

It is clear that childbirth has become hospitalised and removed from community hands (the average community midwife now attends no more than three home deliveries per year, and a GP one every 6–7 years). Antenatal care by contrast is still shared to a large extent. Trends to hospitalise childbirth have not been entirely unopposed.

Important debating points include:

•   the place of birth (home confinements or not?);
•   the cost-effectiveness of GP maternity units;
•   the antenatal routine (is it streamlined and efficient, or a waste of available resources?).

Home confinements or not?

There has been a tendency to explain the decline in PNM in terms of more and safer hospital confinements. A 1980 report found that PNM was, respectively:

•   6 per 1000 in GP maternity units (low-risk cases);
•   18 per 1000 in consultant units (higher-risk cases);
•   23 per 1000 at home.

It was recommended that home deliveries should be phased out even more. This can be contrasted with the experience in the Netherlands (the only country in Western Europe where home confinement is still common—34% in 1981):

•   the percentage of instrumental deliveries is the lowest in Europe;
•   the morbidity and mortality figures are *lower* amongst the home group, and amongst the lowest in the world.

Proponents of home confinement argue that:

1   The headline figures on outcome are misleading. Fifty per cent of all home deliveries are not planned, but due, for example, to precipitate labour; some occur despite contrary medical advice. The PNM for home deliveries booked for hospital care is very much higher than for those booked for home care (e.g. 45–54/1000 compared with 1.6–1.9/1000 in the Northern Region Perinatal Mortality Survey Co-ordinating Group's study (1996)).

2   Continental experience proves alternatives are safe and feasible.

3   A less interventionist policy (fewer inductions, less instrumentation and technology, fewer caesarean sections) should be promoted:

   (a) childbirth is a unique emotional experience and should not be spoiled;

   (b) the differing caesarean section rates of countries like the UK and the US argue that childbirth approaches are influenced more by expediency and opinion than necessity.

3 People have the right to a free choice.

Opponents of home confinement say:

1 7% of so-called low-risk pregnancies produce potentially life-threatening situations (neonatal asphyxia; postpartum haemorrhage).

2 GPs see insufficient intrapartum work to maintain their expertise with, for example, obstetric forceps. (This is really a false argument since it applies only for the time that home confinement is rare!)

'Active birth' movements appear to be on the increase so this debate may assume more importance in the future.

GP maternity units or not?

There are at least three aspects to this: costs, standards (PNM) and patient preference.

Costs

In 1981 the average GP unit delivery cost £395 and the average consultant unit delivery £485. Of course this does not compare like with like (as the higher-risk consultant patients are offered a high-technology service) but the question is, would a lower technology service suffice and save money? At present the specialist hospital sector receives more than 80% of the total maternity budget. It has been estimated that savings of 40% could be made simply by postnatal transfer to cheaper GP units. In 1981 a Joint Working Committee of the Royal College of Obstetricians and Gynaecologists and the Royal College of General Practitioners recommended expanding the GP units attached to specialist hospital units.

PNM

This is lower amongst the selected low-risk cases in GP units than the higher-risk cases of consultant units suggesting, given proper selection, that standards are acceptable.

Patient preference

A 1985 Oxford study found that patients booked for delivery in a GP unit:

- saw their GPs more often in the antenatal period;
- saw fewer midwives;
- received less conflicting information;
- were admitted a little later in labour;
- more often had their GP present at their birth;
- were more likely to breast-feed immediately after birth.

However, a high level of satisfaction was expressed with the care received in both types of unit.

Is antenatal care a waste of resources?

Two particular areas have come under scrutiny recently: the role of midwives and the antenatal routine.

Concern has been expressed over a needless duplication of resources in the antenatal routine. Nearly two-thirds of midwives work in clinics where GPs carry out an abdominal examination, even when this has already been done by a midwife. This is part of a more general complaint, namely that the skills of midwives are underused: they tend to assemble information, not to make decisions they are well qualified to make.

The antenatal routine: dogma or necessity?

The traditional schedule of antenatal visits was laid down in the 1920s, when the risks of pregnancy were very different from contemporary risks.

1   According to a survey by Hall *et al.* (1980), routine antenatal visits are not very productive in detecting new obstetric problems e.g.:

   (a) the rate of first detection of growth retardation varies from 0.2 to 0.7%;

   (b) the rate of detection of breech presentation after 32 weeks is 0.1–0.9%;

   (c) the rate of detection of hypertension only exceeds 1% after 34 weeks.

2   Marsh (1985) examined his antenatal routine and found it was possible to reduce the number of antenatal attendances for low-risk primiparae from 15 to 8, and for low-risk parous women from 15 to 6 without problems. Indeed, benefits counted include:

   (a) more time per patient and a pleasanter working atmosphere;

   (b) more opportunity for patients to ask questions, and hence more satisfied customers.

3   A randomised controlled trial in low risk pregnancies comparing traditional frequency and reduced frequency schedules of antenatal attendance has shown in the latter group fewer investigations, interventions and false alarms, but more maternal anxiety and dissatisfaction (Sikorski *et al.* 1996);

4   Finally, a trial comparing shared care with practice-only care in low risk pregnancies has shown no benefit from costly hospital attendances (Tucker *et al.* 1996).

Few of our routines (or those of hospitals) have been subjected to critical review. It is quite likely that antenatal care is not the only area subject to arbitrary and wasteful policies.

4.7 THE MANAGEMENT OF CORONARY CASES IN GENERAL PRACTICE

Background

In the UK there are 108 000 deaths per year from myocardial infarction (MI). On the average GP's list this means about 9 cases per year, of whom:

- 2–3 will die within the first 30 min;
- 2–3 will have MIs in public places (whereupon ambulances are usually called);

So a management decision has to be made on only 3–5 cases per year.

Most deaths occur within the first hour (some 60% of all deaths), but 60–75% of cases are visited after this high-risk time (the mean delay before medical assessment is 3 h, largely because of patients' diffidence). In other words, GPs generally see a subgroup of likely survivors. In view of this, and the small number of cases involved, the question of home care has been examined.

Advantages
Possible advantages of home care include:
1 Avoidance of transport risks (there is some evidence that tachycardia, arrhythmias and hypotension are more common in transit).
2 Continuity of care.
3 Comfort and familiarity of the home environment.
4 Psychological benefits to the partner, who is a carer and not a helpless onlooker.
5 Improved compliance in rehabilitation.
6 Financial savings for the NHS (home care is much cheaper than high-technology coronary care units).
7 It is good for the professional morale of GPs and district nurses.
8 It is possibly less stressful for the patient (one study suggested a disproportionate number of deaths after ward rounds!).

Disadvantages
Possible disadvantages of home care include:
1 80% of patients have arrhythmias—some suffer ventricular fibrillation and are potentially retrievable with immediate care — preventable deaths. The cause of home deaths is often unknown, so it is difficult to know how many deaths could have been prevented.
2 Home care is inappropriate for patients with complications: left ventricular failure, shock, persistent chest pain, bradycardia, etc.
3 Not all patients or their partners can cope with the uncertainty of home care—some like the comfort of high technology around them: the patient's expectations are important.
4 Although the number of cases per year is small, the number of visits per patient is high.
5 Home care may deny patients the opportunity to receive modern thrombolytic therapy (see below).

Trials on home care: the pre-thrombolytic era
There have been three major UK trials (Table 4.5), all conducted before the advent of thrombolytic agents. The Bristol study (Mather *et al.* 1976) was criticised by the Royal College of Physicians because only

Table 4.5 Major UK trials on home care after myocardial infarction.

Trial	Results	
	Deaths at home	Deaths in hospital
Bristol study (Mather *et al*. 1976): 455 patients under 70 years seen within 48 h and randomised	12% at 1 month 20% at 1 year	14% at 1 month 27% at 1 year
Teeside study (Colling *et al*. 1976): 2000 patients allocated one-third to home; one-third to a CCU bed; one-third to a general medical bed	8.8% at 1 month	12.9% at 1 month (CCU bed) 18.7% at 1 month (general bed)
Nottingham study (Hill *et al*. 1978): 349 patients assessed by a cardiac team at home. After 2 h stabilisation, randomised	13% at 6 weeks	11% at 6 weeks

CCU, coronary care unit.

an ill-defined minority of cases were randomised. The Nottingham study (Hill *et al*. 1978) also involved stabilisation by a cardiac team and the exclusion of 24% of patients from randomisation due to complications or social conditions.

However, these studies suggested home care was a credible alternative to hospital referral, and in 1974 the Royal College of General Practitioners published criteria for deciding on home vs. hospital care. The situation now needs to be re-thought in the light of new evidence.

Thrombolytic therapy for myocardial infarction

The advantage of these agents has now been confirmed in several large-scale trials (Table 4.6). Streptokinase, the most commonly used agent, can reduce deaths by about 25% in the first 24 h. The best results come from the earliest possible treatment.

Aspirin has a synergistic benefit (a further 20–25%) and must be given routinely in the absence of contraindications; and continued (as its benefit probably derives from preventing thrombus extension over days or weeks, rather than acute thrombolysis).

The major risk of thrombolysis is haemorrhage. Other problems include:
- allergy;
- hypotension;
- prolonged intravenous infusion route (streptokinase);
- cost (the newer agents);
- a small increase in the risk of ventricular fibrillation.

These risks were quantitated in the ISIS-2 study (Table 4.7). The later ISIS-3 trial, which compared the side-effects and efficacy of alternative thrombolytic regimens, identified streptokinase and aspirin as the probable treatments of choice (Cobbe 1992).

Table 4.6 Important trials of thrombolytic therapy in myocardial infarction (MI).

Trial	Regimen	Patients and controls	Principal results	Comments
ISIS-2 (Second International Study of Infarct Survival) (*Lancet* 1988; **ii**, 349–60)	Streptokinase alone vs. aspirin alone vs. both vs. neither (1.5 million units of streptokinase given i.v. over 1 h; 160 mg aspirin per day)	17 000 patients within 24 h of a suspected MI Placebo controls	At 5 weeks: • Streptokinase reduced mortality by 25% • Aspirin reduced mortality by 23% • Both together reduced mortality by 42% Early improvements were maintained at 15 months	• Streptokinase and aspirin had independent additive effects • The earlier the treatment, the better the outcome (50% reduction in mortality if given within 4 h) • Equally effective in the over-70s
ASSET (Anglo-Scandinavian Study of Early Thrombolysis) (*Lancet* 1988; **ii**, 525–30)	Altepase (100 mg over 3 h) vs. placebo (All received a heparin bolus and infusion)	5011 patients within 5 h of a suspected MI	At 4 weeks: • Treatment reduced mortality by 26%. Benefits were maintained at 6 months	• The benefit was confined to those with ECG evidence of infarction
ISAM (Intravenous Streptokinase in Acute Myocardial Infarction) (*New England Journal of Medicine* 1986; **314**, 1465–714	Streptokinase (1.5 million units i.v. over 1 h) plus heparin infusion vs. placebo	17 000 patients within 6 h of a suspected MI Double-blind randomisation	At 3 weeks: • Mortality in the streptokinase group was lower, but the difference was not significant	• The ISAM study also assessed infarct size and myocardial function and found a slight improvement in the treated group
GISSI (Gruppo Italiano per lo Studio della Streptochinasi nell' Infarto Miocardico) (*Lancet* 1987; **ii**, 871–4)	Streptokinase vs. placebo	11 700 patients within 12 h of a suspected MI. Controls were randomised to a 'usual care' group	At 3 weeks: • Mortality in the thrombolytic group was reduced 18%. At 12 months the benefit was maintained	• The earlier treatment was given, the greater the benefit

ECG confirmation was sought, except in the ASSET trial where it was non-mandatory. Patients with bleeding tendencies were excluded in all trials.

Experts would exclude from treatment those with a predisposition to bleed, e.g.:
- bleeding diathesis;
- haemorrhagic cerebrovascular accident;
- recent haemorrhage;
- recent surgery, subclavian puncture or other invasive procedure;
- peptic ulcer;

Table 4.7 Complication rate from thrombolytic therapy (ISIS-2 Trial 1988).

Complications (%)	Streptokinase (1.5 million units i.v. over 1 h)	Placebo controls
Haemorrhage	0.5	0.2
Haemorrhagic strokes*	0.1	0
Embolic strokes*	0.6	0.8
Allergic reactions	4.4	0.9
Transient hypotension	10.0	2.0

*Most of the trials show a small increase in haemorrhagic cerebrovascular accidents (CVAs) with thrombolysis, offset by a fall in embolic CVAs. The overall CVA rates in treated and untreated groups are comparable.

- suspected aortic dissection;
- uncontrolled severe hypertension.

Should GPs give immediate thrombolytic treatment?

Since immediate treatment confers a large survival benefit, the question arises: should GPs give pre-hospital thrombolytic treatment? Because of the risks of treatment and misdiagnosis the British Heart Foundation Working Group (1994) recommends that GPs who do so will need to have a defibrillator available, and to take a confirmatory ECG prior to treatment. Benefit has been shown for patients with ST elevation or left bundle branch block, but not for those with ST depression or normal ECGs. Several practical problems arise for the GP:

1 He would need to carry and be able to use an ECG machine, and to read the tracing, and to maintain these skills although only seeing three to five cases a year. He would also need a defibrillator.

2 He would need to carry a relatively expensive stock of medicine for occasional but vital use.

3 He would obviously prefer to administer a single bolus injection rather than a prolonged infusion. At present this is a more expensive option.

4 He would need to ensure skilled after-care and supervision.

Set against these problems is evidence from two large randomised controlled trials of significant benefits from pre-hospital treatment (Table 4.8), most evident in those whose journey time to hospital was prolonged (e.g. those in rural areas). The British Heart Foundation Working Group recommended that practices should develop policies that expedite urgent treatment, for example:

- educating high risk patients to seek help at the earliest possible stage;
- training practice staff to respond rapidly to patients with chest pain;
- planning a rapid GP response time;

Table 4.8 Trials of pre-hospital thrombolytic treatment in acute myocardial infarction.

Trial	Design	Main findings	Notes
European Myocardial Infarct Project (*N Engl J Med* 1993; **329**, 383–9)	Randomisation between i.v. antistreplase and placebo; and between before and in-hospital administration	Cardiac deaths were 16% lower in the pre-hospital group (but all-cause mortality was not significantly lower)	The median treatment delay was 55 mins less in the pre-hospital group. In those treated ⩾90 mins earlier, mortality was 42% less
GREAT Group Study (*BMJ* 1992; **305**, 548–53)	Randomised double blind parallel group trial of i.v. antistreplase vs placebo, given at home or in hospital	Mortality was 49% lower in the early treatment group	The median delay was 139 mins less in the pre-hospital group (—the study area was rural)

- urgent liaison with ambulance staff (e.g. a rendezvous at the patient's home with resuscitation equipment);
- a plan, appropriate to local circumstances, for early thrombolytic treatment (in areas with ready access to hospital, a direct fast track referral system; in remote areas the equipment and training to administer thrombolytics at home).

It also highlighted the responsibility of hospitals to process and treat obvious MIs speedily; and suggested that HAs co-ordinate locally agreed policies between GPs and specialists.

Ideally the 'call to needle' time should not exceed 60 min, although currently it is two to three times as long.

How does this influence the criteria for home management of coronary cases?

The implication is that all patients likely to benefit from treatment (excluding those for whom thrombolysis is contraindicated) should be admitted as soon as possible.

There is evidence that GPs' attitudes to home care have changed in response to this new therapeutic option. Thus, in 1975 21–39% of GPs were prepared to consider home care in an uncomplicated coronary in a 45-year-old man (Hampton *et al.* 1975); in 1990 only 3% would do so (Pell *et al.* 1990).

Attitudes change with the age of the patient. Two-thirds would still manage patients over 80 at home, although there is evidence that age is not a contraindication to therapy, and in fact the greatest benefit is seen in the elderly.

Trials on home treatment cannot of course assure the GP that in the individual case the correct decision is made. GPs who cannot accept the death of a home-managed MI case without self-recrimination should not be attempting it, irrespective of these considerations.

A number of longer term interventions are likely to be beneficial in patients who have suffered and survived an MI, e.g.:

- the management of hypertension, if present;
- the control of diabetes, if it exists;
- quit-smoking advice;
- advice on weight reduction and the benefits of regular, moderate exercise;
- the prescription of a cardioselective beta-blocker or angiotensin-converting enzyme (ACE) inhibitor;
- recent evidence from two large studies suggests that lipid-lowering therapy has a powerful impact on later cardiovascular mortality, even in MI patients with reasonable cholesterol levels (Table 4.9);
- aspirin therapy.

In 1988 the Antiplatelet Trialists' Collaboration published an overview of 25 randomised, placebo-controlled trials of the use of antiplatelet agents in some 29 000 patients who had recovered from some vascular event (these included thrombotic stroke, transient ischaemic attack and unstable angina as well as MI). Most trials were of the aspirin vs. placebo type. The collaborators found that allocation to the antiplatelet group:

1 reduced vascular mortality by 15%;
2 reduced non-fatal vascular events (strokes and MI) by 30%.

The results were similar in all categories of vascular event, and aspirin therapy was especially impressive in unstable angina. It was also highly effective in preventing first MIs in those presenting with cerebrovascular accidents and vice versa. However, they make the case for aspirin treatment in the secondary prevention of coronary artery disease. (Some of the factors that need to be weighed in this decision are described below.)

Although much can be done in the secondary prevention of coronary heart disease, the evidence suggests that doctors pay insufficient attention to this aspect of care. For example, a survey of 2583 MI

Table 4.9 Large-scale trials of lipid-lowering drug therapy in the secondary prevention of coronary heart disease.

Trial	Study subjects	Main findings
Scandinavian Simvastatin Survival Study (4S)	>4000 patients with a history of MI or stable angina	• 30% fall in total mortality risk • 42% fall in CV mortality risk • 34% fall in major coronary events
Cholesterol And Recurrent Events (CARE) Study	>4000 MI survivors with mildly elevated cholesterols	Pravastatin therapy led to: • 24% fall in the risk of CV death or non-fatal MI • 37% fall in the risk of a fatal MI.

MI, myocardial infarction; CV, cardiovascular.

survivors indicated that blood lipids had been measured in fewer than 40% (in fact 75% had a raised cholesterol); 20% were not on aspirin; and there were many instances of treated but uncontrolled hypertension and hyperlipidaemia (ASPIRE Steering Group 1996).

4.8 WHO SHOULD TAKE ASPIRIN?

The background
The bleeding tendency induced by aspirin has been recognised for years, and the suggestion that prevention of clotting in the right place (e.g. skin cuts) might be put to advantage in preventing clots in the wrong place (e.g. coronary arteries) was first made in the 1950s by Laurence L. Craven, an American family doctor.

Pharmacologically aspirin inhibits cyclo-oxygenase, a key enzyme in the conversion of arachidonic acid to prostacyclin and thromboxane. Two opposing effects are induced:

1 *In the platelets* — reduced thromboxane synthesis, reducing their tendency to aggregate.

2 *In the vascular endothelium* — reduced prostaglandin synthesis, encouraging vasoconstriction.

In practice the endothelial effect is thought to be transient and that on the platelets more prolonged. The net result is an antithrombotic predominance.

In the 1960s, following a better understanding of these processes randomised therapeutic trials began and the last two decades have proved most exciting in the history of this ancient medicine.

The evidence of benefit
In secondary prevention of vascular disease
• The ISIS-2 trial (1988) confirmed that low-dose aspirin given in the early stages of a myocardial infarction reduces the risk of death by about a quarter (Table 4.6).
• The Antiplatelet Trialists' collaboration paper reported a substantial effect on cardiovascular mortality and non-fatal cardiovascular events, as described above.

These trials indicate a clear benefit for aspirin (unless contraindicated) in patients who have had a primary vascular event.

In the primary prevention of vascular disease
Two large, expensive primary prevention studies have reached differing conclusions:

1 A study of 5000 male British doctors, taking 500 mg aspirin daily was negative. Although total mortality was 10% lower in the treatment group the difference was not statistically significant, and the incidences of non-fatal stroke and MI were not reduced (Peto *et al.* 1988).

2 The American Physicians' study (1988) also sought to study the effects of beta-carotene on cancer incidence. Thus, 22 071 male doctors aged 40–84 were randomised between combinations of aspirin (325 mg), beta-carotene and placebo. The aspirin part of the study was terminated prematurely because of the large reduction in fatal and non-fatal MI in those taking aspirin (an overall 47% reduction).

It has proved difficult to reconcile these differences, though they may conceivably be related to a lower dose of aspirin in the American study, or to the use of beta-carotene, although it is not presently known to have an effect on vascular disease.

The potential for harm

1 Aspirin can worsen any bleeding condition. Thus, in patients with a haemorrhagic stroke it has the potential to worsen intracranial bleeding (and this itself poses practical problems as only two-fifths of health districts in England and Wales had a computerised tomography scanner in 1988). If used in primary prevention an increased risk of intracranial bleeding would need to be offset against potential benefits.

2 It can cause gastrointestinal bleeding and induce or worsen peptic ulceration.

3 It can exacerbate asthma and induce allergic reactions.

Who should take aspirin?

Those who have suffered a primary vascular event, including those with:

- a non-haemorrhagic stroke;
- transient ischaemic attacks;
- unstable angina;
- MI (at the earliest possible time).

Who should not?

Aspirin is contraindicated in patients with a bleeding tendency, e.g.

- known bleeding diathesis;
- haemorrhagic cerebrovascular accident;
- recent haemorrhage;
- recent surgery, subclavian puncture or other invasive procedure;
- suspected aortic dissection;
- uncontrolled hypertension.

It should not be used in those with peptic ulcers or a known aspirin sensitivity, and only with extreme caution in those with asthma.

The advantages and disadvantages of treatment may need to be weighed on an individual basis, as a balance of risks is likely to exist.

At the present time the role of aspirin in the primary prevention of vascular disease is uncertain, so a blanket suggestion that we should all take an aspirin a day cannot be supported.

4.9 THE CHRONIC FATIGUE SYNDROME

Features

Chronic fatigue syndrome (CFS), also called myalgic encephalitis (ME) and epidemic neuromyasthenia, has the following epidemiological and clinical characteristics:

1 *Occurrence* — sporadic and in epidemics. The prevalence is estimated at 0.1–3% (depending on the criteria employed).

2 *Sex ratio*—10 times more common in women than in men.

3 *Social class*—no clear link with social class or occupation (although specialist referral is more common for upper social classes and for medical personnel).

4 *Symptoms*—typically follows an upper respiratory tract infection with incomplete recovery. Symptoms are protean (Table 4.10), but profound fatigue, worsened by minimal physical or mental exertion, is the cardinal feature. Consensus case criteria have been proposed to aid recognition (Sharpe *et al.* 1991).

5 *Signs*—usually non-specific.

6 *Laboratory tests*—usually non-specific.

7 *Diagnosis*—by exclusion.

8 *Outcome*—in three camps: full recovery, chronic illness and relapsing and remitting ill health.

Aetiology

This remains controversial with some evidence supporting a psychogenic origin and some favouring an organic one.

1 Epidemics have occurred with all the characteristics of mass hysteria (e.g. the Royal Free outbreak in 1955). An increased incidence of pre-existing neurosis has been reported in sufferers, and the majority of cases display features consistent with other psychiatric conditions —chiefly depression, anxiety and somatisation disorder.

2 However:
    (a) some patients do have neurological signs;
    (b) some routine laboratory tests have been abnormal;

Table 4.10 Common symptoms seen in the chronic fatigue syndrome.

Profound muscle fatigue*	Fainting attacks
Myalgia	Poor memory
Headache	Poor concentration
Paraesthesiae	Poor sleep
Dizziness	Mild dysphasia
Urinary frequency	Hyperacusis
Cold extremities	Emotional lability
Bouts of sweating	

*Excessive muscle fatigue is generally regarded as the cardinal symptom.

(c) abnormal lymphocyte function and immunological changes have been described (although the data have been heavily criticised);

(d) some evidence of hypocortisolism;

(e) higher central 5-hydroxytryptamine mediated responses;

(f) lower brain-stem perfusion (in one study, but not in others);

(g) muscle biopsies have found necrosis and type II fibre predominance (but inconsistently);

(h) abnormal potentials have been described in electromyogram tracings;

(i) nuclear magnetic resonance abnormalities suggest intracellular acidosis at an early stage in exercise.

Many viruses have been investigated as possible causes — varicella, influenza, the Epstein–Barr virus, and especially the Coxsackie virus. However, a prospective study found no more fatigue after 6 months in patients presenting with viral illness than in those consulting with other problems (Wessely *et al.* 1995), and there is little credible evidence of transmissibility.

There is obviously a problem in lumping together cases with a wide variety of non-specific symptoms and treating them as if they are a single disease entity. This problem besets research into CFS.

Experts' views fall into two camps: those who support the psychogenic hypothesis and those who believe the condition to be organic. Alternatively the condition may be *triggered* by organic factors, but *sustained* in vulnerable individuals by psychiatric or psychological ones. A comprehensive review of CFS has recently published by the Royal Colleges of Physicians, Psychiatrists and General Practitioners.

Management

This is also problematic. Patients with genuine psychiatric illness may become mislabelled; other conditions may mimic CFS; many patients are reluctant to accept psychiatric treatment and are worried by the lack of a firm diagnosis. An outbreak of CFS is likely to prove a taxing management problem!

A variety of treatments have been attempted, including: immunoglobulin G injections; oral antifungal agents; steroids, azathioprine, interferon and acyclovir; carbamazepine (for myalgia); pizotifen (for headaches); and exclusion diets and dietary supplements. There is no clear evidence of benefit over placebo treatment.

Cautious, planned, mutually agreed increase in activity forms the cornerstone of treatment. Excessive rest and over-ambitious activity programmes are likely to be counterproductive. Cognitive behaviour therapy has been shown to help in three randomised controlled trials. Otherwise the approach is symptomatic, with analgesia, anxiolytics, antidepressants and supportive counselling. The latter in particular is necessary as these patients suffer considerable distress.

Background

The discovery of the association between *Helicobacter pylori* and peptic ulceration has provoked a good deal of discussion about the management of dyspeptic patients in general practice.

1   *H. pylori* is a Gram-negative spiral-shaped bacterium which colonises the stomach. The likelihood of infection increases with age (and half of over-50 year olds are infected).

2   Only a small percentage of infected people develop peptic ulcers. Conversely, 95% of those with duodenal ulceration and 80% of those with gastric ulceration are infected.

3   The organism's exact role in peptic ulceration is unclear. Other factors, such as hypersecretion of acid, smoking and genetic predisposition are probably important.

4   However, in randomised controlled trials treatment of *H pylori* infection has proved particularly effective in curing peptic ulcers. Compared with conventional ulcer treatment (H-2 antagonists and proton pump inhibitors) antimicrobial treatment may:

(a) increase ulcer healing rates from 78% to 93%;

(b) decrease first year recurrence rates from 66% to 9%;

(c) generally eliminate the need for long-term maintenance therapy.

5   The preferred treatment is triple therapy. One cheap, well-established regimen involves a 2-week course of bismuth subcitrate, metronidazole and tetracycline. This eradicates *H. pylori* in 95% of cases. (Patient compliance is higher with dual therapy, but eradication rates are much lower.)

6   *H. pylori* infection has also been linked with coronary heart disease and risk of gastric cancer.

Screening tests for *H. pylori*

1   *IgG antibodies* against *H. pylori* can be detected using inexpensive practice-based test kits. The sensitivity and specificity of the test are high (95%), particularly in patients under 45 years of age. However, seropositivity may reflect past colonisation rather than current infection.

2   *Urea breath test*: urea is hydrolysed by *H. pylori* urease to give carbon dioxide and ammonia. Following ingestion of urea labelled with C^{13} or C^{14}, isotopically labelled carbon dioxide can be detected in breath. The test is sensitive and specific, and indicates current infection; but it is dearer and less convenient than serology (the patient has to fast overnight; the test takes 30 min, and is normally performed in outpatients). The dose of radiation is much smaller than for a chest X-ray, though still considered inadvisable in the very young and in pregnant women.

3   *Endoscopy*: if there are other indications for endoscopy, the pres-

ence of *H. pylori* can be established by mucosal biopsy with culture, or a slide test for urease.

159
Chapter 4
Clinical
Dilemmas

Management options in dyspeptic patients

H. pylori infection can reliably be detected and eradicated. Failure to treat may have serious consequences; but failure to treat specifically may result in expensive and unnecessarily prolonged treatment. What approach then should be taken to the patient presenting with dyspepsia?

Four different approaches have been suggested:

1 Endoscope and perform test 1 or 2 above on all patients; give eradication therapy if peptic ulceration and *H. pylori* infection co-exist.

2 Perform the non-invasive screening tests; endoscope those who are *H. pylori* positive; treat as in the first option.

3 Perform the non-invasive screening tests; give eradication therapy to those who are *H. pylori* positive without endoscopy.

4 Prescribe eradication therapy on the basis of symptoms alone; only investigate those whose symptoms are not helped.

It is not clear at present which of these options should be preferred, although recent guidelines from the British Society of Gastroenterology have come down in favour of the first option. The more invasive, costly and inconvenient approaches enable a more precise diagnosis, and the identification of other serious pathology; but treatment based on symptoms or limited investigation will often result in unnecessary treatment (even amongst *H. pylori* positive patients with dyspepsia only a quarter have an ulcer; and 40% of those taking triple eradication therapy experience some side-effect).

The decision on whether to endoscope a patient also depends on his age (the risk of cancer rises in older patients), and the presence or absence of symptoms of concern (e.g. weight loss, rectal bleeding).

Randomised controlled trials are currently examining the alternatives. However, GPs should act now in patients receiving long-term maintenance treatment for proven peptic ulcer, and offer them a trial of eradication therapy.

4.11 MEASURING QUALITY OF CARE

There exist wide variations in the quality of care and range of services offered in general practice. Thus:

• three large descriptive studies by the Department of General Practice at the University of Manchester (Wilkin *et al.* 1984) established variations in consulting, prescribing, investigating, referral and average consultation time that could not be accounted for by the characteristics of the population studies;

• referral rates between doctors vary between 5 per 1000 per month and 115 per 1000 per month (Last 1967);

• visiting rates may vary 32-fold (Fry 1973);

• the ability to detect psychiatric illness varies nine-fold between London GPs (Shepherd *et al.* 1966).

Factors contributing to the variation in referral and prescribing rates are reviewed in Chapter 2. Interpretation of such statistics is not straightforward—in particular, 'above average' does not mean 'excessive' or 'profligate', and average is not necessarily the desired endpoint. Costs and effort must be related to outcome, and this is a far harder exercise. However, such variations have generated demands to promote greater consistency in the range and quality of services and several developments and initiatives have followed (some of a legislative nature):

1   The Royal College of General Practitioners was established in 1952 to promote standards within the profession.

2   The postgraduate examination in general practice (MRCGP) followed in the 1960s.

3   In 1973 a system was developed for the selection and reselection of trainers based on the practice visit.

4   Vocational training was introduced in the 1970s and became a 3-year mandatory programme in 1981. Several valuable spin-offs have evolved from this (the development of teaching practices; a clearer definition of the content of general practice; the promotion of small group learning; a more rigorous end of training assessment and so on).

5   Over the last 25 years there has been a great deal of fundamental research within primary care.

6   Government requirements (e.g. the introduction of annual reports and practice charters).

7   College initiatives. In 1983 the Royal College of General Practitioners launched its 'Quality Initiative' (Royal College of General Practitioners 1983) which encouraged doctors to introduce the principle of quality assessment into their everyday practice. In 1985 it developed the 'What Sort of Doctor?' projects (RCGP 1985c), a study in which participating practices subjected themselves to voluntary quality assessment in the form of structured practice inspection by a visiting team of peers. A subsequent policy statement, 'Quality in General Practice' (RCGP 1985d), reiterated the college's ambition to promote quality assessment and professional development from within by voluntary initiative. Other innovative suggestions include:

• the concept of protected time for study;

• further education for young principals in their early years of practice (a voluntary extension of vocational training);

• regular reassessment of established principals;

• a voluntary system of continuing medical education (CME).

The Government too has had an influence. As part of its 'Citizen's

Charter' initiative GPs have been required to produce their own prac-tice charters, detailing services and minimum standards, and to publi-cise them in annual reports; and in some instances, such as cervical screening and immunisation, remuneration has been linked to explicit numeric targets.

Admirable though the voluntary initiatives have been (less palat-able some of the legislative ones), a fundamental question remains: what is good quality of care and how does one measure it?

As Clark and Forbes (1979) point out, this is an emotive subject. Quality of care means different things to different people at different times. From the *patient's* perspective it presumably relates to his per-sonal needs and if his expectations are met he is more likely to be satisfied, even if from the medical viewpoint the treatment was inap-propriate. From a *doctor's* perspective, quality of care relates to accu-racy of diagnosis and efficient treatment; and from the *community's* viewpoint it must include just and accurate rationing of resources: a doctor who offers prolonged counselling to one patient and denies six others an early consultation is offering high-quality care to the former patient at the expense of the others.

There are other problems: quality assessment is fine as long as activities can be easily counted (the number of BP checks, the number of smears, the percentage vaccinated) but a number of highly desir-able qualities are not easily counted, e.g.:

- approachability of staff and doctors;
- a sympathetic ear;
- compassion and dedication;
- the ability to inspire confidence in patients.

Attempts to measure these qualities are beset with difficulties and open to the charge of subjectivity.

Furthermore, in many circumstances GPs cannot agree on the best policy anyway; formal protocols may not be flexible enough to reflect individual circumstances. Even when there is a consensus view on good management, this has seldom been subjected to rigorous valida-tion; there is a danger in identifying practices which we *think* are beneficial and calling them good practice without showing objective benefit.

Recently great emphasis has been placed on evidence-based medi-cine and the search for measurable, objective health outcomes. There are now proposals to develop general practice performance indicators and to publicise league tables of performance. But unless great care is taken, interpretation will be bedevilled by differences in case mix, and the essential subjectivity of measures of disease status, functional ability and quality of life.

There are problems in conducting research in general practice, both from the point of view of methods and that of ethics (see Section 1.3 and Section 7.11). Finally it is important to appreciate that many practices (inner city ones particularly) function under difficult circumstances and any system of assessment must recognise this in its accounting methods.

To its credit the Royal College of General Practitioners has proposed ways in which subjective aspects of good practice can be measured. Principal amongst these is the concept of peer review, and although it remains a difficult exercise to measure quality in a field which is still as much an art as a science, this is not an excuse for refusing to try.

5 Social Medicine

5.1 SOCIAL CLASS

The Registrar General's classification of social class is based on *occupation*:
- for men and single women on their own occupation;
- for married women on their husband's occupation;
- for children on their father's occupation;
- for the retired and unemployed on their last significant period of employment.

This system is widely accepted and is comprehensive for the whole population, although it is clearly not precise to label people on the basis of their job alone, and even less precise to label women on the basis of their spouse's job. The classification has five divisions, as shown in Table 5.1.

Social inequalities related to class

Various studies (e.g. those by the Office of Population Censuses and Surveys (OPCS) and by the Department of Employment and the Royal Commission on the Distribution of Income and Wealth) have highlighted class inequalities in areas like wealth, income, living and working conditions. Typical findings are illustrated in Table 5.2.

In wealth terms the gap between rich and poor is widening. Thus, according to the *1987 Social Trends* the income of the bottom two-fifths of households fell from 10 to 6% of the total, while the top one-fifth's share rose from 44 to 49%.

Health inequalities related to class

Unfortunately there is no perfect measure of health: self-reported symptoms are often unreliable and, while death is an unequivocal event, it does not help in the measurement of minor and chronic illness. Field-workers have attempted to circumvent this problem by examining a variety of parameters. In fact, as Table 5.3 illustrates, the relationship of health to social class is so clear that it is borne out for *all* the parameters considered. Similar gradients have been shown for nearly all leading causes of death, and for common chronic musculo-skeletal, circulatory and respiratory complaints; and there is a clear gradation through the classes which applies to all ages and both sexes: class 5 has the worst health, class 1 the best, and the other classes are in between, in the exact order that they appear in our class structure. This is equally true in international and prospective studies; when the comparison is between geographical units of comparative affluence and deprivation; and even after account is taken of smoking (see Delamothe 1991; Eachus *et al.* 1996; Smith 1996; Watt 1996).

Table 5.1 Registrar General's five divisions of social class.

Social class	Description	Population (%)*
1	Professionals (e.g. doctors, lawyers)	4
	Larger employers and businessmen	
2	'Lesser' professions and trades (e.g. teachers, shopkeepers)	16
3 N	Skilled non-manual (e.g. clerical workers, secretaries)	33
3 M	Skilled manual (e.g. electricians)	21
4	Semi-skilled manual (e.g. machinists, farmhands)	18
5	Unskilled manual (e.g. labourers)	7

*OPCS: General Household Survey 1994.

Table 5.2 Social inequalities related to class (from the Royal Commission on the Distribution of Income and Wealth 1980; OPCS 1996; Department of Employment 1977).

Item	Upper classes	Lower classes
Personal wealth	Top 1% own 25% of the total	90% are left with the remaining one-third
	Top 10% own two-thirds	
Income	Top 10% receive 25% of the total	The bottom 50% also receive 25%
Unemployment (%, in 1995)	4% (class 1)	26% (class 5)
Living conditions:		
1 Official overcrowding (more than 1.5 persons per room)	Virtually unknown	10% (class 5)
2 Central heating	95% (class 1)	81% (class 5)
3 Car	95% (class 1)	55% (class 5)
4 Telephone	99% (class 1)	75% (class 5)
5 Home environment	Generally good areas	Close to heavy industry and pollution; more often lacking private garden, etc.
Diet		*Less* fruit and vegetables, meat and dairy products
		More refined products, e.g. bread and sugar
Working conditions:		
1 Shift work	Less than 5% (class 1)	25% of all manual workers
2 Holiday	Usually 4–6 weeks	Typically 3–4 weeks
3 Working hours		7 hours/week longer on average
4 Job content		Less varied; closer supervision; more disciplinary activity (e.g. more than 90% 'clock-on')

On the 10th anniversary of the Black Report commentators pointed out that socio-economic differences in health, like those in wealth, were widening (Davey *et al.* 1990). Similar patterns can be seen in all industrialised countries collecting relevant data (Lynge 1981).

Table 5.3 Health inequalities related to social class (OPCS 1986, 1995, 1996; ONS 1996).

Parameter	Social class 1	Social class 5	Approximate relative risk
Stillbirth rate (deaths/1000 total births)	4.9	8.6	1.8 : 1.0
Infant mortality rate (deaths in first year/1000 live births)	4.3	6.6	1.5 : 1.0
Standardised mortality ratio*:			
• for 1–15-year age group	77	165	2.1 : 1.0
• for adults (men aged 20–64; women aged 20–59)	70–75	135–165	2.1 : 1.0
Acute sickness rate (number of restricted activity days/person each year)	17–24	27–42	1.6 : 1.0
Prevalence of chronic sickness (%)	27–29	37–42	1.4 : 1.0
Age-standardised patient consulting ratios for serious illness (age 16–64)	(I & II) 81–90	(IV & V) 115–120	1.4 : 1.0

*Standardised mortality ratio is the ratio of observed mortality in a population subgroup to that expected as average for the whole population. It is multiplied by 100, so that a standardised mortality ratio of 100 denotes average risk, less than 100 below-average, and more than 100 above-average risk.

Two contradictory theories have been proposed to explain these findings:

1 *Health determines social class*: e.g. sickly individuals fail to hold down good jobs, or ill health over several generations produces a similar social drift—there is no great evidence to support this theory.

2 *Social class determines health*: e.g. exposure to disease-producing agents and access to medical resources is class-related. There is some evidence in favour of this model:

(a) lower social classes use the preventive services less than classes 1 and 2;

(b) lower social classes are more likely to indulge in unhealthy habits like smoking;

(c) the lower classes live in less healthy environments and suffer more deprivation.

The distinction between these two theories is of more than academic importance: if social class *does* determine health it suggests that health inequalities are best combated by tackling social inequalities, and this approach would be socio-political rather than medical. (Many commentators and epidemiologists indeed believe this to be true.)

Inequalities of access to health care

Tudor Hart (1971) argued that the 'inverse care law' applies in the UK: i.e. the *provision* of health care is inversely related to the need for it. He attributes this to market forces in a free economy: prosperous areas attract more resources and more highly skilled personnel.

There is some evidence in favour of this 'law':

• some depressed areas with high morbidity receive poorer facilities than the so-called affluent areas;

- the higher social classes, who appear to be the least in need of preventive services like cervical screening, are the highest users of the service;
- according to OPCS surveys, the upper social classes are more likely to be referred to hospital than their working-class counterparts in the event of chronic handicapping illness;
- according to Cartwright and Anderson's survey, practices in middle-class areas are more likely to employ doctors with higher qualifications, and less likely to use deputising arrangements than practices from working-class areas; they are also more likely to have extra equipment like an ECG machine;
- on average, middle-class patients have longer consultations with their GP (6.2 min) than working-class patients (4.7 min); they ask more questions and cover more problems; doctors in working class areas have heavier surgeries.

Deprived areas

Nowhere is the inequality of access to health care more clearly illustrated than in inner cities, where there are problems in the recruitment of health care personnel because of high overheads, vandalism, vagrant or highly mobile populations and social problems like alcohol and drug addiction. This has also led to GPs who live outside their practice areas, to the heavy use of deputising services, and to the use of hospital casualty departments by patients for basic primary care problems.

To redress this problem a deprivation payment exists for GPs whose areas are officially 'deprived'. These areas are identified using the Jarman Index, a scoring system based on factors identified by a panel of GPs as contributing to increased workloads (Table 5.4) (To obtain the Jarman Index, each factor is weighted according to its perceived impact on workload, and scores are linked to census data for each electoral ward in England and postcode in Scotland. Deprivation payments are made at three levels according to the score.)

The need for a deprivation payment has generally been acknowledged. Critics of the current arrangements point out, however, that:

- the score at which payment is accepted is far higher than Jarman himself intended (with many fewer wards qualifying);
- the Jarman Index is based on historic census data and lags major demographic changes in employment and housing;

Table 5.4 Factors scored in the Jarman Index of deprivation.

Elderly living alone	Single-parent households
Under-fives	Overcrowded households
Unskilled	House-movers
Unemployed	Residents in ethnic minorities

- small differences in the score around payment bands translate into big differences in income.

167

Chapter 5
Social
Medicine

5.2 ILLNESS BEHAVIOUR

The clinical iceberg
Many minor conditions are extremely common and it is normal for people to feel ill a lot of the time, e.g.:
- in one survey more than 90% declared themselves to have been ill in the last 2-week period (only 20% consulted their GP);
- another survey found that patients only take about one in 37 symptom episodes to their GP (and only one in 109 gastrointestinal upsets, one in 184 headaches and one in 456 energy level changes; Banks *et al.* 1975).

The level of self-care is very high. According to a study by Dunnell and Cartwright (1972), in a 2-week period:
- 80% of all adults and 55% of all children had taken at least one medicine;
- the average number of medicines taken was 2.2 for adults, and 1.1 for children (two-thirds were non-prescription medicines).

It is clear from these data that a clinical iceberg exists and the majority of symptom episodes do not reach medical attention.

Social definitions of illness
It is a basic tenet of medical sociology that definitions of illness and health *vary*, depending on socially determined perceptions; for example, whether you regard tension headaches, hypertension, alcoholism or premenstrual tension as illnesses depends on your viewpoint: doctor and patient may disagree, and one generation may disagree with another.

Illness behaviour
Given the foregoing comments it is interesting to consider what prompts a person to consider himself in need of medical advice; a complex decision which sociologists call illness behaviour. Factors shown to be important include:

1 *Culture*: e.g. Italians, Jews and those of Mediterranean origin have been shown to have lower thresholds for reporting pain.

2 *Symptom presentation*: symptoms presenting in a striking way are more readily perceived as illness, as are those deemed to be 'severe'.

3 *Lay beliefs*.

4 *Sex and social class*: women and social classes 4 and 5 consult more often.

5 *Stress levels*: e.g. mothers who have high scores on anxiety-depression rating scales consult more often, for themselves and for their children (Leach 1993).

6 *Accessibility of medical care*: e.g. as the distance between home and the surgery increases, the likelihood of consultation decreases.

7 *Learned behaviour*: much anecdotal experience suggests that high usage of medical services runs in families, perhaps because members learn their illness behaviour from one another and pass them on to future generations.

8 *Trigger factors*: Zola (1973) identified five triggers that influenced the timing of decisions to consult:

(a) another interpersonal crisis;

(b) perceived interference with personal and social relations;

(c) perceived interference with job or leisure activities;

(d) the pressure of other family or friends (approximately 75% conduct lay consultations prior to the professional one);

(e) the setting of an arbitrary deadline ('If I feel the same next week.').

The Health Belief Model, developed by a group of social psychologists in the 1950s, proposes that people vary individually, and for different conditions, in:

• health motivation;
• perceived vulnerability;
• the perceived seriousness of the condition;
• the perceived costs and benefits of obtaining medical care;
• cues for action (new symptoms, TV article, friend's advice, etc.).
   The decision to consult does *not* correlate with:
• the true seriousness of the illness;
• the doctor's perception of a need to consult.

In other words, patients are poor judges of illness and take decisions often at variance with what doctors believe to be the correct use of the service. According to Dunnell and Cartwright (1972) 20% of GPs felt half or more of their consultations were trivial, unnecessary or inappropriate. Perceptions have not changed 25 years on. It is, however, fortunate that only one in 37 symptom episodes receives medical attention, as the health service would otherwise surely be overwhelmed!

5.3 STRESS

Stress rating scales

Several attempts have been made to quantify the amount of stress attached to important life events. Holmes and Rahe's Social Readjustment Rating Scale (SRRS) was obtained by asking a large sample of people to score 42 life events, pleasant and unpleasant, according to the amount of readjustment needed (Holmes & Rahe 1967). Taking marriage as the midpoint (50) on a scale of 1–100, typical ratings were:

• death of a spouse   100
• divorce   73

- marriage   50
- major change at work   29
- change of house   20
- holiday   13

Stress and physical illness

The SRRS shows a crude correlation with physical illness, e.g.:

- one study classified doctors into high-, medium- and low-risk groups, based on their stress scores: the ratio of self-reported illness over the next 9 months was approximately five-times greater (49%) in the high-risk than in the low-risk group (9%);
- another study found a linear relationship between stress scores and illness in naval personnel (Holmes & Masuda 1974).

Other studies suggest that major life events can affect physical problems like peptic ulceration, urticaria and diabetic control.

Stress and psychiatric illness

There is a relatively poor correlation with the SRRS here, but much empirical experience in general and psychiatric practice indicates that stress is a vital precipitant of psychiatric ill health. The failure of the SRRS has been blamed on the relative crudity of a scale that ascribes the same rating to an event without examining the individual and the context of the event.

Brown and Harris (1978), investigating depression in women, found that stresses mattered only if they were believed to have long-term threatening implications (major loss or potential loss of health, marriage, job, etc.). Painful but self-limiting stresses were less important. The same authors were able to identify predisposing vulnerability factors in the women's environment or past history, e.g.:

- lack of a confiding relationship at home;
- no employment outside the home;
- three or more children under 15 years old at home;
- loss of mother before age of 11 years.

Studies like this further emphasise the importance of social factors and life events in the course of a mental illness.

Important stress factors

Bereavement

Parkes' studies (Parkes *et al.* 1969) suggest a much higher morbidity and mortality in the recently bereaved, e.g.:

- widowers aged 55 years or over have an increased mortality of about 40%, in the first 6 months after their wife's death and there is still an effect at 1 year;
- although deaths from suicide are increased, much of the effect is from cardiovascular disease;
- the risk is greater for men and greater for close relationships than distant ones.

Work

The relationship between health and stress factors at work is unclear. Thus:

• manual workers paid by result have higher catecholamine levels than other workers, and stressed air traffic controllers have high blood pressure on duty, but these findings do not correlate with cardiovascular disease or psychiatric breakdown;

• ambitious, rapidly promoted employees of big companies fail to show an excess of cardiovascular disease despite heavier responsibilities.

Lack of work

Retirement does not appear to be a major stress factor, assuming it is planned; redundancy by contrast is a great source of stress. Thus:

• self-reported illness, including chronic ill health, is more common;

• in the short term, blood pressure and serum cholesterol can be raised;

• loss of work, or threat of it, is associated with markedly higher consultation rates, both for the individual and the spouse (and GPs in areas of high unemployment can therefore expect to have higher caseloads);

• longitudinal mortality studies from 1971 to 1981 showed, after adjustment for social class, an excess of mortality of 20–30% among the unemployed (Moser *et al.* 1987);

• important effects on mortality have also been described in Italy, Denmark and Finland. In Finland the effect was still evident after adjustment for background variables; and it showed a dose–response relation — mortality increased with duration of unemployment (Martikainen 1990);

• deaths from suicide, lung cancer and ischaemic heart disease are more common; so too are depression and parasuicide.

Unemployment is concentrated in the lower social classes and this may partly account for the observed class inequalities in health.

Marriage

Clearly this can be a positive or a negative force, e.g.:

• the married have a lower mortality rate than the unmarried, widowed or divorced (this effect is greater for men than women);

• however, marital problems are a well recognised precipitant of alcoholism, suicide, accidents and psychiatric illness, and the constrained role of mother and wife, in particular, may cause depression in housewives.

Family problems

Problems within the family are a potent source of stress that can affect more than one generation, e.g.:

- child-battering and alcoholism are often passed from parents to children;
- loss of a parent in childhood by death, divorce or separation has been associated with diverse effects such as suicide, tuberculosis and serious accidents in later life (Chen & Cobb 1960);
- Laing and others have proposed that schizophrenia is a rational response to an abnormal family environment;
- maternal deprivation seeds many emotional disorders of childhood.

Social upheaval
Migrant and other studies suggest major upheaval can predispose to physical and mental ill health.

The role of personality
Friedman and Rosenman (1974) proposed two types of personality related to cardiovascular risk:
1 *Type A* people show:
   (a) impatience;
   (b) competitiveness;
   (c) a sense of the pressure of time and responsibility.
2 *Type B* people do not exhibit any of these traits.
   Some studies suggest that type A men have twice the risk of heart disease when compared with type B men.
   Attempts have been made to link physical illness to personality type for other conditions like peptic ulceration but the results have not been scientifically validated. Vulnerable personalities are certainly a well established concept in psychiatric illness (e.g. the schizoid personality is linked to schizophrenia, and the cyclothymic to bipolar depression).

The value of social support
Social integration
Integration into a social community or family is generally protective, e.g.:
- lower mortality rates in married men;
- lower death rates in Mormons and Seventh Day Adventists.

Family support
Support of a family can:
- reduce the impact of stress (e.g. following enforced redundancies men supported by family and friends experience fewer stress-related symptoms);
- influence the course and outcome of physical illness (e.g. orthopaedic patients rehabilitate more quickly if they are married and have children at home);

- influence the course and outcome of mental illness (e.g. Brown's studies suggest relapse in schizophrenia is higher when patients come from families with high expressed emotion);
- provide vital care for those with chronic illness and handicap (e.g. Harris *et al.* (1971) found 37% of the *very* severely handicapped elderly, often senile, bedfast, or doubly incontinent, receive only family support and no community service input; other surveys indicate that only one-tenth of the physically disabled in the UK are in homes or hospital).

Families can also constitute a *pathological* influence (as described earlier).

The structure of family life is changing (more divorces, more single-parent families, working women and mobile populations). This threatens to undermine the supporting role of the family, especially with respect to their ageing relatives.

5.4 ETHNIC MINORITIES

Historically much of the immigration to the UK was encouraged by the British Nationality Act 1948, the poverty and poor prospects of the colonies and Britain's demand for labour in the 1950s and early 1960s.

There are two main patterns of migrant-community relationship:
1   'Integrated' or 'assimilated' (e.g. West Indian communities).
2   Culturally separate and isolated (e.g. Asian communities).

There is strong evidence that racial prejudice places immigrant groups in a position of social inequality (Table 5.5).

As in the case of social class, social inequalities are mirrored by inequalities in physical and mental health:
1   *Physical health.* Migrants have:
    (a) lower birth weight babies;
    (b) a higher perinatal mortality rate;
    (c) more anaemia (sometimes dietary, sometimes due to ethnic diseases like sickle cell and thalassaemia);
    (d) more rickets;
    (e) more imported and tropical diseases.
2   *Mental health.* It is sometimes difficult to distinguish between cultural beliefs that seem bizarre to the western mind and true mental illness. However, some studies on West Indian migrants suggest that the stress of social upheaval, alien culture and racial discrimination cause more mental breakdowns.

The inequality in health is in part explained by behavioural traits (e.g. less use of antenatal and postnatal services; restrictive diets), in part by genetic vulnerability, and in part by social disadvantages like unemployment, poor housing and discrimination.

Cultural differences also pose problems in the *doctor–patient relationship*, e.g.:

Table 5.5 The influence of racial factors on social status and employment (adapted from Smith 1976).

Nature of job	Whites (%)	West Indians (%)	Indians (%)
Professional/white collar	40	8	20
Social class 4 and 5 jobs	18	32	36
Professional jobs with equivalent qualifications	79	31	

- language barriers;
- completely different values and beliefs;
- different (culturally determined) patterns of illness behaviour;
- taboos concerning the physical examination of women.
    It is therefore difficult to ensure that these patients are not also disadvantaged in the medical care they receive.

5.5 THE ELDERLY

The size of the problem
1   The percentage of the population over 65 years of age is now approximately 16%, comprising:
    (a) 12% in the 65–79 years age group;
    (b) 4% aged 80 years or over.
2   This represents a considerable growth in the elderly population (the percentage of over-65s was only 6% in 1901).
3   The percentage of very elderly (over 80 years old) is growing faster than that of the elderly as a whole.
4   There are three reasons for this growth:
    (a) a slight increase in life expectancy;
    (b) a fall in birth rates (which means the young are a relatively smaller percentage of the whole);
    (c) a present glut of elderly produced by the dramatic decline in perinatal mortality at the turn of the century.

Characteristics of the elderly
1   More often women than men:
    (a) mean life expectancy of women is approximately 6 years greater than men;
    (b) 80% of the over-85s are women and there are twice as many women as men among the over-75s.
2   Multiple physical problems.
3   Drug problems:
    (a) polypharmacy and drug interactions;
    (b) impaired drug handling and clearance;
    (c) sensitivity to drug effects.
4   Financial status. On the *plus* side the elderly gain:

(a) a statutory retirement pension;

(b) certain exemptions and concessions, e.g. on prescription charges and travel fares.

On the *debit* side of course they lose their earning power. On balance the latter is not compensated for and studies suggest about 50% of the over-65s live below, or occasionally far below, the official poverty level.

Although state benefits may help in part, they are under-claimed because:

(c) the benefits system is complicated and confusing;

(d) the elderly fear the humiliation of means testing and the stigma of 'scrounging'.

5 Other problems:

(a) inadequate housing;

(b) subnutrition;

(c) social isolation and apathy;

(d) physical handicap.

A combination of these factors renders the elderly population prone to an increased risk of hypothermia.

Support for the elderly

1 Family trends (fewer children, a more mobile population, more working women) mean fewer carers nowadays. Also society's current values place the elderly in relatively low esteem when compared with the right of other family members to exercise their independence. Studies in London in the 1950s showed that 70% of the elderly received regular family help, and 15% were kept out of hospital only because of it, but in the 1980s more elderly people lived alone for the reasons described. Thus:

(a) 40% lived with an elderly spouse;

(b) 30% lived alone;

(c) 12% lived with their children;

(d) 12% were in other households;

(e) 6% were in residential care or hospitals.

The proportion who live alone rises with age (e.g. to two-thirds in over 85 year-olds).

2 Where family support is provided, there is a cost, e.g.:

(a) loss of paid work, social life and holiday opportunities;

(b) family discord;

(c) impaired health of the carers.

3 Alternative support systems are provided through the Social Services departments:

(a) *Home helps.* For more than 700 000 elderly, who pay according to their means, home helps perform many important services — cleaning, washing, shopping, collecting prescriptions and pensions. They also provide companionship and are an early warning system for the primary health care team.

(b) *Meals on wheels*. Hot meals provided from central kitchens to the home on a subsidised basis. Voluntary organisations also contribute to this service.

(c) *Social Services day centres*. These provide a more stimulating environment and a social outlet for the isolated elderly and day relief for their carers.

4 These support systems are considerably under-used in relation to the need; for example, in one study 6% of the 65–75-years age group and 19% of the over-75s used these services, but this supplied only one-quarter of the perceived need for home helps and one-sixteenth of the need for meals on wheels. Similarly there is evidence that aids and adaptations for the home are under-provided, under-used and under-maintained.

Under-use of aids and support services arises because of:

(a) ignorance regarding their availability;

(b) the reluctance of a largely stoical elderly population to ask for help;

(c) the limited provision of resources;

(d) the high level of commitment of many carers, despite personal difficulties and stress.

Institutional care

Options include:

- private nursing homes;
- private residential care;
- Social Services Part 3 accommodation;
- voluntary association non-residential homes;
- local authority sheltered housing (including warden-controlled and other flats for the elderly).

The provision made by local authorities is determined by Part 3 of the National Assistance Act 1948, which imposes a duty to 'provide for those who by reason of age or infirmity need care and attention not otherwise available'. The level of provision is set at 25 per 1000 over-65-year-olds, but standards vary widely. Many homes include a short-stay bed quota for trial periods and relief admissions.

Only 6% of the elderly live in residential or hospital care, and these are divided up as follows:

- 50% in homes for the elderly;
- 17% in geriatric beds;
- 17% in psychogeriatric beds;
- 9% in acute hospital beds;
- 6% in private nursing homes;
- 2% in homes for the handicapped.

Unfortunately there is poor provision for the care of common nursing problems in the elderly, like incontinence, confusion and poor mobility, which often overspill into acute hospital beds (approximately 50% of general beds are occupied by the over-65s). It is feared that this problem will escalate as the numbers increase in line with predictions. The division of resources between NHS, Social Services and local authorities has also been criticised as a fragmented and poorly co-ordinated service.

5.6 DISABILITY AND HANDICAP

Problems of the disabled
The disabled encounter various problems which include:
- poor mobility (and hence reduced leisure opportunities);
- difficulties with basic self-care;
- disadvantage in employment and difficulties in education;
- the need for a modified environment at home, at work and in public places;
- poverty;
- the stigma label and other psychological problems.

Mobility and the disabled
Resources that are available include:
- physiotherapy;
- the provision of walking aids;
- home adaptations (handrails, stairlifts, etc.) through the advice of a domiciliary occupational therapist;
- the provision of a wheelchair;
- disability working and living allowances;
- sometimes a grant towards a specially adapted car;
- advice, for example from the Directory for the Disabled, on the help that travel agencies, car-hire firms, British Rail and the airlines can provide;
- voluntary or paid visitors, home helps and day centre attendance to combat the problem of isolation.

Employment and the disabled
Unemployment levels are higher amongst the disabled (e.g. in 1981 when the general level of unemployment was 10.1%, unemployment among the disabled was at 15.3%).

Various Disabled Employment Acts have endeavoured to correct the problem, e.g.:
- under earlier rules an employer of more than 20 employees was legally obliged to employ at least 3% of his workforce from those registered disabled under the Act;
- sheltered workshops are provided by local authorities and voluntary bodies;
- under the Sheltered Placement Scheme a host company provides an opportunity for disabled workers to integrate with able-bodied ones: the host company provides tools and training and pays accord-

ing to output, with the balance of salary provided by an employing sponsor;

- the Government provides PACTs (Placement Assessment Counselling Teams) and residential retraining courses to help the disabled find work;
- grants are available for adaptation of premises and equipment to meet the needs of the disabled, assistance with fares to work (when inability to use public transport incurs extra expense) and a 'job introduction' grant to promote trials of employment;
- a Government-sponsored company, Remploy, provides about 8000 jobs for the disabled;
- certain groups of visually handicapped people can be helped at the cost of engaging a sighted reader at work for their assistance.

The 1995 Disability Discrimination Act made it illegal to discriminate against disabled job applicants and those who become disabled in the course of employment, providing reasonable accommodation can be made for their condition. This may have far-reaching consequences, but has not yet been tested in courts and tribunals.

Poverty and the disabled

Surveys indicate that the disabled often suffer financial hardship, e.g.:

1 *OPCS survey (1971):* over 30% of disabled people were on supplementary benefit, while a further 7% were eligible but were not claiming (Harris *et al.* 1971);

2 *General Household Survey (1978):* approximately 50% of homes where the head was disabled came close to the state definition of poverty (Royal Commission on the Distribution of Income and Wealth 1978).

The *reasons* for greater financial hardship among the disabled include:

- restricted employment;
- extra expenses (special diets, higher fuel bills, transport costs, home adaptations, etc.).

Although welfare benefits are available (see below) they do not adequately compensate because:

- the claim system is complicated and off-putting;
- the rates are not very high (and combinations are not always additive);
- patients miss out through diffidence, embarrassment or ignorance.

Housing and the disabled

The Disabled Persons Act requires local authorities to consider the housing needs of the registered disabled and to provide assistance with structural alterations and adaptations (e.g. ramps, rails, adapted bathrooms, widened doorways).

5.7 WELFARE BENEFITS

About £170 billion was paid out in 1993/4 on social protection benefits — half of this on pensions for the elderly. The welfare system is very complicated and subject to regular review. Although the details change from time to time, the principles change more slowly, so this discussion will concentrate on principles. The areas of most interest to general practice are those benefits arising from:

1 sickness;
2 handicap and disability;
3 industrial injury and diseases.
    (Other important benefits are summarised in Table 5.6.)

Sickness

The major sickness benefits are:

1 *Statutory Sick Pay (SSP)*. Paid by employers to employees who have made qualifying class 1 National Insurance (NI) contributions. This covers them for 28 weeks.

2 *Incapacity Benefit*. Paid at three rates:

   (a) *Short-term Incapacity Benefit at the lower rate*. Paid for the first 28 weeks to those who do not qualify for SSP (e.g. the self-employed, unemployed and non-employed) who have made qualifying class 1 or 2 NI contributions.

   (b) *Short-term Incapacity Benefit at the higher rate*. Starts at 28 weeks, i.e. when the previous two benefits expire, and runs until a year.

   (c) *Long-term Incapacity Benefit*. Paid after a year to those below retirement age who are unfit to work.

   Eligibility for all categories is decided by an adjudication officer. In the first 28 weeks GP medical certificates are accepted as evidence that the claimant is not fit for his usual work ('the *own occupation test*'); after 28 weeks a form Med 4 is requested from the GP and a Benefits Agency doctor may conduct 'an *all-work test*' (patients with illness that is severe and obviously in capacitating, e.g. dementia, tetraplegia, terminal illness are exempted from the test). The all-work test is intended to provide a common, more objective assessment of physical, sensory and mental capability for work (and may result in some claimants being declared fit, and advised to claim Unemployment Benefit instead of Incapacity Benefit).

   People who have not made the qualifying contributions (e.g. housewives) are covered by a scheme which parallels Incapacity Benefit and pays a *severe disablement allowance*. To qualify the claimant must be:

1 aged 16–65 years;
2 incapable of work (as assessed in an all-work test) for at least 28 weeks;
3 excluded from the contributory benefits already described;

Table 5.6 Some important welfare benefits.

Category	Benefit	Qualifying conditions
Low income	Income support	Age 18 years or over. Working less than 16 h/week. Low income. Means tested (savings must not exceed £3000 for the full benefit)
	Family credit	People working more than 16 h/week bringing up children on low wages. (Related to family income, number and age of children.) Means-tested (see above). Tax-free
	Housing benefit	Paid to those finding it hard to pay their rent (a council tax benefit is similarly available). Means tested. Depends on income, family size, savings and level of rent. Tax-free
	Social fund benefits	Exceptional expenses that cannot be met out of income, e.g.: • maternity expenses • funeral expenses • cold weather expenses • community care grant • budgeting and crisis loans Savings over £500 taken into account
Unemployment	Unemployment benefit	Up to 1 year for unemployed people who have made Class 1 National Insurance (NI) contributions and are available for work. Taxable
Maternity*	Statutory maternity pay	Paid by employers who deduct payments from their NI contributions. Women must have worked at least 26 weeks up until the 15th week before birth, and paid NI contributions for 8 weeks before this. Payments are available for 18 weeks. (The self-employed may claim a maternity allowance from the DSS if they have made enough NI contributions. Also paid for 18 weeks)
	Incapacity benefit	In the last 6 weeks of pregnancy and for 2 weeks afterwards the maternity certificate is accepted as evidence of incapacity for work, and incapacity benefit can be claimed by those who cannot claim statutory maternity pay or the maternity allowance
Children	Child benefit	Tax-free cash payment to anyone who has a child under 16 years, or 16–18 years old in full-time education up to A-level standard. (Not means-related)
	Guardian's allowance	Weekly payment on top of child benefit if you take on orphaned child into the family. Tax-free
Single parents	One-parent benefit	Paid independent of income and in addition to child benefit
	Tax allowances	Personal allowance may be increased to the value of a married man's allowance
Widows*	Widow's payment	A lump sum to widows under 60 (or those over 60 whose husbands had not received a retirement pension). Tax-free, but dependent on husband's qualifying NI contributions
	Widowed mother's allowance	Paid to widows who still receive child benefit
	Widow's pension	Age 45 or over when their husband died or their widowed mother's allowance ended. A taxable benefit paid in addition to the husband's pension

* Additional exceptional circumstance payments also possible—see Social fund benefits, above.

4 at least 80% disabled (if first incapable of work after their 20th birthday).

Handicap and disability
The benefits for the handicapped and disabled are subdivided into:
1 Those received by the patient (patient benefits), e.g.
   (a) attendance allowance;
   (b) disability living allowance;
   (c) disability working allowance.
2 Those received by the carers (carer benefits), e.g. invalid care allowance.

Patient benefits
1 *Attendance Allowance.* To qualify a person must be aged over 65 and require a lot of supervision or personal care because of severe physical or mental disability. Although normally available only if conditions are likely to be met for 6 months, an exception is made in the case of those with terminal illness (i.e. those expected to die within 6 months). At two rates: daytime only (lower rate) or day and night (higher rate). Tax-free and can be added to other benefits.
2 *Disability Living Allowance.* A similar allowance in those aged 5–65. Has two components:
   (a) a *care* component — e.g. help washing, dressing, using the toilet. (Paid at three rates.)
   (b) a *mobility* component—for those over 5 who are unable (or virtually unable) to walk. (Paid at 2 rates.) To qualify the claimant must have been affected for at least 3 months, and be expected to need the benefit for at least 6 months more (except in terminal illness).
3 *Disability Working Allowance.* An allowance for disabled people in employment but receiving low incomes. The claimant must be aged 16+, work at least 16 hours/week, have a significant disability/illness, and be in receipt of one of the other disability allowances. The benefit is tax-free, but income-related and means tested.

Carer benefits
Invalid Care Allowance is paid to carers giving up work to look after a handicapped dependant. Carers must be:
• of working age (16–65 years old);
• looking after someone in receipt of an Attendance Allowance, Disability Living Allowance or Constant Attendant Allowance
• spend at least 35 hours/week as a carer, and as a result earn no more than £50 per week.

Welfare allowances are not always generous. Furthermore the qualifying conditions may be exacting, confusing or non-additive with other benefits. They may also be means-related or limited in supply.

Concessions for the disabled are numerous, e.g.:
- road tax exemption;
- council tax relief;
- assistance with travel fares (to hospital and work);
- health benefits (free prescriptions and glasses, free dental treatment, etc.);
- assistance from Social Services (concessionary bus fares, day nurseries, aids and home adaptations, home help, meals on wheels, day centres, laundry, provision of a telephone, etc.).

Charitable assistance is also available in many forms outside the welfare system, e.g.:
- the loan of a wheelchair for travel on airlines or railways or for use in major shopping areas or theatres;
- advice on holidays for the disabled and other facilities through productions like *The Directory for the Disabled*;
- hire-cars adapted for disabled customers.

Industrial injury and diseases

The major benefits are:

1 *Sickness benefits*. These are SSP and Incapacity Benefit, paid as for acute illness except that qualifying contributions for Incapacity Benefit may be waived.

2 *Industrial Injuries Disablement Benefit*. Paid for injuries arising during the course of work or for prescribed industrial diseases. Related to the degree of disablement and paid even if the person continues (or returns) to work. Those people requiring daily care and assessed to be 95% disabled are entitled to a *Constant Care Allowance* (which is similar to the attendance allowance payments for severe non-occupational disablement); those assessed at 100% may qualify for an *Exceptionally Severe Disablement Allowance*.

3 *Industrial death benefits*. A pension is paid to the spouse or children in two instalments: a short-term pension (first 26 weeks), then a permanent pension.

4 People who contracted their industrial disease or injury before 5 July 1948 may be able to claim:

    (a) various prescribed disease benefits (e.g. for pneumoconiosis or byssinosis);

    (b) a workmen's compensation supplement.

    (The Industrial Injuries Act is outlined in Section 7.3, which also lists those industrial diseases that are notifiable by law.)

Other welfare benefits

Some of the other principal welfare benefits are briefly described in Table 5.6. For information on the benefits available to war veterans, widows and pensioners, or for that matter a fuller discussion of any of the benefits described here, those interested are referred to the Benefits Agency pamphlet *Which Benefit?*—FB2.

Health benefits

In addition to the welfare benefits a range of health benefits are available to dependent groups such as:

- pregnant women and mothers in their first postnatal year;
- children under 16 years old;
- low-income groups (those on income support or family credit);
- the retired (men and women over 60).

Benefits include:

- free NHS prescriptions, dental treatment; hearing aids on free loan (if prescribed by a consultant); help with the cost of glasses;
- free milk and vitamins (expectant and nursing mothers, children under school age from low-income families);
- hospital travelling expenses (means-tested).

Additional prescription charge exemptions

Certain other groups are exempt from NHS prescription charges by virtue of the chronic nature of their illness. These include:

1 Epileptics.

2 Those with continuing physical disability to the point where the patient cannot leave home without the help of another.

3 Patients with fistulae.

4 Those undergoing replacement/maintenance treatment, e.g. patients suffering from:

   (a) Addison's disease;
   (b) hypopituitarism;
   (c) myxoedema;
   (d) hypoparathyroidism;
   (e) myasthenia gravis;
   (f) diabetes mellitus.

5 War and service pensioners.

Exemptions are obtained either by age declaration or by Health Authority or DSS exemption certificates.

Prescription 'season tickets' are also available but are not free. They are pre-payment certificates which can be purchased from the Health Authority (HA) (application forms supplied by the DSS and post offices); but they only save money if more than about 14 scripts are needed in 12 months (or five scripts in 4 months for the shorter 'season').

Help for the visually handicapped

About two people per 1000 are registered as blind and a further one per 1000 as partially sighted. These figures greatly underestimate the true prevalence of visual handicap and it is thought that a further three people per 1000 have reading difficulties and four per 1000 severely limited distance vision.

Blind registration

For the purposes of registration the main factor is poor visual acuity (usually 3/60 or less for those registered blind and 6/60 or worse for the partially sighted), although allowance is also made for field loss. Registration requires a consultant's signature and is carried out through the Director of Social Services. Benefits of blind registration include:

- an extra income tax allowance for those earning;
- additional supplementary benefit for those already qualifying for payments;
- entitlement to the severe disablement allowance for those of working age;
- a slightly reduced TV licence;
- parking concessions;
- concessionary travel fares;
- free postage on items specifically related to their incapacity;
- assistance through the Social Services with rehabilitation (mobility and orientation training), daily living skills (aids and training) and communication (e.g. learning Braille).

Other services available include:

- large-print books (through public libraries and the National Library for the Blind), talking books (through public libraries and the British Talking Book Service for the Blind) and Braille books (loaned by the National Library for the Blind);
- radios (on free extended loan from the British Wireless for the Blind Society);
- telephones (through the Blind Fund);
- advice from the Royal National Institute for the Blind.

Partially sighted

For the partially sighted most of the additional financial benefits are not available. However, younger individuals may be entitled to education at special schools for the visually handicapped.

Help for the deaf

Deaf people may be entitled to some benefits through the Chronically Sick and Disabled Persons Act 1970. In particular it may be worthwhile registering with the local employment office and at the local Social Services department. The former department may assist through its PACT scheme (see Section 5.6). The local authority Social Services department may help with personal problems and may be able to provide a range of special aids, including:

- louder doorbells, extra doorbells, visual doorbell systems or tone-modified doorbells;
- flashing-light alarm clocks and alarms that activate a vibrator pad placed underneath the pillow or mattress;
- sound-activated visual indicators (devices that flash in response

to a predetermined sound, e.g. ringing phone, doorbell or crying baby);
- TV adapters (e.g. headphones, induction loops and infrared transmissions);
- amplified telephones;
- travel concessions;
- holidays for old age pensioners.

These aids are available provided that there is a real need and the individual is formally registered with the department. In addition anyone who has a hearing problem and could benefit from using a hearing aid is entitled to one through the NHS free of charge (through the ear, nose and throat consultant's outpatient clinic).

The Royal National Institute for the Deaf provides an information service, a wide range of reading material, a list of teachers of lip-reading, rehabilitative and longer-term residential care services, and training courses on behalf of the Department of Employment.

5.8 DEATH AND DYING

Attitudes to death

In the Middle Ages, when life expectancy was only 30 years or so, death was readily accepted as an everyday event. But with increasing life expectancy a taboo grew up around the subject.

Doctors' attitudes

Doctors' attitudes are complicated by uncertainty (of true diagnosis, of accurate prognosis, of whether the patient really wants to know). Questionnaires of the early 1960s and late 1970s suggest a complete reversal of doctors' attitudes from compounding the taboo to fighting it. In practice, however, and in part because of the uncertainty element, the strong tendency is still *not* to tell.

Patients' attitudes

Patients' attitudes are complex. Most patients harbour suspicions. Thus, Hinton (1980) interviewed patients in the 10 weeks prior to death and found that:
- 66% recognised death as a possibility;
- 8% were non-committal;
- 26% talked only of recovery.

In some studies two-thirds did not really want their suspicions confirmed and most wanted only messages that reinforced an optimistic view of their condition. These are of course generalities in the very individual experience of dying. Other interesting generalisations have been made about the so-called *awareness patterns* and *stages of dying* (Table 5.7).

Table 5.7 Patterns of dying.

The four awareness patterns	
1 Closed awareness	The patient does not recognise death, although everyone else does
2 Suspected awareness	The patient suspects that others know and tries to confirm it
3 Mutual pretence	All sides know but pretend the others do not
4 Open awareness	Everyone knows and openly admits it

Stages of dying (Kubler Ross 1970)	
1 Denial and isolation	Shocked and numbed: 'It can't be me'; It's a mistake'; intense isolation
2 Anger	'Why me?' Anger may be displaced or projected on to staff
3 Bargaining	A phase of good behaviour to try and postpone death
4 Reactive depression	Due to physical suffering or impending loss (of health, life, family, etc.)
5 Acceptance	

The place of death

Increasingly death has been removed from the community and hospitalised. However, much of the terminal illness is still spent at home, e.g. Ward (1974) found in 279 cancer deaths the mean stay in hospital was only 8.7 days.

Home care is still considered natural and preferable to the majority of patients, relatives and families, once they share the problem. Prior to this they often experience various worries in isolation:

1   The patient often prefers the home but worries that he will be a burden.

2   The relatives often prefer the home but worry they will be unable to cope.

3   The GP prefers the home but worries about both these things!

It is a balanced judgement since good-quality terminal care depends on:

1   Available resources (GP time, nursing time, aids and appliances, the ability to provide 24-h care).

2   The nature of the problem.

3   The attitudes of patient and carers.

Communications

During terminal illness patients, families and doctors tend to endure unpleasant feelings which they fail to share and which hinder effective communication.

The patient's feelings

Common reactions are:

  1 *Anxiety*:

  (a) for himself ('What is it like? Will there be pain and suffering? Will I lose control?');

  (b) for his family ('Will they cope? Will they suffer and feel abandoned?');

(c) about his disease (ignorance and fear of the unknown).

This anxiety is totally understandable, but it may also become maladaptive and hence pathological.

2 *Depression*: a mourning reaction for loss of health, life, family, station, etc.

3 *Anger*:
   (a) 'Why me? Can't the doctors do more?';
   (b) frustration born of impotence;
   (c) anger displaced on to the family or medical staff.

4 *Guilt*: at letting dependants down or being a burden.

5 *Denial*: 'There's been a mistake; I need a second opinion'.

6 *Dependence and regression*.

7 *Bewilderment* and the search for meaning.

8 *Withdrawal*.

9 *Paranoia*: patients who cannot cope with 'I'm dying' sometimes substitute 'They're killing me'.

10 *Isolation*, loneliness and loss of worth.

Family problems

1   All of the reactions felt by the patient may be experienced by the relatives in their own right or observed in their loved-one. Inevitably they cause distress, particularly the upsetting tendency of some patients to withdraw from their family.

2   Attempts from both sides to protect their loved-ones from stress actually exacerbate the situation: deceit and tension disrupt family bonds.

3   Relatives particularly feel the sense of impotence and frustration.

4   A long terminal illness is exhausting.

5   Bereavement forces new roles on to the survivors.

6   Guilt feelings are very common:
   (a) guilt if illness occurs at a juncture when relationships were strained;
   (b) guilt in wanting a terminal illness to end;
   (c) guilt because of the human but selfish tendency to dwell most on one's own problems, etc.

7   Practical problems:
   (a) financial hardship;
   (b) time off work;
   (c) loss of the family driver, etc.

The doctor's problems

1   Should I tell?
   (a) Does the patient really want to know?
   (b) Do the relatives agree?
   (c) Will they cope with the information?
   (d) If I hold back and don't tell, it will be hard to live the lie; and

what will happen to my relationship with patient and family when the truth can no longer be hidden?

2   Do I really know?

   (a) uncertainty of diagnosis;

   (b) uncertainty of prognosis.

3   Can *I* cope? Terminal illness highlights to doctors:

   (a) their own failure and impotence;

   (b) their own mortality. It also brings out their own defence mechanisms, e.g. *avoidance* by:

- the detached scientific approach;
- limiting contact to ritualistic conversational gambits;
- false cheeriness.

On top of these psychological problems there are the physical ones like:

- symptom control;
- 24-h availability;
- resource provision (aids, nursing time, access to a hospice, bereavement follow-up).

Management of death and the dying

The *objectives* of care are to:

- promote the patient's self-esteem (emphasise value and role);
- promote the patient's emotional comfort (relieve anxiety, depression and guilt);
- promote mutually supporting family relationships.

Needless to say these objectives are easier said than done and require a deft touch, but certain management pointers are probably valid:

1   Listen to the patient:

   (a) this shows the patient he is valid (understood and not abandoned);

   (b) it allows him to ventilate unpleasant feelings (anger, frustration, guilt, shame, fear);

   (c) it enables the GP to gain a sense of what the patient knows and what he wants to know.

2   Encourage him to retain his role and responsibilities and to participate in decision-making. This emphasises he still has worth and importance, undiminished by illness. Try to preserve his dignity above all.

3   Work with the family:

   (a) encourage openness;

   (b) promote insight into the family's own feelings and those of their loved-one;

   (c) allow the family to vent their feelings;

   (d) encourage family care where this is possible;

   (e) prepare the family members for their new roles and responsibilities;

4   Control physical symptoms.

5   Remember practical problems; for example, if the patient is the family breadwinner, financial hardship may require the social worker's attention.

Bereavement

Normal grief

Normal grief reactions are said to encompass the phases of:

1   Shock; numbness; blunted emotion; incomprehension (this lasts up to 2 weeks).

2   Physical distress; restlessness; withdrawal and grief. At this stage the dead person is to all intents and purposes still with them, to the point whereby the bereaved person may search for the departed, set the table for him, talk to him, hear his footsteps and even see him. There is a preoccupation with memories and idealisation and emotional reactions (depression, insomnia, anorexia, guilt) are common.

3   Gradually a more realistic memory develops, depression lifts and a process of disengagement occurs.

Normal grief reactions may last up to 6 months.

Abnormal grief

Abnormal grieving is said to apply when:
* grieving is *prolonged* (more than 6 months);
* the *intensity* of depression is extreme (patients who isolate themselves from family and friends, take a lot of time off work, attempt suicide).

Post-bereavement mortality

Bereavement has a mortality which Parkes highlighted in his classic studies:
* morbidity and mortality are high in the first year and raised even after 2–3 years;
* widowers aged 55 years or more have an increased mortality of about 40% in the first 6 months and overall 20% of widowers die in the first year compared with 4% of matched controls;
* men are affected more than women and the risk for close relationships is greater than for distant ones.

Management of bereavement

The management of bereavement really begins with the preceding terminal illness:
* ensuring the family members are prepared and recognise their new enforced roles;
* making the terminal illness as painless as possible by promoting harmony, comfort and mutual support;
* encouraging family care: the family should be there at the end and see the body afterwards.

Afterwards the GP must be an available and sympathetic ear. A desire to vent feelings and to search for meaning are common sequelae, as are visits with emotional problems and minor ill health. Close contact with the family also allows the pathological grief reaction to be recognised at an earlier stage. Referral to a self-help organisation (e.g. The Compassionate Friends or Cruse) may be valuable.

Cot deaths

Cot death is a particular variant of the 'death and dying' theme which deserves attention in its own right. (It is also a topical examination subject.)

Cot death or *sudden infant death syndrome* (SIDS) has been defined as the sudden unexpected death of an infant or young child, unexplained by post-mortem.

Epidemiology

1　There are about 400 cases per year, i.e. approximately 0.7 per 1000 live births or one case for a GP every 6 years on average. The incidence fell by two-thirds between 1989 and 1993 following a health education campaign (see below).

2　Relative risk is increased by:

(a) *sleep position*: the risk in babies that sleep prone or on their sides is nine times that of babies sleeping on their back;

(b) *racial characteristics*, e.g. it is more common in American Blacks; less common in Israelis;

(c) *birth order*: 50% are second-born children, 25% first and 25% third or later;

(d) *genetic similarity*: the risk in twins is doubled and thought to be increased three to four times if a sibling has already died of it.

It also depends on:

(e) *time of year*: 70% of SIDS occur between October and March;

(f) *the child's age*: nearly 80% occur between 1 and 6 months;

(g) *the child's sex* (by a slight margin: the male/female ratio is 1.4:1.0);

(h) *maternal and paternal smoking*: odds ratios of 2.1 and 2.5, respectively.

3　All social classes are affected but it is more common in the illegitimate and the poorly housed.

Aetiology

Aetiological theories are numerous. Sleep apnoea, abnormality of the larynx or surfactant, viral infection, and toxins from PVC mattresses have all been championed, but the breakthrough came when attention was paid to the ethnic variations in incidence. The excess risk in babies who sleep prone rather than supine emerged as one explanation for the low incidence of SIDS in Hong Kong where the practice is common. It has been suggested that babies who sleep supine radiate more body heat, protecting against febrile apnoea due to overheating. In view of the seasonal pattern, some commentators have suggested that low levels of daylight exposure increase the risk.

The exact cause of SIDS, however, eludes precise definition. Many believe it to be multifactorial and research continues.

Prevention

The recent 'back to sleep' health education campaign has proved remarkably effective in reducing the incidence of disease. Parents should be advised to:

- place babies on their back to sleep;
- avoid overheating;
- give up smoking and avoid smoky atmospheres at home; and to
- contact their doctor if the baby appears unwell.

Similar advice has prevented many cot deaths in Australia, New Zealand and other countries.

Supportive management in a case of SIDS

When questioned afterwards, 70% of people say initial GP support was good, but 30% say they found no real support and 10% claim that no contact was made at all.

Initial management includes:

1 Confirming death.
2 Offering sympathy and allowing venting of feelings.
3 Advising:
  (a) the cause is unknown;
  (b) the parents are *not* to blame;
  (c) police enquiry and a post-mortem are painful but inevitable.
4 Making arrangements:
  (a) the removal of the body;
  (b) an anxiolytic?
  (c) the care of the siblings;
  (d) a follow-up visit.

Follow-up care includes:

1 Being available as a counsellor.
2 Monitoring the grief response.
3 Advising on post-mortem findings, on SIDS, on support groups, etc.
4 Referring the family to a paediatrician for counselling (do siblings need an apnoea monitor?).
5 Fostering a positive attitude to further pregnancies.
6 Attention to detail, e.g.:
  (a) 5% receive immunisation appointments for their dead child;
  (b) remember the siblings: a high percentage undergo grief reactions, often manifesting as behavioural problems.
7 Referral to the Foundation for the Study of Infant Deaths.

6 Social Diseases

This chapter considers a number of conditions that are all produced by modern patterns of social behaviour. They are:
- smoking;
- alcohol abuse;
- obesity;
- drug abuse (including the misuse of tranquillisers);
- child abuse;
- acquired immune deficiency syndrome (AIDS).

These social diseases form an important proportion of the modern doctor's workload and are important exam topics. For some of them the government has set explicit health improvement targets (see Table 3.4 (pp. 94–95)).

6.1 SMOKING

The problem
Smoking is:
- responsible for 50000–100000 deaths per year with an average reduction in life expectancy of 10 years;
- the single greatest cause of premature death (e.g. 90% of lung cancer deaths and 75% of chronic bronchitis deaths in men under 65 years);
- the number one preventable cause of ill health (World Health Organization definition).

The overall cost to the NHS of smoking-related illness runs into hundreds of millions of pounds.

The known medical health *risks* are summarised in Table 6.1. The *benefits* of stopping smoking are equally clear-cut: all risks are significantly reduced and this effect is particularly rapid in the case of ischaemic heart disease.

Changing patterns
Recognition of the risk–benefit situation is slowly gaining ground, as reflected in the changing pattern of cigarette smoking:
1 More people are giving up, e.g. smoking among men aged 16 years or over fell from 52% to 27% between 1972 and 1994, and amongst women in the same age group from 41% to 27% (*General Household Survey 1994*).

The effect is largely class-related, e.g.:
(a) in the 1960s smoking was equally common in all social classes; now it is three times less common in class 1 than class 5;
(b) 80% of doctors do not smoke (40% are ex-smokers).

Table 6.1 Medical health risks of cigarette smoking.

To the patient	To others
Lung cancer	*To the fetus*: growth retardation *in utero*
Cancers of oropharynx and bladder	*To the infant/young child*: recurrent upper respiratory tract infections
Bronchitis and emphysema	*To the child in later life*: a greater likelihood of smoking (because of parental example)
Ischaemic heart disease	*To innocent bystanders:* risk from passive smoking (lifetime exposure increases the risk of lung cancer by 10–30%)
Peripheral arterial disease	
Aggravation of peptic ulceration	

2   Health-conscious public attitudes and legislation have:
   (a) reduced the tar yields on all cigarettes;
   (b) increased the proportion of filtered cigarettes to more than 90%;
   (c) banned the overt advertising of tobacco on TV;
   (d) expanded the non-smoking facilities in public places.
3   In surveys:
   (a) at least 70% of smokers have tried to give up at least once;
   (b) 80% claim they 'would if told'.
   In some countries (e.g. Norway) all tobacco advertising has been banned by law, a stance supported by overwhelming public opinion.
4   However, among older schoolchildren 31% of boys and 28% of girls are regular smokers by their final year.

Continuing obstacles

Political barriers

Political barriers are still considerable however:
1   Biting legislation is unlikely because of its unpopularity with a sizeable voting faction of the public.
2   Tobacco taxes raise a revenue of £5000 million in the UK and 50 000 people are employed in the tobacco industry.
3   Tobacco lobbies are very influential.
4   Tobacco companies spend more on promoting cigarettes than the anti-smoking lobby could ever raise to oppose them. Covert sponsorship advertising also still operates though there is a European plan to ban this.
5   While considerable savings could be made by the NHS if there were less smoking-induced disease, pension expenditure would have to rise if effective no-smoking policies were pursued.

Personal barriers are no less important. As discussed in Section 3.1, before surrendering their cigarettes, people carry out a personal cost–benefit appraisal. Amongst the sacrifices they count:

- the pleasurable pharmacological effects of cigarettes and their anxiolytic qualities;
- the social role they fulfil (relaxation rituals, social activities performed in groups, conversation fillers);
- the unpleasant withdrawal craving they face.

Appraisal of benefits depends on *knowledge* and *objectivity*. Some people are genuinely ignorant of the relative magnitude of risks in their life ('I'm just as likely to be knocked over'), and the health benefit of giving up ('It's too late now: the damage is done'). Others are not receptive to objective information: they belong to the fatalist school, the 'will of Allah' school or the 'someone else's problem' school.

What can the GP do?

Fowler (1982) proposed the following plan for GPs:

1 Record every patient's smoking habits in the notes.
2 Use every opportunity to advise them on how to stop and reasons why they should.
3 Supplement advice with a leaflet (e.g. the GUS or Give Up Smoking kit).
4 Follow up the patient's attempts.

Advice should cover certain basic ground:

(a) the health hazards of smoking;
(b) the benefits of giving up (and not just on life-span but on quality of life, social acceptability and bank balance!);
(c) possible coping strategies (Table 6.2);
(d) formulating a plan, starting date and review interval.

Does advice help?

Russell *et al.* (1979) found that advice given as part of a routine

Table 6.2 Some coping strategies for those giving up smoking.

1 Recruit a fellow and tell other people. Enlist family support
2 Avoid others who smoke
3 Record all cigarettes: where, why and whether enjoyed. Much smoking is habitual: cut out first the cigarettes smoked by rote and not really enjoyed
4 Look for alternative activities: something to nibble or chew; occupying the hands with something; relaxation exercises; deep breathing or yoga
5 Three commonly tried patterns of withdrawal are:
   (a) the saturation method: smoking 2–3 times the usual amount for 2–3 days, until thoroughly sick of smoking
   (b) the sudden withdrawal approach
   (c) the gradual withdrawal approach: one cigarette less each day or taking the first cigarette 1 h later each day
6 Nicorette chewing gum

consultation (and supplemented with leaflet and warning of follow-up) persuaded about 5% of smokers to give up. This does not sound a great deal, but with more than 600 smokers per GP's average list this would represent 500000 people per year if the effort were made nation-wide.

Does Nicorette chewing gum help?

Controversially Nicorette is not available on NHS prescription, since the Advisory Committee on Borderline Substances advised that it was 'not a drug'. It is thought to act by relieving the withdrawal effects due to nicotine dependence. Early trials (e.g. Raw *et al.* 1980) were very impressive and studies from specialist smoking clinics suggest 47–50% initial success rates. Nicorette:

- was better than placebo in five trials;
- produced blood levels of nicotine and fewer withdrawal effects.

   Long-term abstinence seems to depend on the degree of support:

- with intensive specialist support it is 27%;
- with minimal GP support and some follow-up 21%;
- with minimal GP advice and no follow-up 10% (in some studies lower, say 4–9%).

It is difficult to translate the results obtained on the highly motivated clientele of specialist smoking clinics into everyday experience where motivation levels are often lower, and there are a lack of controlled trials in the ordinary general practice setting. Nevertheless, a case can be made for making Nicorette available on the FP 10 prescription, particularly since we are in the paradoxical position of being able to prescribe on the NHS for other forms of addiction (e.g. heminevrin for the alcoholic, and methadone for the drug addict).

6.2 ALCOHOL ABUSE

Size of the problem

1   7.5% of consumer outlay goes towards buying alcohol (equivalent to 9 pints per adult each week, and over £10 billion annually).

2   In 1994 30% of men and 14% of women drank more than the recommended limits (*Health Survey for England 1994*). The Government's *Health of the Nation* target is about half this.

3   Figures from the Office of Population Censuses and Surveys have indicated that:

   (a) 0.4% of the population are alcohol-dependent;

   (b) 2% have alcohol problems;

   (c) 8% are heavy drinkers.

4   Wilkins (1974) interviewed patients from general practice with at-risk characteristics, and found in a practice of 12000:

   (a) 250 'abnormal drinkers' (2%);

   (b) 155 problem drinkers or addicts (1.3%).

5   Alcohol is responsible for 5000–40000 premature deaths per year.

6   Only the tip of the iceberg has been recognised: in some studies one-fifth of 'healthy' men attending screening programmes have abnormal liver function tests, and probably one in 10 heavy drinkers is known in general practice.

The physical, psychological and social problems associated with alcohol abuse are summarised in Table 6.3. Several points are worth emphasising:

1   Alcohol withdrawal is a serious and unpleasant condition, comprising tremor, nausea, insomnia, sweating, mood disturbance, hallucinations, hyperacusis, perceptual disturbances and convulsions.

2   Alcohol abuse probably causes brain damage long before gross deficits are seen: computerised tomography scans show sulcal widening/ventricular enlargement in 40–50% of apparently unimpaired male alcoholics.

Table 6.3 Harmful effects of alcohol abuse.

(a) Physical

System affected	Complication	Comment
Gastrointestinal	Carcinoma of the oesophagus	Increased three-fold
	Carcinoma of the oropharynx	Increased four-fold
	Oesophageal varices	
	Peptic ulceration	
	Gastritis	
Hepatobiliary	Cirrhosis	Deaths from this increase 10-fold
	Alcoholic hepatitis	In 10–30% of cases
	Pancreatitis	25% of all causes
Neurological	Peripheral neuropathy	In 10% of cases
	Convulsions	In 10% of cases
	Korsakoff's psychosis	
	'Brain damage'	? in 40–50% on CT scanning
	Alcohol withdrawal reactions	
Cardiac	Alcoholic cardiomyopathy	
Respiratory	Pneumonia and tuberculosis	
Metabolic	Obesity	
	Vitamin deficiencies	Especially thiamine
Fetus	Fetal alcohol syndrome	

(b) Psychological and social

Problem	Comment
Depression and suicide	Eighty-fold increase in men; the overall risk is about 15%
Sexual problems	
Family and marital	High incidence of divorce and wife-battering
Employment problems	e.g. two and a half times as many working days lost
Accidents	Common, e.g. 14% of fatal driver accidents involve significant alcohol abuse
Crime	

3 Alcohol abuse affects more than one generation: children grow up in an environment affected by social, family and marital strife and are more likely to become or marry an alcoholic themselves: alcoholism in pregnancy may produce a baby suffering from the fetal alcohol syndrome, the risks of which are

(a) 17% neonatal mortality;
(b) mental subnormality and poor growth;
(c) craniofacial, limb and cardiovascular defects;
(d) premature delivery.

Identifying the problem drinker

GPs are well placed to spot problem drinkers since two-thirds of their patients see them in a year, nearly 90% in 5 years, and the alcoholic probably sees his GP twice as often as other patients. Acres (1979) has highlighted several other advantages the GP has in this respect:

1 A long-standing and detailed knowledge of many of his patients and their families.
2 An opportunity to observe changes in behaviour, attitudes and attendance patterns.
3 A chance to visit and see the patient's home environment.

Barriers to recognition of the problem drinker

1 *Definitions.* There is no acceptable and universal definition of alcoholism, problem drinking or alcohol abuse, and no consistency of advice on 'safe' drinking levels:

(a) Anderson (1984) distributed a questionnaire to 70 people engaged in alcohol research, asking 'What is safe?': answers varied from less than 7 units per week to a maximum of 55 units per week.
(b) the Health Education Council (1983) recommended 21 units per week for men and 14 units per week for women;
(c) these limits were endorsed in 1995 by the BMA and a working party of the Royal Colleges. Controversially, however, a Department of Health working party advised that a 'benchmark' 50% higher in women, and a third higher in men would not incur significant health risk. (Several studies had suggested that moderate alcohol intake had a beneficial effect on risk of heart disease in older men and women.)

If expert advice is contradictory, is it so surprising GPs find difficulty in recommending limits to their patients?

2 *GPs' attitudes.* There are many problems:

(a) on average GPs themselves consume more than they should (standardized mortality ratio from cirrhosis 311) so they may not be best placed to advise;
(b) GPs often lack the experience of handling problem drinkers, and the sensitive counselling skills needed have been neglected in traditional medical school training;

(c) it is easier to avoid potential conflict and embarrassment in a consultation which is, in any case, too short to deal with the problem;

(d) alcoholism will be exacting to deal with, problems will be difficult and time-consuming, GPs are generally pessimistic about outcome, and alcoholics are help-rejecting complainers, leaving most GPs feeling helpless and frustrated;

(e) doctors are taught at medical school to distrust the drinking history they obtain — given a sensitive line of questioning and dubious returns it is simpler not to ask;

(f) the diagnosis is not straightforward — vague and protean patterns confuse the unwary, and making a connection between apparently unrelated events requires a methodical record system (when often there is none).

3 *Patients' attitudes.* Patients face many problems in common with their doctor:

(a) ignorance regarding safe drinking levels;

(b) a variety of vague effects that may not be linked with alcohol;

(c) psychological barriers (anxiety, guilt, shame, embarrassment) that result in denial;

(d) the perception of a negative, censorious or uninterested attitude in the family doctor;

(e) underestimation of true consumption: due to tolerance or cognitive impairment (if volunteers drink in simulated restaurant surroundings, the heaviest drinkers tend subsequently to underestimate their drinking by up to 12%).

4 *The unknown drinker.* Not all problem drinkers present to their doctors:

(a) teenagers may be better known to the police;

(b) professional people in competitive jobs may drink away from home;

(c) the elderly may drink in complete isolation.

The tools of detection

Unfortunately there is another barrier to detection: the absence of a cast-iron diagnostic test. The main tools of detection are:

1 *The honest question*: useful only if you get an honest answer in return.

2 *Blood tests*: these are markers, but they are not particularly sensitive and have a high false-positive rate (Table 6.4).

3 *CAGE and MAST questionnaires*: these simple questionnaires are reproduced in Table 6.5. Their advantage is that they are quick, simple to administer and generally well received. Mayfield *et al.* (1974) have shown they have a useful discriminating power, greater in fact than the best laboratory tests. Thus:

(a) the brief MAST questionnaire (scores ⩾6) has a sensitivity of 85% and a specificity of 86%;

Table 6.4 The value of gamma glutamyl transferase (γGT) and mean corpuscular volume (MCV) in assessing alcohol consumption (Chick *et al.* 1981).

	γGT ≥50 iu/l	MCV ≥98 fl	Both raised
True positives (men drinking more than 56 units/week)	50%	23–32%	62%
False positives (men drinking less than 56 units/week)	15%	5%	11.5–22.0%

(b) the CAGE test (scores ≥2) has a sensitivity of 93% and a specificity of 76% (Bernadt *et al.* 1982).

(It is likely, despite the value of these quick, convenient screening questionnaires, that they are little used in general practice; a small personal straw poll of local training practices indicated that very few trainers, principals and trainees knew even in general terms what problem the questionnaires addressed.)

4 *Postal questionnaires.* Potential shortcomings of this type of screening are:

(a) the possibility of a poor response rate;

(b) the administrative cost and effort;

(c) the validity of the results, the main fear being that the people most in need of help are the least likely to respond honestly.

In practice, however, the postal questionnaire is surprisingly effective. Wallace and Haines (1985) distributed a postal questionnaire to 3000 patients in practices in north-west London asking:

(a) whether people felt they had a drink problem;

Table 6.5 The CAGE and MAST questionnaires.

(a) The CAGE questionnaire (Mayfield *et al.* 1974)

Have you ever felt you ought to **C**ut down on your drinking?
Have people **A**nnoyed you by criticising your drinking?
Have you ever felt bad or **G**uilty about your drinking?
Have you ever had a drink first thing in the morning to steady your nerves or get rid of a hangover (**E**ye-opener)?

(b) The brief MAST questionnaire (Pokorny *et al.* 1972) Circle correct answer

Do you feel you are a normal drinker?	Yes	No (2 pts)
Do relatives or friends think you are a normal drinker?	Yes	No (2 pts)
Have you ever attended a meeting of Alcoholics Anonymous?	Yes (5 pts)	No
Have you ever lost friends because of drinking?	Yes (2 pts)	No
Have your ever got into trouble at work because of drink?	Yes (2 pts)	No
Have you ever neglected your obligations, your family, or your work for 2 or more days in a row through drink?	Yes (2 pts)	No
Have you ever had delirium tremens (DTs), severe shaking, heard voices, or seen things that were not there after heavy drinking?	Yes (5 pts)	No
Have you ever gone to anyone for help about your drinking?	Yes (5 pts)	No
Have you ever been in hospital because of your drinking?	Yes (5 pts)	No
Have you ever been arrested for drunken driving?	Yes (2 pts)	No

Total score:

(b) for an estimate of drinking levels;

(c) the questions of the CAGE screening test.

Positive responders were people who thought they had a drink problem, who gave at least two positive CAGE responses, or who admitted a consumption in excess of 42 units per week for men, or 21 units per week for women. Responders attended for further discussion and estimations of mean corpuscular volume, gamma glutamyl transferase and breath alcohol. They found that:

(a) the response rate was 72%;

(b) 7% of men and 3% of women expressed concern and thought they might have an alcohol problem;

(c) 10% of the practice were identified as positive responders—a substantial number of these were previously unknown;

(d) postal questionnaires were a viable alternative to other screening methods, with a high degree of sensitivity and specificity amongst respondents.

5 *The GP's checklist.* Many authors argue that early recognition of problem drinking depends on a low index of suspicion, and that GPs should be armed with a checklist of common alcohol presentations that prompt closer enquiry. Wilkins (1974) suggests an alcohol at-risk register based on a series of at-risk indicators (Table 6.6). Using his checklist, Wilkins noted in 1 year that 5% of his adult population consulted with one of the at-risk characteristics. Of these 546 patients, 28% were found to have alcohol-related problems or addiction, while the frequency in control patients was only 3%.

What can GPs do about alcoholism?

Several simple recommendations bear consideration for the GP who wishes to undertake screening:

1 It is feasible on an opportunistic basis to ask all patients about their drinking habits and to make a record of this. After a defined interval a computer-generated prompt would then enable further enquiry. The aim should be 100% knowledge.

2 Self-administered questionnaires have a high response rate and yield about 10% of people expressing concern about their level of drinking. At present no tool of detection is much better than this, and the advantage to the GP is that patient self-administration makes no inroads into GP time, excepting of course the problems unearthed.

3 The CAGE and MAST questionnaires are quick, simple and fairly accurate screens, easily administered by nursing staff (e.g. in the context of a well-person clinic).

4 Practices could benefit from an at-risk checklist and register.

5 It focuses the mind to have some clear targets in mind. The *Health of the Nation* target, for example, is to reduce the proportion of men drinking 21 units/week from 28% (1990) to 18% (in 2000); and that of women from 11% to 7%, respectively.

Table 6.6 Wilkins' suggested at-risk indicators for detecting alcoholism (after Wilkins 1974).

Categories	Subcategories	
Physical diseases	Pancreatitis, cirrhosis, peptic ulcer, gastritis, peripheral neuritis, tuberculosis, congestive cardiac failure (unknown origin), epilepsy (for the first time after age of 25 years), malnutrition/obesity, haematemesis/melaena	
Mental diseases	Anxiety, depression, attempted suicide, other psychiatric illnesses, sexual problems	
Symptoms of alcohol addiction	Morning shakes, blackouts/memory loss, delirium tremens, hallucinations, fugue states, morbid jealousy, withdrawal fits	
Blood tests	Mean corpuscular volume ≥98 fl, gamma glutamyl transferase ≥50 iu/l	
Occupations	Liver cirrhosis mortality (standardized mortality ratio, average = 100)	
	Publicans and innkeepers	1576
	Ships' officers	781
	Barmen, barmaids	633
	Fishermen	595
	Hotel proprietors	506
	Restaurateurs	385
	Medical practitioners	311
Work problems	Three or more jobs (over the last year), multiple short spells of absenteeism (over the last year), dubious sick note requests	
Accidents	e.g. road traffic accidents, accidents at work and at home	
Criminal offences	e.g. drunk and disorderly, drink-driving convictions	
Family and marital problems		
Marital status	Single males ≥40 years, married ≥ once, divorced or separated	
Family history of alcohol abuse		
Smelling of alcohol in the consultation		

Is screening for alcoholism worthwhile?

In general, changing a patient's behaviour is one of the least rewarding areas of practice in terms of effort and returns. GPs are particularly pessimistic when it comes to the alcoholic, so is there any point to screening?

Available data tends to deal only with severely dependent individuals for whom the prognosis is clearly bad. However, detection at the earlier pre-dependent, heavy drinking stage is more beneficial. Several studies suggest screening for problem drinking can be rewarding (Table 6.7). Furthermore a well known study by Edwards *et al.* (1977) comparing intensive conventional treatment (Alcoholics Anonymous referral, psychiatrists, social workers, drugs to cover withdrawal, etc.) with simple advice (and no significant follow-up) found no significant difference between the two groups at 12 months, suggesting that GPs do not require extensive time and facilities to help.

If we do not seek, we will not find. It is likely in the management of

Table 6.7 Studies of prognosis in alcohol abusers.

Study	Format	Results
Vaillant (1980)	456 Bostonian teenagers followed over 35 years	110 developed symptoms of abuse, but of these: • 48 later achieved abstinence for at least 1 year; • 22 returned to social drinking
Polich (1980)	758 men admitted to an American alcohol unit—a 4-year follow-up	14% had died. Of the survivors: • 28% were abstainers; • 18% were non-problem drinkers
Pollak (1978)	69 alcohol-dependent patients given several short therapeutic sessions. Independent assessment by relatives and a research worker	19% were sober at 2 years; 45% had 'improved'. Only three patients had sought help other than from the family doctor in that time
Costello (1975)	Analysed the results of 58 other studies involving 11 000 patients	After 1 year: • 1% were dead; • 25% had no current problem; • 53% were drinking continuously; • 21% were lost to follow-up

alcohol-related problems that the best dividends are realised when detection is early.

6.3 OBESITY

The problem

Obesity is measured in a variety of ways including:
- simple weight measurements;
- corrected weight (weight as a percentage of ideal weight for similar height, age, sex and build: 'ideal' according to insurance data);
- skinfold thickness.

The preferred method for classifying body weight is the Quetelet index or *body mass index*. This is calculated by dividing weight (in kilograms) by the square of height (in metres; Table 6.8).

Many people are overweight:
- 12% of men and 16% of women are obese (BMI 30+);
- 42% of men and 29% of women are overweight (BMI 25–30);
- 10% of children are overweight;
- on an average GP's list more than 300 individuals have a weight problem;
- at any one time 65% of British women and 30% of British men are trying to lose weight.

The risk to *mortality* has been debated. The Seven Nations Study found after other risk factors were considered (e.g. high blood pressure, hyperglycaemia, hyperlipidaemia), knowledge of adiposity *per se* did not help in the prediction of a future heart attack (Keys *et al.*

Table 6.8 Classification of body weight using the body mass index.

Weight:height ratio	Category
20	Underweight
20–24.9	Normal (grade 0)
25–29.9	Overweight/plump (grade I)
30–39.9	Moderate obesity (grade II)
40+	Severe obesity (grade III)

1972). However, others have argued that obesity *causes* some of the other risk factors (reversible associations with weight gain have been demonstrated). There is in any case considerable *morbidity* due to mechanical and metabolic effects (Table 6.9). *Psychological sequelae* are also common in this stigmatising condition.

Aetiological theories

Many theories have been put forward including:

1 *Psychological/behavioural models*, e.g.:

(a) emotional conflicts in childhood;

(b) inability to distinguish the arousal of hunger from fear, anger, anxiety;

(c) food received as a reward in childhood;

(d) learning to eat by the clock and leave the plate clean;

(e) eating when bored, lonely or miserable.

2 *Social models*, e.g.:

(a) the 20th century diet—over-rich in refined carbohydrates and fats;

(b) lack of exercise due to 20th century transport and labour-saving tools.

3 *Developmental/biochemical models*, e.g.:

(a) a disturbance in the long-term weight control system of the hypothalamus;

Table 6.9 Morbidity attributable to obesity.

Osteoarthritis—hips and knees; backache; flat feet	Abdominal surgery—postoperative difficulties with deep venous thromboses, pulmonary embolisms, chest infections, wound dehiscence, etc.
Impaired respiratory function; chronic bronchitis	
Reduced exercise capacity (fitness)	
Varicose veins; varicose ulcers	
Haemorrhoids	Childbirth; more chance of pre-eclamptic toxaemia, fetal loss, postpartum haemorrhage; reduced fertility
Gallstones	
Diverticulitis	
Ventral hernias	Diabetes
Increased risk of carcinomas of colon, breast and uterine body	Gout
	Coronary artery disease
	Cirrhosis
	Hypertension
	Psychological problems: teased, ridiculed, and treated by society as the model of unattractiveness

(b) an increase in the number of brown fat cells inherited;

(c) the perpetuation of childhood obesity.

As usual when there are many theories to choose from, no one is entirely satisfactory.

Management

The pros and cons of whether a self-limiting minor disorder like obesity should occupy medical time need to be considered. It is obviously difficult not to be sympathetic when approached for help by patients trying to do something positive to promote their own health. However, many authors have argued that:

1   Obesity is not a disease but a social/behavioural problem with medical complications, and hence the solution is not necessarily a medical one; perhaps the onus should not be put on doctors to treat.

2   The risk to mortality is much less than previously thought (this is crucial, but controversial).

3   The condition is so common that an undertaking to treat all obesity would be a great drain on medical resources.

4   Many other problems are seen on a large scale, the treatment of which may be more deserving of medical time (e.g. smoking and hypertension, a reduction of which would probably have a greater impact on morbidity).

5   Long-term results in medical hands are fairly poor (about 1–12% in studies). There is no evidence that doctors achieve better results than self-help groups like Weight-Watchers.

There is less debate that obesity should be tackled in the following *medical* conditions:

- maturity-onset diabetes;
- hyperlipidaemia;
- hypertension (a 5 kg weight loss reduces BP by 8–16/4–8 mmHg);
- medical conditions aggravated by obesity, e.g. angina.

Assuming treatment is undertaken, the major options are: dietary advice and counselling; exercise; drug therapy; behavioural methods; group therapy and alternative medicine-type approaches.

1   *Dietary advice.* This consists largely of common sense measures, e.g.:

(a) using artificial sweeteners;

(b) choosing the low-calorie version where available (low-calorie drinks, low-fat cheese, skimmed milk, etc.);

(c) increasing fruit and vegetable intake;

(d) substituting white meat for red, wholemeal flour for white, and grilling for frying;

(e) cutting out snacks, nibbles and notoriously high-fat foods.

2   *Exercise.* This has been under-rated as a method of weight reduction, since calculations based on their respective calorie equivalents suggest that considerable exercise produces only modest fat losses. However, we now know that after exercise the basal metabolic rate

may be raised for several hours, so that true weight loss is probably greater. Regular activity has other beneficial effects too — in reducing the risk of heart disease, strokes, oesteoporosis and diabetes. But presently 70–80% of adults take insufficient exercise.

3 *Drug treatment.* Appetite suppressants are now much out of favour because of their potential hazards, in particular the risk of addiction. In general, they should:

(a) never be used in patients with known addiction/drug abuse tendencies;

(b) only be used in the plateau phase when the rate of weight loss has slowed;

(c) only then be used for a limited period to aid motivation, prescribing an exact number of tablets, and with regular (e.g. 2-weekly) review.

4 *Behavioural methods.* The main reason for failure to diet successfully is failed motivation. Various behaviour-modifying tips have been suggested to help maintain the all-important motivation element, e.g.:

(a) eat only when hungry;

(b) leave food on the plate;

(c) use a smaller plate, knife and fork;

(d) be last to start and first to finish;

(e) eat only at the table and then leave it;

(f) keep food out of sight;

(g) keep a record;

(h) have a reward system.

5 *Group therapy.* This also depends on the principle of stimulating motivation. Weight-watching groups use devices like:

(a) competitions, prizes, rewards or fines;

(b) pairing of individuals for mutual support;

(c) the example of successful group leaders. They claim a better-than-average success rate.

6 *Starvation and very low calorie diets (VLCDs).* Starvation has been used for many years under medical supervision in the treatment of massive obesity. It is no longer considered acceptable because:

(a) sudden unexpected deaths have occurred linked to K^+ depletion;

(b) weight loss in starvation is 50% fat and 50% lean (fat-free), whereas the excess weight comprises 75% fat and 25% lean: the inappropriate loss of lean in starvation lowers metabolic rate, making it harder to sustain weight loss. (Crash diets and self-imposed semi-starvation suffer the same drawback.)

VLCDs (diets supplying less than 600 kcal/day) have become popular. They are formulated to be nutritionally complete except for energy, and produce rapid weight loss with minimal loss of lean. However, concern has been expressed regarding their safety and efficacy. The Committee on Medical Aspects of Food Policy (COMA) report (1987) recommended that they were not a preferred option for weight loss, and were particularly unsuitable for people with a relatively small amount of weight to lose (body mass index <30), for children, the elderly and pregnant women.

Success rates in general practice are disappointing (1–12%), and there is no evidence that GPs are any more successful than anyone else (indeed weight-watching groups claim a 30%, success rate). The Government's stated aim is to reduce the prevalence of obesity to 6% in men and 8% in women (half the present level) by the year 2005. However, the proportion considered obese has been rising steadily in successive surveys.

6.4 DRUG ABUSE

The scale of the problem

Home Office notifications are rising, with a trend towards multiple drug abuse; for example, in 1960 there were 437 registered opiate users, but in 1978 the figure was 4122; and in 1994 the Home Office received 34000 notifications, including 13500 new cases.

This is probably the tip of the iceberg:
• one-third of addicts attending accident and emergency departments are not officially registered;
• a national survey of college students revealed that 20% were regular cannabis users and a third had experimented with other drugs (Webb *et al.* 1996);
• glues and solvents have been inhaled by a fifth of 15- and 16-year olds and 1.5–3% have tried heroin, cocaine or crack (Miller *et al.* 1996).

The price of illicit heroin has increased 15- to 35-fold over 10 years.

Epidemiology and aetiology

1 *Sex*. Male to female ratio is 4:1
2 *Age*. The peak is 20–35 years of age.
3 *Social class*. All social classes in the UK.
4 *Associations*. There is a higher chance of:
  (a) family disharmony;
  (b) alcoholism;
  (c) peer group pressures and imitative behaviour;
  (d) ready availability (witness the problem in the medical profession!).

These associated circumstances are thought to play a part in the *aetiology*. Reinforcement of drug-taking behaviour is then obtained from the stimulating or sedating properties of the drug.

Drugs of addiction can be subdivided according to their properties into stimulants, depressants and hallucinogens: physical dependence is a feature of the depressant group.

Detection
Recognition of drug abusers in general practice depends on a high index of suspicion and sensitive history-taking.

Physical clues
Nausea, malaise, sweating, stupor, constipation, pinpoint pupils, ataxia (the exact constellation depending on the drug abused); and other external signs, e.g. self-neglect, needle marks, facial/perioral rash (solvent abusers).

Psychological and social clues
Moodiness, irritability and personality change, inappropriate euphoria, confusion, hallucinosis and psychosis, furtiveness, drug-seeking behaviour, unexplained debts, criminal behaviour, parental concern ('something is wrong').

Legal obligations placed on the GP
See Section 7.2.

Management of drug abuse
The management of drug abuse requires expertise. Legal restraints on the prescribing of certain drugs and the inadvisability of blindly prescribing others pose some practical constraints on GP involvement. Nevertheless, the GP is, as always, able to offer support and counselling and referral as indicated. The ingredients of a treatment programme include:
1 The therapeutic contract (what is on the table and why; the duration and conditions).
2 The treatment of withdrawal symptoms (for depressant drugs).
3 Non-prescribing support (for stimulant drugs).
4 Long-term maintenance (under specialist supervision).
5 Specialist services — group and individual psychotherapy; social skills retraining and work rehabilitation; family/marital therapy; rehabilitation houses and therapeutic communities.

Prognosis
The prognosis depends on the drug abused, but approximately 50% of opiate abusers develop long-term dependence and 2–3% die annually. Intravenous drug abusers who share contaminated syringes may also contract AIDS—in some areas of the UK, such as Edinburgh, infection rates of up to 80% have been reported, making a higher mortality rate likely.

Solvent abuse
Solvent abuse differs from 'hard drug' abuse in a number of important ways:
• it is very much a group activity;

- it involves a younger age group (14–16 years);
- it carries a much better prognosis (psychological dependence may occur but physical dependence is rare).

About 1 in 10 secondary school children try sniffing experimentally, but only 1% are thought to be long-term abusers.

In general, misusers are more likely to come from a broken home, a large family or have an unemployed parent; and more likely to be involved in smoking, drinking, fighting, vandalism and regular truancy than non-users.

Agents abused included glues, modelling cements, petrol, cleaning solvents, paint cleaners and aerosols. The available concentration can be maximised by inhaling from a plastic bag or crisp packet (viscous products), or a handkerchief or plastic bottle (liquids). Mixtures usually contain acetone and toluene and produce a euphoria–drowsiness pattern that simulates drunkenness (but is achieved faster).

Rare toxic effects include:
- aplastic anaemia;
- polyneuropathy;
- cerebral and hepatorenal damage.

Large doses cause central nervous system depression with ataxia, nystagmus, dysarthria, drowsiness and coma. Perioral eczema and chronic upper respiratory tract infection may result from repeated contact with adhesives, and those inhaling petrol additionally risk lead poisoning. More important is the risk of fatal accident or serious injury while intoxicated. There is also a fire risk, especially when sniffing and smoking are combined. Occasional deaths have occurred from arrhythmias, and from asphyxiation after cold aerosol sprays have induced laryngeal spasm. A few solvent abusers progress later on to alcohol and other drugs.

Misuse of tranquillisers and hypnotics
Another familiar example of drug abuse is enacted daily in the surgery when tranquillisers and hypnotics are prescribed to dependent patients.

Although physical dependence on benzodiazepines was first reported in 1961, the risk was considered low until an article in the *British Medical Journal* suggested otherwise in 1980. Since then the pressure to curtail prescribing has been building. In 1983 the legal profession began exploring the possibility of a patient compensation scheme and in 1987 the Council for Involuntary Tranquilliser Addiction was formed. Against this background, the number of prescriptions in England fell from 29.7 million in 1982 to 21 million in 1989.

Why do people take tranquillisers?
1 Foremost as a pharmaceutical crutch with anxiolytic and hypnotic

properties at times of personal strain (stresses come in all forms — sexual, financial, marital, interpersonal).

2   However, a significant number commence taking tranquillisers to relieve a somatic symptom (not always related in their minds to stress), or under the strain of chronic ill health, or because of free-floating anxiety, anxiety-prone or inadequate personalities. In surveys people taking tranquillisers for the first time gave as the initial reason:

(a) a somatic symptom in 53% of cases;

(b) recognisable stress *alone* in 30% of cases;

(c) 'internal tensions' in 19% of cases.

The most common strains and conflicts mentioned by women centred around their roles as wife, mother and houseworker, while men tended to discuss problems in their work or work performance.

3   Ready availability and ready prescribing compound the problem. Prescriptions are offered for social reasons (see Section 2.2), in place of counselling, or because problems taken to a doctor tend to become 'medicalized'.

Are tranquillisers effective?

Initially tranquillisers are effective, but:

•   Kales (1974) found their hypnotic effect can fall off or disappear over periods as short as 2 weeks;

•   the Committee on the Review of Medicines (1980) pointed out that there is little convincing evidence that anxiolytics are still effective after 4 months' continuous treatment;

•   Tyrer *et al.* (1988) found that when anxiolytics are used for more than 4 weeks they are less effective than antidepressants and psychological procedures.

Does tranquilliser taking matter?

Benzodiazepines are a very safe group of drugs, much safer than barbiturates. As a result the drawbacks of prescribing have been recognised late in the day.

1   *Withdrawal syndromes.* The overall incidence of the withdrawal syndrome is unclear: estimates vary from 30 to 100% depending on the population studied, the definition of abuse, duration of use, rate of withdrawal and length of follow-up (Pertusson *et al.* 1981; Tyrer *et al.* 1983). There is also evidence that withdrawal problems can occur after as little as 4–6 weeks' regular treatment. The syndrome appears within 3 days of stopping a short-acting drug and within 7 days of stopping a long-acting one. It usually lasts about 2 weeks but can go on for several months. It includes:

(a) anxiety;

(b) perceptual disturbances (including heightened sensitivity to all forms of sensory stimuli);

(c) a feeling of continuous movement;

(d) depersonalisation and derealisation;

(e) weight loss;

(f) electroencephalogram changes and epileptic seizures;

(g) psychotic behaviour (paranoid delusions, visual hallucinations).

2 *Psychological impairment*. Short-term usage impairs psychomotor function, and can produce anterograde amnesia. Chronic usage impairs performance in psychological tests, and abnormal computerised tomography scans have been found more commonly in chronic benzodiazepine users than in matched controls. Furthermore, it is likely that a significant number of accidents in the elderly are attributable to excessive sedation.

The implication is that it does matter that people take tranquillisers. Patients who have been taking a benzodiazepine for a long time should have their medication slowly withdrawn over 4–12 weeks, if at all possible (perhaps substituting a long-acting drug for a short-acting one in the first instance). People commenced on benzodiazepines for the first time should have treatment (preferably *intermittent* treatment) for periods less than 4–6 weeks. A firm decision on duration at the outset and a definite review date help to avoid the common pitfall of repeat prescribing by default.

In many cases the precipitating stress is still unresolved, which perpetuates drug-seeking behaviour. Non-drug-related approaches— counselling and relaxation — have more to offer, but demand more from the doctor in time and stamina.

6.5 CHILD ABUSE

Child abuse has received much publicity of late. It may truly be more common or simply recognised more often.

Incidence
A GP sees one case every 2 years typically, but the true incidence is believed to be much higher:
• perhaps 10–15% of all 'accidents' in children under 2 years old;
• perhaps 20% of all children are sexually abused.

Epidemiological features
1 *The home background*:
   (a) very young parents, often unmarried or with marital problems;
   (b) lower socio-economic class (though not invariably);
   (c) financial problems and/or poor housing;
   (d) lack of support at home;
   (e) large family already;

(f) parents who themselves had troubled childhoods and were battered;

(g) step-parents.

2   *The circumstances of the pregnancy*:

(a) termination requested but turned down;

(b) poor antenatal attendance; difficult pregnancy;

(c) a baby with physical handicap or prematurity;

(d) a baby requiring Special Care Baby Unit care after birth.

Nearly 90% of abused babies are the first or last in birth order. Mothers abuse more often than fathers. Meal times and bedtime are particular 'flashpoints'.

3   *The postnatal period*:

(a) early maternal separation;

(b) early signs of poor bonding;

(c) lack of preparation at home; delay in choosing a name;

(d) poor attendance at child health/immunisation clinics;

(e) unusual feeding practices (e.g. 'bottle-propping').

4   *Suspicious injuries*:

(a) a history not consistent with the injury;

(b) delayed reporting;

(c) multiple injuries at different stages;

(d) characteristic injuries (e.g. cigarette burns, fingertip bruises, strap marks, bite marks, black eyes, pull-injury with epiphyseal separation).

5   *The demeanour of the child*. 'Frozen awareness' is also said to be characteristic, and such children are unusually obedient in behaviour and often fail to thrive.

6   In childhood sexual abuse look for:

(a) a clear statement from the child;

(b) sexualised behaviour in the child at an inappropriately young age;

(c) recent tears or bruising in the anogenital region.

A report from the Cleveland enquiry concluded that anal dilatation was a suspicious sign meriting investigation, but not in itself evidence of anal abuse.

Management of child abuse

Ethical dilemmas abound, e.g.:

• whether to breach confidentiality;

• when to involve the police;

• whether children should be taken into care for their own good, or left supervised at home for the parents' good;

• how to distinguish between rigid discipline and cruelty/criminal abuse?

There is no simple answer but several general points of advice may help:

1   Have a low threshold of suspicion.

2 Get another opinion (colleague, health visitor, local police surgeon, paediatrician).

3 Try to confirm the diagnosis (e.g. skeletal survey showing multiple fractures of different ages).

4 Consider whether the child needs to be immediately removed to a place of safety. Hospital admission may avoid confrontation, otherwise a Place of Safety Order is obtained from a magistrate on application by the police, Social Services or NSPCC, and gives authority to remove a child to a place of safety (hospital, police station, community or foster home) for up to 28 days.

5 Consider calling a case conference (involving medical, social and perhaps psychiatric disciplines) and registering the child as 'at risk'.

6 Offer the family the support and care needed.

The most difficult decision on management is whether to attempt to reunite the child with his family, and work with them to repair the family unit, or whether the risk to the child is too great, when alternative arrangements (e.g. fostering) will need to be explored.

Prevention of child abuse

Prevention entails recognising the needs of high-risk groups in advance of the event. They need to be seen often. The social worker may be able to improve home circumstances and provide the necessary support (e.g. childminders or play groups). Unnecessary separation in the postnatal period must be avoided, and medical and Social Services follow-up is needed. The health visitor is a key figure in the prevention of child abuse, and will need to visit frequently in high-risk situations.

6.6 AIDS

The size of the problem

AIDS was first described following a handful of cases of *Pneumocystis* pneumonia and Kaposi's sarcoma among homosexual men and intravenous drug abusers in California and New York in 1981. From that tiny base the pool of infection swelled in the most dramatic fashion:

• by the end of 1987 the World Health Organization (WHO) had been officially notified of 73 747 cases of AIDS from 129 countries;

• by December 1995 in the UK 11 872 AIDS cases had been described, of whom 64% had died;

• in 1994–5 the prevalence of human immunodeficiency virus (HIV) infection among injecting drug users in London was about 4%, and that in pregnant women as a whole 1 in 580.

These figures probably display only the tip of the iceberg: we know the pool of HIV seropositive individuals is much greater — at least 5 000 000 world-wide (WHO) and 30 000–40 000 according to conservative estimates in the UK (Department of Health): and many of these (20–30% on current views) will also develop AIDS.

The economic consequences of the AIDS epidemic have also been highlighted, e.g.:

• in the UK the 3000 new cases in 1988 cost the Exchequer £88 million;

• the first 10 000 cases in the USA cost 1.6 million hospital days, $1.4 billion in health costs and $4.8 billion in lost economic activity.

Part of the problem with AIDS is the extent of our ignorance. While short-term extrapolations may be quite accurate, the long-term view is hazy and incomplete. For example:

• are we dealing with one or several epidemics?

• what are the limits of the incubation period? (The average of 8–9 years conceals a great deal of variation);

• does the infectivity of AIDS vary during that time?

• what is the ease of spread per sexual encounter? (Again there is a variability that suggests unknown biological factors are at work);

• what do we know of the frequency, intensity and types of sexual activity in populations?

• can sexual practices be modified by public education?

This last factor has a critical bearing on the validity of any mathematical projections. There is certainly encouraging evidence that homosexual behaviour has changed due to the AIDS situation, but it is not clear that the heterosexual population will follow suit until the virus becomes more prevalent and awareness levels are raised.

Recently there have been reports of dramatic clinical benefit from combined protease inhibitor and nucleoside analogue therapy in AIDS sufferers, suggestive of an important breakthrough.

Doctors and patients have already been confronted by death and disease in fit adults, young women widowed, young children orphaned, and parents attending their own children's funerals. A large part of the burden of care naturally falls on community-based services: 80% of the AIDS sufferer's time will be spent at home. GPs will in future find themselves more involved in aspects of care and prevention.

Clinical aspects

The presentation and clinical features of HIV infection are outlined in Table 6.10. It is important that GPs recognise the possibility of HIV infection in high-risk groups.

High-risk groups and those in need of the HIV test include the following individuals:

1 People with polyglandular lymphadenopathy (PGL), or features of AIDS-related complex (ARC) or AIDS (Table 6.10).

2 Men who have had sex with another man in the last 10 years.

3 Drug users who have injected drugs at any time in the last 10 years.

4 Haemophiliacs receiving unscreened blood products.

5 Prostitutes.

6 People who have lived in or visited areas of high prevalence (e.g. Africa, North America), and had sex with people living there.

7 Certain recipients of blood transfusions (blood has been screened in the UK since October 1985, but not always abroad).

8 People who may have been accidentally exposed (e.g. by needle-stick injury).

9 Sexual partners of the above groups.

10 Children of infected mothers.

The Department of Health announced in 1988 an extensive programme of testing for HIV of unlinked anonymous samples. After all possible identifying tags have been removed, the residue of blood collected for legitimate tests is randomly screened for HIV, unless the

Table 6.10 Clinical features in HIV seropositive individuals.

1 *Completely asymptomatic*

2 *Persistent generalised lymphadenopathy (PGL)*
Enlarged firm lymph nodes
Sometimes painful
No obvious cause
Present at least 3 months

3 *AIDS-related complex (ARC)*
Acne
Fatigue
Herpes simplex
Herpes zoster
Immunosuppression
Malaise
Mild diarrhoea
Night sweats
Oral candida
± PGL
Pyrexia of unknown origin
Seborrhoeic dermatitis
Weight loss

4 *AIDS*
Dementia
Depression
Diarrhoea
Encephalitis
Fits
Headaches
Kaposi's sarcoma (25%)
Malignancies
Meningitis
Opportunistic infections
PGL
Pneumocystis pneumonia (60%)
Psychosis
Pyrexia of unknown origin
Wasting

patient has spontaneously objected. Data are collected for community benefit, to monitor disease trends. The system is designed to ensure that everyone, including the donor, cannot identify positive cases. The scientific, legal and ethical basis of this programme has been well reviewed (Gill *et al.* 1989).

Aspects of counselling and management

1 Prior to blood testing it is important that these people are appropriately and sensitively counselled. They should know the limitations of the test and have considered the implications of a positive test.

2 Post-test counselling is vital in view of the serious range of psychological reactions (shock, fear and anxiety, isolation, depression, guilt, frustration, obsessive disorders) that accompanies news of a positive result. About 10% of seropositive individuals will need to be referred to a psychiatrist or psychologist, and there is a real risk of suicide in patients left unattended around this time.

3 Follow-up must include common sense advice to patients and their partners (on safer sexual practices; the myths and truth about transmission and infectivity; and such diverse matters as how to cope with spillages of body fluid, and who to tell and what to say).

4 A number of support services exist to provide information and help (e.g. local special clinics and health education departments; AIDS help and advice lines; self-help groups). Doctors need to develop close, effective working links with these bodies.

5 GPs will need eventually to deal with the complications of AIDS and will need to recognise those they can manage and those that require specialist support.

Aspects of prevention

1 Anxiety about AIDS means that doctors have to cope with the 'worried well' (people who remain well but have symptoms they attribute to AIDS), the 'worried ignorant', and the 'worried guilty'. They need to reassure and to educate, to engender appropriate degrees of concern and appropriate responses.

2 They need to give clear and explicit advice to the general public on the prevention of AIDS and safer sexual practices (Table 6.11). Advice must be blunt and clear, but appropriate to the needs of the individual and the context of the consultation. GPs may be better placed than other health care personnel to fulfil this role.

3 GPs (as good employers) need to educate their staff and to protect them from exposure to the virus through appropriate health care measures and protocols (Table 6.12).

Educating the carers

GPs clearly need to think out their advice and to ensure it is accurate and up to date. Fortunately there is no shortage of information to help

Table 6.11 Advice on avoiding AIDS.

(a) The ladder of risk:

No risk
Solo masturbation
Massage away from genital area

Low risk
Mutual masturbation
Dry kissing
Body-to-body contact
Penis-to-body contact (except between thighs and buttocks)

Medium risk
Wet kissing
Fellatio
Urination
Coitus interfemoris
Anilingus
Fingering
Douches and enemas

High risk
Anal and vaginal sex
Fisting
Sharing sex toys and needles
Any sex act drawing blood

Risk *increases* with number of sexual partners
Risk *decreases* with use of a condom in intercourse
Risk *decreases* with the additional use of a water-based spermicide (especially in anal
   sex)

(b) Using a condom:

7% failure rate (half due to incorrect use). Advice needs to be specific and full, e.g.

Before
• Use before every act and put on before the penis touches the partner's vulva or
rectum
• Wait until the penis is erect, then pinch the top of the condom with one hand;
with the other put the sheath on the end of the penis and unroll it all the way down

After
• Withdraw the penis from the vagina or rectum, holding the condom on the penis
as you do so
• Take the condom off, taking care not to spill the semen, and dispose of it carefully
• Use a fresh condom next and every time

(c) Advice for the drug abuser:

Scale of increasing risk
Abstinence
Using drugs but not injecting them
Using sterile equipment only
Using but not sharing equipment
Using and sharing cleaned equipment
Using and sharing unclean equipment

Cleaning equipment
Aim: to flush the virus out
Method: rinse with hot water and washing-up liquid immediately; rinse in clean
   water

Table 6.12 Control of infection advice.

1 *Specimen-taking and handling*
- Adequate training first
- Wear gloves and disposable plastic apron
- Use minimum volume of blood
- Avoid spillages
- Dispose of sharps into a puncture-proof bin
- Do not re-sheathe needles
- Put specimen in robust leak-proof container in sealed bag and use biohazard labelling
- Notify senior laboratory staff

2 *Hygiene/disinfection steps*
- Do not share between patients devices that can draw blood, e.g. syringes and needles, electrolysis equipment, tattoo/acupuncture sharps
- Use disposable sterile equipment as much as possible
- Otherwise sterilise by heating (autoclave is better than boiling)
- Liquid disinfectants may do as second best, e.g. hypochlorite, gluteraldehyde, alcohol

3 *Coping with spillages*
- Clean up immediately
- Use gloves and apron (as above)
- Use liberal amounts of household bleach diluted 1:10 (with hot water)
- Leave for 30 min
- Wipe up with disposable paper towels
- Carefully dispose of gloves, apron and towels
- Thoroughly wash and dry hands

4 *First aid for staff*
- Body fluid on skin, in eyes or in mouth—wash away as soon as possible
- Penetrating wounds
  (a) encourage bleeding
  (b) wash with soap ans water
  (c) notify employer
  (d) post needle-stick prophylaxis now available

educate the carers, such as:

1 The trade press, the journals and Department of Health circulars.
2 Seminars, symposia and lunch-time meetings at postgraduate centres.
3 Distance learning courses (such as the Royal College CLIPP programme).
4 Information lines.
5 HA local liaison specialists.
6 Public information material for surgeries — display posters, leaflets, advisory material (and free condoms) to present to patients.

Attitudes to AIDS have improved, and this should help. Surveys have suggested that seropositive patients fear a negative reaction from their GP, worry about confidentiality, and often concealed the diagnosis from him (King 1988); but a more sympathetic public and professional image is now being projected to those in need.

7 Legal and Ethical Matters

7.1 THE 1983 MENTAL HEALTH ACT (ENGLAND AND WALES)

Definitions

Mental disorder (Section 1)
Included in the definition of mental disorder are:
- mental illness;
- arrested or incomplete development of mind;
- psychopathic disorder.
  It *excludes* from the definition:
- promiscuity;
- sexual deviancy;
- dependence on alcohol or drugs.

Nearest relative (Section 26)
The nearest relative according to Section 26 of the Act is the first surviving person appearing in the following list:
1 husband or wife (or co-habitee for more than 6 months);
2 son or daughter (if aged over 18 years);
3 father or mother;
4 brother or sister (aged over 18 years);
5 grandparent;
6 grandchild (aged over 18 years);
7 uncle or aunt (aged over 18 years);
8 nephew or niece (aged over 18 years);
9 non-relative living with the patient for 5 or more years.

'Approved' doctor and social worker
Doctor and social worker 'approved' under the terms of the Act as having special expertise and training in the area of mental health.

Principles
1 The *grounds* for admission under the various sections are similar, namely:
   (a) that the patient suffers from a mental disorder of a nature and severity which justify that particular section in the interests of the patient's own health and safety, and the safety of others;
   (b) that treatment has to be in hospital.
2 The applicant must be a social worker or nearest relative.
3 Usually two medical recommendations are needed (an approved doctor and a doctor with prior knowledge of the patient), except in the event of emergency, when one signature gives limited powers of detention.

4 Admission has a limited tenure and there are prescribed discharge powers and rights of appeal.

Details

For details of the main sections of the Act see Table 7.1. (Northern Ireland and Scotland have their own Mental Health Acts but the principles are similar to the English and Welsh Act.)

Table 7.1 The main sections of the 1983 Mental Health Act.

Section number and purpose	Application	Medical recommendations	Other conditions	Duration	Discharge powers
2 Compulsory admission for *assessment*	Nearest relative *or* approved social worker	Approved doctor *plus* doctor who knows the patient	**1** Not more than 5 days between medical examinations **2** Application is valid for 14 days **3** The social worker normally interviews the nearest relative and/or informs him in writing	28 days. Not renewable	Responsible officer (RMO) *or* hospital manager *or* nearest relative. (The patient can also appeal to the Mental Health Review Tribunal)
3 Compulsory admission for *treatment*	As above	As above	As above	6 months (renewable for a further 6 months and then yearly)	As above. (If the patient does not appeal, the hospital managers *must* appeal on his behalf after 6 months)
4 Compulsory admission for *assessment in an emergency.* Compliance with Section 2 conditions would cause an undesirable delay	As above	*Either* approved doctor *or* doctor with prior knowledge of patient	**1** The medical referee must have seen the patient in the last 24 h **2** Application valid for 24 h only	72 h. Not renewable	RMO *or* hospital managers. (Patient cannot appeal)

Other sections sometimes required

1 Section 5: the emergency detention of informal *inpatients* by the RMO or his nominated deputy for 72 h so that a Section 2 or 3 can be considered

2 Section 7: reception into guardianship

3 Section 115: right of entry of approved social worker into premises so he can remove a patient to a place of safety. (Section 135 is the same, with a police constable)

4 Section 136: removal of a patient from a public place by a constable to a place of safety (e.g. cell or hospital) for up to 72 h to allow medical examination

Much legislation now exists regarding the use and misuse of controlled drugs, e.g.:

- Dangerous Drugs, Notification of Addicts Regulations 1968;
- Misuse of Drugs Act 1971;
- Misuse of Drugs Regulations (Notification, and Supply to Addicts) 1973;
- Misuse of Drugs Regulations 1985.

Under the 1971 Misuse of Drugs Act three categories of controlled drugs were defined:

1 Class A: including opium, heroin, morphine, most opiates, pethidine, LSD and other hallucinogens, cocaine and methadone.
2 Class B: including cannabis, amphetamines and barbiturates.
3 Class C: including benzphetamine, chlorphentermine and diethylpropion.

These categories relate broadly to the degree of harm caused by misuse. The classification has limited significance for doctors and is used mainly in setting the penalties for unlawful possession and intent to supply.

Of greater importance to the medical profession are the Misuse of Drugs Regulations 1985 which define five groups of drugs (Schedules 1–5) and describe those regulations governing import, export, production, supply, possession, prescribing and record-keeping of controlled drugs.

- Schedule 1: including drugs like cannabis and LSD which have no therapeutic use. Possession and supply are prohibited and availability is solely by Home Office license for research purposes.
- Schedule 2: including the opiates and major stimulants. GPs can possess these drugs for approved medical use but there are strict rules regarding safe-custody, record-keeping and the format of prescriptions (see below).
- Schedule 3: including barbiturates, diethylpropion and pentazocine. The format of the prescription is regulated and invoices must be kept for 2 years.
- Schedule 4: including benzodiazepines (except temazepam, which has been moved to Schedule 3). Control requirements are minimal.
- Schedule 5: controlled drugs combined with other drugs in amounts so small that they are not liable to produce dependence. Invoices must be kept for 2 years and manufacture is regulated by the Home Office.

The other Points of relevance to the GP are as follows:

1 Anonymised information on the trend in drug misuse is collected by the Home Office from treatment agencies. (Formerly GPs had to supply the names of addicts they had attended, but this requirement has been withdrawn.)
2 Doctors need a special licence (issued by the Home Secretary) to

prescribe heroin, morphine or cocaine in the treatment of drug addiction (a special prescription form, FP 10 (MDA), has been introduced for this purpose).

3   Doctors must keep controlled drugs within a locked compartment, or if on their person, within a locked receptacle. (Note that a locked car boot is insufficient — it must be a locked case in a locked boot.)

4   Doctors must keep a register of the use they make of their controlled drug supply, and the police have the right to inspect this register.

5   It is an offence to issue an incomplete prescription for a controlled drug and the pharmacist will not dispense under these circumstances. The legal requirements are:

(a) scripts should be written in indelible ink;

(b) they should be signed and dated personally by the prescriber;

(c) the prescriber should write in his own hand the name and address of the patient, the dose, the form of the preparation, the strength to be dispensed and the total quantity;

(d) all numbers must be in words and figures;

(e) the address of the prescriber must appear on the script.

6   If controlled drugs need to be disposed, this should be done in the presence of a witness and formally recorded.

7   Controlled drugs cannot be prescribed for patients leaving the country, and doctors cannot carry controlled drugs abroad unless endorsed by a licence from the Secretary of State.

Careless or improper use of drugs must also lay the GP open to a charge of professional misconduct or incompetence. Note that there is a black market for the resale of drugs obtained from GPs by deception, and also a black market for stolen blank scripts which can be forged to obtain drug supplies.

7.3 INDUSTRIAL INJURIES

Patients can claim for injuries 'arising out of and in the course of their employment' even if due to their own foolhardiness or carelessness. The Industrial Injuries Act lays down 47 'prescribed' industrial diseases which are recognised for compensation purposes, and a schedule for prescribed degrees of disablement from trauma.

Compensation becomes payable through:

1   The State Industrial Injuries Scheme: this contributes *disablement benefits* (on a 1–100% scale assessed by a medical board), and *industrial death benefits* (see Section 5.7);

2   An individual's private action against his employer (if he can demonstrate negligence).

State claims can be made up to 5 years retrospectively.

In addition there are a group of diseases that are compulsorily *notifiable* by employers to the Health and Safety Executive when they occur in an industrial setting. Industrial diseases notifiable under the Reporting of Injuries, Diseases and Dangerous Occurrences Regulations (RIDDOR) 1995 include:

- poisoning by a number of industrial agents, e.g. arsenic, benzene, beryllium, cadmium, carbon disulphide, lead, manganese, mercury, phosphorus;
- chrome ulceration;
- skin cancers;
- folliculitis and acne (induced by tar, pitch and oils);
- occupational asthma;
- extrinsic allergic alveolitis;
- pneumoconiosis;
- byssinosis;
- compressed air sickness;
- vibration white finger;
- a number of occupational infections, e.g. leptospirosis, tuberculosis, hepatitis, anthrax, work with human pathogens;
- a number of occupational cancers (e.g. from ionising radiation or asbestos).

Notes

1 The lists of *reportable* and *prescribed* diseases associated with occupation are similar but not identical. They are drawn up for separate and quite distinct purposes: the one to allow investigation and enforcement under the Health and Safety at Work Act 1974, the other to allow state compensation under the industrial injuries provisions of the Social Security Act 1975.

2 The obligation to report under the RIDDOR Regulations falls on the employer, not the doctor (except in respect of his *own* staff). However, if the employer is to do so, the doctor must make the diagnosis clear to him.

3 Other health and safety at work obligations imposed on GPs as employers (safety policies, accident books, insurance, etc.) are described in Section 7.9.

7.4 THE CORONER

Notifiable deaths

Deaths that should be reported to a coroner include:

- all sudden or unexpected deaths, suicides and deaths where the cause is not known;
- deaths which appear suspicious, violent or unnatural;
- deaths where the doctor has not attended within the prior 14 days;
- deaths within 24 h of hospital admission (in most areas—some personal variation);
- accidents and injuries;
- industrial disease;

- medical mishaps (specifically including anaesthetics, operations and drugs, either therapeutic or addictive);
- deaths arising from ill treatment, starvation or neglect;
- poisoning;
- abortions;
- stillbirths (when there is doubt as to whether the child was born alive);
- service disability pensioners;
- prisoners.

All alcohol-associated deaths used to be notifiable, even if due to alcoholic cirrhosis in the chronic alcoholic, but death due to chronic alcoholism is no longer notifiable, unless associated with one of the above circumstances (thus, the drunk who falls and fractures his skull qualifies for notification under the 'accidents and injuries' clause). Deaths from human immunodeficiency virus (HIV) and acquired immune deficiency syndrome (AIDS)-related illness do not normally require referral.

The Scottish system

In Scotland a slightly different system applies: deaths are reported to a procurator fiscal, in the same circumstances as for the coroner in England, with the addition of deaths of foster children and the new-born.

7.5 NOTIFIABLE DISEASES

Under the Public Health (Control of Disease) Act 1984 and Public Health (Infectious Diseases) Regulations 1988 the following infectious diseases in England and Wales must be notified to the local authority's Medical Officer for Environmental Health:

Anthrax	Food poisoning
Cholera	Lassa fever
Diphtheria	Leprosy
Dysentery (amoebic or bacillary)	Leptospirosis
Encephalitis	Malaria
Marburg disease	Scarlet fever
Measles	Smallpox
Meningitis	Tetanus
Mumps	Tuberculosis
Ophthalmia neonatorum	Typhoid fever
Paratyphoid fever A and B	Typhus fever
Plague	Viral haemorrhagic fever
Polio	Viral hepatitis
Rabies	Whooping cough
Relapsing fever	Yellow fever
Rubella	

In Scotland and Northern Ireland (where notifications are to the chief administrative medical officer) the list of notifiable conditions is amended.
1 In *Northern Ireland* it *includes*:
   (a) gastro-enteritis (in those aged under 2 years);
   (b) infective hepatitis.
However, it *excludes*:
   (a) food poisoning;
   (b) leprosy;
   (c) malaria;
   (d) ophthalmia neonatorum;
   (e) tetanus.
2 In *Scotland* it *includes*:
   (a) continued fever;
   (b) erysipelas;
   (c) leptospiral jaundice;
   (d) membranous croup;
   (e) puerperal fever.
However, it *excludes*:
   (a) encephalitis;
   (b) tetanus;
   (c) tuberculosis.
A small fee is payable for each notification.

AIDS is not notifiable by statute. However, doctors are urged to participate in a voluntary confidential reporting scheme.

7.6 THE ABORTION ACT

Under the Abortion Act 1967 and the Abortion Regulations 1991 termination of pregnancy is allowable if there is a risk:
1 To the woman's life (greater than if the pregnancy were to continue).
2 Of grave permanent injury to the woman's physical or mental health.
3 To her physical or mental health (greater than if the pregnancy were to continue).
4 To the physical or mental health of her existing children.
5 Risk of a handicapped child (rubella-damaged, Down's syndrome, etc.).

Clauses 3 and 4 can be employed only when the pregnancy does not exceed 24 weeks.

Two medical referees must sign the 'blue form' (form HSA 1).

Approximately 180 000 legal terminations are performed annually in England with an approximate mortality of 2.6 per 100 000.

The Abortion Act represents a middle ground between the extreme views of 'no abortion at all' and 'abortion on demand'. It does not place an absolute value on human life (human suffering coming higher in priority), but it places a *high* value—fetal destruction must be justified. Critics of the legislation point out that it is arbitrary and its application is inconsistent, e.g.:

• the 24-week time limit is based on notions of fetal viability which arguably occurs much sooner than this;

• under clause 5 Down's syndrome pregnancies are routinely terminated, but in a legal test case a life-saving operation was ordered on Down's syndrome baby Alexandra against the parents' wishes;

• clauses 3 and 4 are open to wide and subjective interpretation: practice varies widely throughout the country and from one doctor to another;

• the death rate from legal termination is lower than that for pregnancy, so it could be argued under clause 1 that *all* women should receive a termination on request.

(Exam candidates may be quizzed on their own attitudes to abortion. Obviously this is a question of convictions and belief rather than right and wrong answers, but you need to consider all the practical implications of your views. If, for example, you regard termination as 'murder through a legal loophole', what do you do when faced by the patient requesting an abortion? Do you refer her to a colleague or a consultant? If you refuse to help her, are you within the terms of your service or within the ethical code of medical practice as a whole? And how do you stand with your colleagues? And what about post-coital contraception or the fitting of coils?)

7.7 THE DATA PROTECTION ACT 1984

Users of computer-held data must register with the data protection registrar on a triennial basis. 'Users' obviously includes GPs with a practice computer, but may also include computer bureau services from Health Authorities (HAs) or accountants, for example. The key point is the *control* of personal data—automatically provided information which identifies individual patients.

Users need to comply with several principles. Data should be:

• obtained and processed lawfully;
• held for a specific lawful purpose;
• not otherwise used or disclosed;
• no more than required for the purpose;
• dispensed with when no longer necessary;
• protected against unauthorised access.

More taxing, perhaps, is the obligation for information to be accurate and up-to-date and—more significant for GPs—the principle of subject access. A 1987 amendment of the Act conceded that doctors could restrict access to personal health information when serious physical or mental harm might ensue. However, in view of the relent-less march of computer systems into the surgery it is important to con-sider these problems and to get it right. Failure to register under the Act is a criminal offence.

7.8 ACCESS TO MEDICAL RECORDS

Access to Medical Reports Act (1988)

This Act allows patients to see medical reports prepared for prospec-tive employers or insurers. Doctors must allow those patients who wish to see the report 21 days to do so before it is dispatched. A copy of the report must be provided on request by the patient and a copy (to which the patient has access) kept for 6 months. Patients are allowed the opportunity to discuss the report with their doctors and to attach a codicil if they feel the report is inaccurate. The GP, however, is not obliged to alter his comments if there is still a difference of view. Ulti-mately the patient can refuse to allow the report to be sent, so if access is requested a further consent should normally be obtained prior to dispatch.

Access to Health Records Act (1990)

This Act allows patients aged 16 or over access to their medical notes (manual or computerised), but only notes written after 1 November 1990. It includes reports written by allied professionals (e.g. nurses, dentists, midwives). A copy must be provided, normally within 40 days of a written request, at nominal charge.

Doctors keen to avoid the pitfalls of these acts need to modify their working practices, for example to:

- ensure they receive (and keep) a written informed consent;
- date-stamp all requests for reports and correspondence;
- keep a dated record book and copies of all reports.

GPs can withhold information from the patient if they believe it is likely to risk serious physical or mental harm to the individual or others.

7.9 HEALTH AND SAFETY AT WORK LEGISLATION

The Health and Safety at Work Act 1974 applies to the GP employer and places on him the obligation 'so far as reasonably practicable' to ensure a safely maintained workplace. He must also display a state-ment of safety policy and notify certain categories of accident to the Health and Safety Executive. An accident book must be kept, insur-ance should be taken out against accidents to staff, and the inspec-torate is entitled to enter and inspect premises to ensure they comply with the Act. (Employees too have an obligation to comply with safety practices and it is an offence under the Act to put themselves or others at risk.)

The Control of Substances Hazardous to Health Regulations 1994 and Management of Health and Safety at Work Regulations 1992 require employers to make a formal assessment of risk to employees arising from materials in the workplace and adequately to control and monitor that risk. This might for example include the risk of dermatitis from biocides and sterilising agents and the risk of staff contracting infection from patients and biological samples and waste; electrical safety; proper storage of drugs; and adequate sterilisation procedures.

There are clear implications for the counselling and training of staff, and policies are required for the cleaning of medical equipment and the safe disposal of drugs, contaminated needles, dressings and appliances. A written risk assessment is required.

7.10 MEDICAL CONFIDENTIALITY

Confidentiality has been a basic tenet of medical ethics for 2500 years and is embodied in the Hippocratic Oath, the International Code of Medical Ethics and the Declaration of Geneva (1947). There are several obvious *reasons* for confidentiality:

1   We set store by personal autonomy, the right of individuals to control their own lives and to control disclosures about them.

2   Consultations have an assumed privacy built in to them. Indeed, although there are no legal precedents, there may be an implied *legal contract* of confidentiality, and patients could theoretically obtain redress for breaches through the courts or through the General Medical Council Professional Conduct Committee.

3   Reciprocal respect and confidence are essential to obtain an honest history and meaningful doctor–patient relationship. This is to the mutual benefit of both parties and in some cases frankness may also serve the community best.

Exceptions

There are three general circumstances in which confidentiality may be breached:

1   *In the patient's own interests.* Sometimes doctors share with close relatives and friends some private details of a patient's illness that the patient himself may not be ready to receive (e.g. news of terminal illness).

2   *When required by law.* Statutory disclosures include:
   (a) terminations under the Abortion Act;
   (b) drug addiction under the Misuse of Drugs Regulations;
   (c) notifiable infections under the Health Service and Public Health Act;

(d) industrial injuries and diseases under the Reporting of Injuries, Diseases and Dangerous Occurrences Regulations;
(e) road traffic accidents under the Road Traffic Acts;
(f) births and deaths registration;
(g) coroners' cases.
   Bodies with the power to order disclosures include:
(a) a court of law;
(b) an enquiry appointed by the Secretary of State;
(c) an NHS tribunal;
(d) the Health and Safety Executive.

3 *In the greater interest of the community at large.* This is a grey area, but includes the murderer who will not give himself up, the epileptic who risks serious accident by driving illegally when fit-prone, the child abuser, etc.

It is a source of concern among consumer groups that exceptions to the code of confidentiality are so numerous, in particular that much information on individuals is collected for administrative purposes, e.g.:

• the community health register and recall system collects birth information and distributes it to health visitors;
• many forms of hospital activity analysis are regularly performed;
• the Prescription Pricing Authority collects prescription details;
• the Department of Health and drug companies are informed about patients with suspected drug interactions;
• many authorities have access to child at-risk registers.

Ensuring confidentiality

Practices need to develop policies that safeguard the processing of confidential information e.g.:

1 Store it in a secure fashion; restrict computer access to password holders.

2 Make sure that staff who have access to the records understand the code of conduct (write it into their contracts).

3 When disclosure is required, only give as much information as strictly necessary for the purpose.

4 When assessing a patient for a third party (e.g. employer or insurance company) ensure the patient understands at the outset the purpose of the assessment and that this may necessitate disclosure of personal information or a health opinion (with written consent).

5 When dealing with a lawyer, establish which party he represents.

6 Remember that the obligation continues after a patient's death.

A fuller discussion of these issues exists in the GMC guidance document *Confidentiality*.

The discovery at the Nuremberg War Trials that Nazi doctors had perpetrated atrocities under the guise of medical research led to the declaration of a 10-point code identifying the main ethical principles on which true research should be founded. These principles were further refined in the Declaration of Helsinki (1964), which insists that:

1 Research must conform to generally accepted scientific principles and should be based on adequate laboratory and animal experiments.

2 The experimental protocol should be reviewed by an independent ethical committee.

3 Research should always be supervised by competent and qualified workers.

4 The importance of the objective should be in proportion to the inherent risk to the subject.

5 The health of the patient should be the prime and foremost consideration and should always prevail over the interests of science and society.

6 There should be informed consent regarding aims, methods, risks and possible benefits.

7 There should be no duress to participate and patients should be free to abstain or withdraw at any time.

Despite these caveats medical research is littered with ethical problems.

1 Some authorities believe that 'informed consent' is an unobtainable ideal. It may be impossible to convey every facet of knowledge and judgement to patients who vary in their interest in and capacity to comprehend complicated medical information. (In chemotherapy trials 40–50% of patients are unable to explain the purpose, nature and major complications of a procedure the day after they have been counselled, while informed consent for some cancer patients may result in an unpalatably blunt discussion of their prospects, or disclosures of uncertainty that may undermine their faith in medical care.)

2 Many patients cannot give informed consent, e.g.:
   (a) children;
   (b) the mentally handicapped;
   (c) the mentally ill;
   (d) embryos.

Problems then arise when their basic human right to self-determination is transferred to someone else.

3 Although medical research is undertaken to improve the lot of individuals and society it does not necessarily result in unmitigated good; for example, perinatal expertise may help to preserve damaged babies—is this truly in the best interests of patient or society?

4 Doctors experience ethical qualms in conducting controlled and scientific research when they have reason to believe beforehand that one trial treatment is superior to another. This problem arose in the

Medical Research Council study undertaken in 1982 to establish whether vitamin supplements prevent spina bifida. Persuasive but inconclusive evidence had already suggested that this was so; under such circumstances randomisation causes much soul-searching. However, is it ethical to prescribe *any* treatment without doing everything possible to assess its true worth?

5   Expensive medical research diverts funds from more easily treatable conditions; given limited resources someone must suffer in the short term in the expectation that more people will benefit in the longer term.

All medical research (other than simple audit activities) should be subject to the scrutiny of properly constituted local research ethics committees who, before granting their approval, weigh up such issues and consider how they might be addressed.

The most difficult dilemmas of all arise when research extends the realms of scientific possibility so far that they outstrip contemporary codes of morality. Embryo experimentation is a good example of this. Society has expressed great concern regarding the ethics of surrogacy, genetic engineering and experimentation on 'spare' embryos. There are many contentious issues, e.g.:

- When does life start?
- When does an embryo acquire rights?
- What are those rights and who speaks for them?
- How do we balance an embryo's rights against those of the prospective parents? And against the potential benefits that research brings to humanity?
- Is it acceptable for embryos to be implanted in a mother who bears no genetic relationship at all to them?
- Is it acceptable for spare embryos to be frozen for future use, or killed, or used as tissue for research?

These ethical waters are so murky that the Warnock committee, appointed by the Government to consider them, was unable to reach a unanimous view, and had instead to publish two minority reports expressing differing views. It seems unlikely that the medical profession alone will resolve these issues. Society as a whole must shoulder the responsibility of deciding where to draw the line.

For interested readers the ethics of medical research and informed consent are discussed in more depth in *Doctors' Dilemmas: Medical Ethics and Contemporary Science* by Phillips and Dawson (see Further Reading).

7.12 GP CONTRACTS

Terms of Service

At the time of writing, GPs are independent contractors to the NHS, i.e. they contract with the HA to provide a particular service to

Table 7.2 The GP's main terms of service with the HA.

Definition of a patient	Recorded by the HA as on the doctor's list (accepted and not cancelled, or within 14 days of application to cancel)
	Allocated to the GP by the Joint Allocation Committee
	Accepted as a temporary resident
	In the practice area and needing 'immediately necessary' treatment in an emergency
	Patients for whom he is acting as another doctor's deputy under terms of service
Number of patients	Not more than 3500 per partner (or up to 4500 for one partner in a group practice with an average ≤3500, temporary residents not included in this limit)
Terminating responsibility	By application to the HA: responsibility stops on the 8th day after application (unless the patient is being treated for something needing close supervision and reallocation is delayed)
	The same applies to accepted temporary residents
	For maternity patients *either* by the woman's consent *or* by representation to the HA who examines the grounds
	GPs may transfer their out-of-hours responsibility to another principal. The HA must agree, but will only refuse permission exceptionally
Service to patients	GPs must render all necessary and appropriate medical services of the type usually provided by GPs
	This includes referral (if needed) but contraceptive and non-urgent maternity services are not obligatory
	The *standard* is that normally exercised by his GP colleagues (i.e. he is expected to make judgements to the standard of a reasonable GP, not a hospital specialist)
	This specifically includes:
	• advice regarding general health, diet and use of tobacco, alcohol, drugs and solvents
	• preventive physical examinations
	• offering immunisation against measles, mumps, rubella, pertussus, polio, diphtheria and tetanus
Newly registered patients·	Must offer within 28 days of registration a written invitation to attend a health assessment consultation of defined content (see Table 8.2, p. 242)
	Patients can refuse
	If undertaken, the findings must be recorded, an assessment made and discussed with the patient
Patients aged 75 and over	GPs must invite those aged 75 and over annually to participate in a health assessment of defined content (see Table 8.2)
	They must include the offer to make a domiciliary visit
Practice premises	Must be 'proper' and open to HA inspection at reasonable times
	HA approval is needed regarding the place and time of any proposed changes to this
	Normally 'availability' is construed as:
	• 42 weeks in any year (for full-time doctors)
	• for not less than 26 h over 5 days in any such week
	• at times likely to be convenient to patients
	This includes time spent in clinics and home visiting, but not simply on call
	Those involved in training and approved health-related activities may be exempted from this rule to the extent of a day per week, while part-time principals may elect to be available to a lesser extent (either <26 h but not <19, or <19 h but not <13 h per week) with a suitable reduction in basic practice allowance

Continued

Table 7.2 *Continued*

	Patients attending the premises at the agreed times must be seen except where an appointment system exists, the patient has no appointment and the GP feels his medical condition can wait
Practice area	Is defined with the HA; further changes require HA approval
	An accepted patient is entitled to treatment at the GP's surgery, his registered address or (as required) elsewhere in the practice area, but not outside it unless the address accepted at registration is outside the boundary
Absences and deputies	GPs must arrange adequate emergency cover and take reasonable steps to ensure continuity of treatment
	They must notify the HA of deputising arrangements and obtain HA consent
	They must also notify the HA of cover arrangements if absent for more than a week
	He must also take reasonable steps to ensure his deputy is not disqualified by an HA or the General Medical Council. (There are also conditions attached to the employment of assistants)
Records	Must be adequate and on HA-supplied stationery
	Are the property of the HA and must be forwarded on request, within 14 days of being told of the patient's death by the HA, or within a month of otherwise knowing
Certification	Certain statutory certificates (e.g. incapacity for work, registered stillbirth, pregnancy certification, etc.) are a contractual obligation, and no separate fee can be accepted
Fees	For most NHS work the GP cannot accept a fee from the patient: private medical reports, examinations and certificates, and immunisations not recognized for reimbursement by the HA are important exceptions
Employees	GPs must take reasonable care to ensure employees are qualified and competent and allow them refresher training opportunities
Change of residence	Principals must notify the HA in writing within 28 days of moving house
Practice leaflet	Doctors on the medical list must compile a practice leaflet containing basic information specified by schedule (see Table 1.4, p. 47)
	This must be updated annually where appropriate, and made available to the HA and to the practice's patients
Annual reports	Doctors on the medical list must supply the HA with a confidential report containing basic information specified by schedule (see Table 1.3, p. 45), drawn up in the year ending 31 March and submitted by 30 June
Optional services	Separate medical lists are maintained for maternity, child health surveillance and minor surgery services
	Doctors must be suitably qualified and HA-approved
	Some activities are stipulated by schedule (e.g. minor surgery; see Table 1.7) while others are dictated on a local basis by HAs (e.g. child health surveillance)
Complaints procedure	Practices must have a local system for handling complaints that complies with national criteria (see Section 7.13); and GPs must co-operate in HA independent reviews when complaints are made against them
Local directory of principals	Doctors are obliged to provide sufficient information to enable HAs to compile and publish a local directory of family doctors, their qualifications, services and consulting arrangements (see Section 1.5)

patients accepted on to their list, but they do so on their own responsibility, and are largely free to run their business as they wish. HAs demands certain safeguards and standards that are defined by statute. The main points are summarised in Table 7.2. In return HAs contract to remunerate GPs in accordance with the nationally agreed Statement of Fees and Allowances (see Table 1.6, p. 56).

The independent contractor status has certain *advantages*, e.g.:
- greater variety and flexibility;
- both doctor and patient have a choice;
- GPs can influence their working conditions to a greater extent than as salaried employees;
- GPs are taxed as self-employed (Schedule D rather than Schedule E).

The chief *disadvantage* is that GPs, as managers, must assume administrative and financial responsibilities as well as clinical ones.

However, the 1996 Primary Care Bill introduced a number of alternative choices, such as a practice-based contract or a salaried contract (perhaps as a direct employee of an NHS trust). Change will require successful pilot schemes, but may herald the end of the independent contractor status, the national contract for GPs and the contractual terms and remuneration system described in Tables 7.2 & 1.6. (The proposals are described more fully on pp. 51 and 60).

Partnership agreements

According to the British Medical Association a sizeable number of practices have no formal written agreement. Partners are liable in law for one another's debts (especially tax liabilities), and practice disagreements are commonplace: on both scores a written contract is advisable.

The ingredients of a good partnership agreement include reference to:

1 The name of the parties.
2 The date their partnership commenced and the circumstances under which it can be dissolved.
3 The profit-sharing basis (ownership of premises and division of profits).
4 The division of expenses (including telephone, car, personal allowances and outside remunerations).
5 Basic working conditions, e.g.:
    (a) workload distribution;
    (b) holiday entitlement;
    (c) sick leave, study leave and maternity leave.
6 Practice policies, e.g.:
    (a) who signs the cheques;
    (b) who the practice solicitors/bankers/accountants are;
    (c) what private work and outside activity is allowable;

(d) how far partners can place restrictions on acceptance of patients.

7   Voting rights of the partners in policy changes.

8   Provision for arbitration.

9   The condition on an outgoing partner that he will not set up practice within a close (defined) radius of the present one. (There has been difficulty in enforcing this last item, and in defining equality of workload, and practices often omit to make provision for arbitration.)

Any working arrangement with third parties (e.g. out-of-hours co-operatives) should also be sealed by means of a formal legal agreement.

Commonly encountered problems include:

1   No written agreement to consult when there is disagreement.

2   A written contract different from the initial verbal offer.

3   Inequalities of workload or income contribution not reflected in partners' profit shares.

4   Unfairly restrictive clauses.

5   Disaffected ex-partners who set up practice down the road, taking their list with them.

Incoming partners can take advice from an independent solicitor and accountant, or seek guidance from the local medical council secretary, British Medical Association or other informed body. A correctly drafted agreement seeks to provide equity for all parties in all conceivable circumstances, and is in the interests of all partnerships with honourable intentions.

7.13 COMPLAINTS AGAINST GPS

The number of complaints against GPs has doubled over the last decade. In 1994, service committees investigated 1862 such complaints: 25% were upheld. The major cause of complaint was delay in or failure to make a diagnosis.

The complaints procedure was overhauled in 1996 to provide a unified system throughout the NHS. GPs are now required to establish a practice-based system for handling complaints that complies with national criteria. The idea is to resolve the majority of minor complaints and misunderstandings without recourse to formal HA investigation.

The practice complaints procedure

The practice complaints procedure must be publicised by means of a waiting room poster and information leaflet. This should identify a named practice complaints administrator, and explain to the patients who to speak to, and what to expect. In the event of complaint:

1   The complaints administrator should interview the complainant and explain:

(a) how the complaint will be dealt with;
(b) the likely timetable;
(c) the rules of confidentiality;
(d) the availability of help from the local Community Health Council;
(e) the possible outcomes;
(f) the availability of HA conciliation services;
(g) how to pursue the complaint with the HA if still dissatisfied;
(h) the time limit for making a complaint (normally within 12 months).

2 The complainant should receive a written acknowledgement within 2 working days.

3 The facts of the case should be established and recorded, together with a note of the action(s) taken.

4 The complaints administrator should share any findings with a designated partner.

5 For straightforward complaints a written response should be made within10 working days of contact. This would:
(a) summarise the complaint;
(b) explain the practice's view of the event;
(c) apologise, if appropriate;
(d) describe the outcome and steps taken;
(e) inform the complainant how to contact the HA if still unhappy.

6 The complaints procedure itself should be periodically audited.

7 Complaint statistics and corrective actions must be included in the practice's annual report. It would also be wise to keep careful individual records, including a patients' complaint register.

If a complainant wishes to pursue the issue beyond this system, GPs are obliged to co-operate with HAs in their complaint procedures.

The Health Authority complaint procedure

If called on, the HA may conduct an independent review. This will first consider whether options for a practice-based resolution have been exhausted; or whether to arrange conciliation; or whether no more can be done. An independent review panel has three members: a lay chairperson, another lay representative (both nominated by the Secretary of State), and a convenor (non-executive director of the HA). In clinical complaints the panel is helped by two Local Medical Committee-nominated clinical assessors.

There is no obligation to hold a formal hearing, or engage in lengthy evidence-gathering; but if dissatisfaction remains after the review, the complainant can make a further appeal to a Health Service Commissioner (Ombudsman).

Disciplinary hearings

If a GP is thought by the HA to be in breach of his terms of service, a separate disciplinary investigation may follow. The panel for this hearing will include a legally trained chairperson, three lay members and three LMC-nominated GPs (from another area). The process will normally be completed within 6 weeks.

The hearing differs from a court of law in that:
- neither side can have a paid professional advocate (though the GP can be represented by his defence union or a friend);
- witnesses can be called, but are not compelled to attend;
- no one is under oath;
- members of the panel can question anyone attending.

If the GP is thought to be in breach of his terms of service, the panel may recommend:
- a caution;
- a fine;
- a restriction on the number of patients on the GP's list;
- referral to the General Medical Council or NHS tribunal (for possible removal from the medical list);
- rehabilitation, retraining or additional support.

The GP has the right of appeal against the verdict, and can make representation to the Secretary of State.

In 1996 the GMC produced a package of related documents identifying good medical practice and spelling out the duties of a doctor (Table 7.3). The guidance highlights some of the issues likely to be considered, and perhaps more important, a wider framework of values to which doctors should aspire ethically and professionally.

Table 7.3 The duties of a doctor (adapted from the GMC document *Duties of a Doctor* (1996)).

A doctor must . . .	Some Clinical requirements	Some Professional/ethical requirements
Provide a good standard of clinical care	Proper assessment, treatment and referral; accurate records; correct prescribing	To take due account of efficacy and resource costs
Provide treatment in an emergency	To the best of his abilities	To treat anyone in immediate danger
Keep up to date	Read professional journals	To participate in Continuing Medical Education and audit
Maintain a proper relation to patients	Listen to patients' views; give them information; respect their right to be involved in decision-making; be accessible	To be polite and considerate; to respond to complaints and criticism; to respect patients' privacy and dignity, and their right to refuse treatment, research and teaching; not to allow personal prejudices to influence treatment

Continued on p. 236

Table 7.3 *Continued*

A doctor must . . .	Some Clinical requirements	Some Professional/ethical requirements
Respect patient confidentiality		
Not abuse his professional position	Not recommend investigation or treatment known not to be in the patient's best interest; or to deliberately withhold necessary treatment, investigation or referral	Not to establish improper personal relationships with his patients; or press patients to donate money or benefits
Protect patients against improper conduct by colleagues	Find out the facts; consult an experienced colleague	To be honest; to remember that patient safety comes first
Consider whether his own health puts patients at risk	Consult an occupational health consultant or other suitably qualified specialist; undertake any necessary tests and act on the advice given	To be honest and to remember that patient safety comes first
Work appropriately with other health care professionals	Keep colleagues well informed when care is shared; work constructively in teams; delegate only to those that are competent for the task; make clear arrangements for hand-over and communication; refer with all relevant information	Not to discriminate against or disparage colleagues; to respect the skills of others; to ensure the whole team is polite, effective and confidential
Ensure equitable access to medical care		To always determine management priorities solely on the basis of clinical need
Display financial probity and avoid conflicts of interest	Grants and hospitality may be accepted if the main purpose is educational and the amount accepted proportionate	Not to ask for or accept inducements/hospitality that may affect (or appear to affect) judgement; to only countersign documents and certificates believed to be true
Advertise fairly and appropriately		(See section 7.15)
Only undertake ethical research	Ensure research is not contrary to the patient's clinical interests and that the protocol has been vetted by a proper research ethics committee; record findings truthfully and not make unjustified claims	To accept only payments approved by the ethics committee; not to allow one's conduct to be influenced by payments or gifts

The Consumer Protection Act makes producers of defective products strictly liable for any harm caused, without need on the part of the injured party to prove carelessness or negligence in a law suit.

Normally in the event of mishap due to defective drugs and medical appliances the onus of liability falls on the *manufacturer*. However, if the manufacturer of personally administered emergency medicine cannot be identified the Consumer Production Act places liability on the immediate *supplier*, i.e. the doctor himself.

The defence unions counsel that GPs should protect themselves through:

- proper container labelling;
- proper patient records;
- a separate personal record of the event, enabling the manufacturer or doctor's supplier to be identified (e.g. a log including data, patient's name, name of the drug, manufacturer's name, batch number and name of immediate supplier).

It is a hard but necessary fact of life that busy doctors need, at anti-social times and in emergency situations, to keep meticulous medico-legal records.

7.15 SHOULD DOCTORS ADVERTISE?

In 1989 the Monopolies and Mergers Commission decided that certain of the restrictions on advertising of medical services were anti-competitive and against the public interest. GPs have been allowed to advertise, subject to two broad caveats:

1 That advertising should not be of a form likely to bring the profession into disrepute.

2 That it should not abuse the trust of patients or exploit their vulnerability or lack of knowledge.

Thus, advertising should not disparage other doctors, or claim superiority over them, or include specific claims of cure. 'Cold calling' and undue pressure from over-frequent advertising are discouraged, and adverts are expected to conform to recognised standards — namely, that they are 'legal, decent and honest'.

Possible outlets for advertising include:

- the local media (newspapers, parish magazines, notice boards);
- yellow pages;
- mail shots.

Potential advantages

1 *To the consumer*: more information available when choosing a doctor.

2   *To doctors*: the opportunity to publicise their hard work and facilities and to be rewarded by higher capitation fees.

3   *To the tax-payer*: competition between doctors may raise standards of care and value for money.

Potential disadvantages

1   *To the patient*: choices made on the basis of this information may be shallow, as patients are not well placed to judge clinical competence. Efforts may be wasted providing gloss rather than substance. It has been suggested that the doctor–patient relationship is an impartial one, sometimes demanding the disclosure of unpalatable opinions, and that this is fundamentally incompatible with self-promotion and self-interest on the doctor's part.

2   *To the doctor*: the profession has misgivings that the code of good conduct will be difficult to police and ripe for exploitation.

3   *To the tax-payer*: the tax-payer ultimately funds advertising by doctors, as costs form part of the practice expenses pool.

A keen debate continues.

8 Schedules and Advice

The purpose of this chapter is two-fold:

1 To present, mainly in tabular form, a lot of basic factual information that may be of help in Paper 2 of the MRCGP examination, as well as the vivas. The first part of the chapter tackles this and is very straightforward.

2 To cover some common clinical situations where GPs are required to give advice.

You can be sure that the examiners will be interested in establishing that you can give sensible and lucid advice to, say, the diabetic or epileptic, the foreign traveller, the driver and the asthmatic. Questions like this crop up in the viva (see Chapter 10). A good answer encompasses not just the traditionally taught physical aspects of the problem, but psychological and social ones, and examples are given to illustrate this point.

It is difficult to know where to begin and end, because effective communication is germane to every clinical contact and likely to appear under many guises in the examination. I would therefore encourage you to supplement the advice section liberally with your own examples.

It is a good principle to consider after every consultation how advice given could have been better phrased and delivered. Probably, if you get into this habit, you will handle this aspect of the examination more competently.

8.1 SCHEDULES

Developmental milestones
Some milestones have well established predictive reliability (e.g. sitting unsupported—90% at 8 months; using 2–3-word combinations—90% at 24 months). Others have a wide range and may follow a particular pattern in families.

Developmental schedules
Developmental schedules widely used include:
• the Mary Sheridan developmental sequence (the 'average child at key ages' approach);
• the Denver screening test (the ages at which 25–90% of normals pass).
    The key areas assessed are:
• vision;
• hearing;
• communication (comprehension and speech);

- social behaviour;
- neurological development (reflexes, gross motor movements, fine control and co-ordination).

Table 8.1 is a simplified description of some of the more memorable developmental milestones in the average child.

Well-person medical assessments

Two particular well-person assessments are required under GPs' Terms of Service. These contractual obligations are described in Section 1.5 and in Table 7.2 (pp. 230–231) and their clinical merit is considered in Section 3.3. Table 8.2 outlines the *content* of these scheduled examinations.

Immunisation

Types of vaccine

1 Toxoids, e.g. diphtheria, tetanus.

2 Inactivated vaccines, e.g. pertussis, typhoid, anthrax and rabies.

3 Live vaccines — all viral (measles, rubella, polio, yellow fever) except BCG.

Spacing and timing of vaccinations

At birth there is some passive immunity acquired when maternal antibodies cross the placenta. At the same time the baby's own immune

Table 8.1 Some common developmental milestones.

Age	Skills
2–4 weeks	Watches mother carefully when she speaks
4 weeks	Able to lift head from a surface
6 weeks	On ventral suspension, head held up on the same plane as body
	When pulled to sitting, marked but not complete headlag
	Can follow objects 1 m away over an angle of at least 90°
	Reacts to loud noises with a startle response
	Has the primitive reflexes (Moro, walking and grasp)
	Smiles (lack of a social smile by 12 weeks needs investigation)
	Gross symmetrical movements, but no fine ones
6–8 weeks	Vocalises when talked to
	Eyes follow a moving person
12 weeks	When pulled to sitting, only slight headlag
	Will hold a rattle placed in the hand
12–16 weeks	Turns head to sounds on a level with the ear
5 months	No headlag
	Able to reach for an object and get it
	When prone, takes weight on forearms
5–6 months	Rolls over (supine to prone)
6 months	Sits supported
	When prone, takes weight on hands with arms extended
	Takes weight on legs if held up
	Begins to imitate
	Transfers a cube from one hand to the other
	Person preference developed

Continued

Table 8.1 *Continued*

Age	Skills
7 months	Feeds self with a biscuit
	Turns head to sounds below the level of the ear
8 months	Sits unsupported (75–90%)
	Picks up a raisin with a raking action (75–90%)
	(50–75% have hand transfer and finger–thumb grasp)
9 months	Crawls on abdomen
9–10 months	Plays 'peep-bo'
	Afraid of strangers
10 months	Creeps on hands and knees
	Pulls himself up to sitting
	Finger–thumb apposition and index-finger approach
	Waves bye-bye
	Plays patacake
	Assists dressing by offering an arm or foot
11 months	One word with meaning
	Walks holding on to furniture or with two hands held
12 months	2–3 words with meaning
	Walks when one hand is held
13 months	Walks unsupported (normal range 12–15 months)
15 months	Feeds himself from an ordinary cup
	Takes shoes off
	Builds a 2-cube tower
18 months	Manages a spoon
	Builds a 3–4-cube tower
	Points to three parts of the body
	Can climb stairs when one hand is held
	10–12 words with meaning
	Jumps using both feet
	Asks for the potty
21–24 months	Joins 2–3 words to make a simple sentence
2 years	Runs without too many falls
	Can kick a ball or stoop and pick an object up while keeping his balance
	Builds a tower of 6–7 cubes
	Points to four parts of the body
	Puts on and takes off shoes and socks
	Speech is intelligible to friends and neighbours
	Tolerates children playing alongside him
2½–3 years	90% can scribble
	15–20% of parents express concern regarding negative behaviour (temper tantrums, breath-holding spells and other outbursts and battles)
3 years	Plays with other children
	Can stand for a short period on one leg
	Can count up to three objects and state age and sex
4 years	Play is highly imaginative
	90% can:
	• jump with feet together
	• pedal a tricycle
	• wash and dry their hands
	• copy a circle
	• give their first and last names
5 years	Can generally hop on one foot and count 10–12 objects

Table 8.2 Requirements of the specified medical assessments.

Newly registered patients
1   Consultation to establish relevant past medical and family history, including:

Medical factors	*Social factors*	*Lifestyle factors*
Illnesses	Employment	Diet and exercise
Immunisations	Housing	Smoking
Allergies	Family circumstances	Alcohol and drug abuse
Hereditary factors		
Screening tests		
Current health		
Medication		

2   Check of height, weight, blood pressure, urinalysis

3   Recording and discussing findings, giving appropriate advice

Over-75s
1   An annual invitation to consult, and offer of a domiciliary visit

2   Assessment, recording and discussion of matters relevant to health, including:
   (a) sensory function
   (b) mobility
   (c) mental condition
   (d) physical condition (including continence)
   (e) social environment
   (f) use of medicines

system is immature, so babies are not vaccinated at birth. (An exception is BCG vaccination given when a close household member has tuberculosis.)

By 6 months passive immunity is lost and host immunity is in the ascendance. Somewhere in between these two dates the first triple and oral polio are given, representing a compromise whereby maximum effect from vaccination is traded against the increasing vulnerability to infection as passive immunity wanes. Pertussis antibody (an IgM antibody) is too large to cross the placenta, so young unimmunised infants are particularly prone to this infection. Measles antibodies are slower to be catabolized and the longer duration of immunity allows vaccination to be deferred.

Until fairly recently it was advised that the optimum immune response for most vaccines required booster doses at approximately 6 weeks and then 6 months. However, the schedule for primary immunisation has been simplified (to start at 2 months with an interval of 1 month between each booster dose) because:

•   experience showed antibody responses to be perfectly adequate when the faster, simpler schedule was used (with fewer adverse reactions);

•   whooping cough and *Haemophilus influenza* Type b infections are most dangerous in the very young;

•   the old regimen was protracted, variable between authorities, and confusing, thus hindering uptake by highly mobile parents with young families.

In general, live vaccines have a prolonged duration of protection because they are more antigenic, and so booster doses are less important. (At first sight polio is an exception, since primary immunisation follows the usual three-dose pattern: in fact three different strains of virus are employed, and so three spaced vaccinations are needed to ensure that antibody responses do not interfere with one another.) It is from these principles that the familiar immunisation schedules are constructed (Table 8.3).

Incomplete courses sometimes cause confusion. Generally speaking:
1   If only one dose is given, a further two doses with a month's gap between them will complete the course.
2   If two doses have been given, the third will still be effective if given within 12 months of the second.

Contraindications to live viruses
1   Acute febrile illness;
2   Pregnancy;
3   Within 3 weeks of another live vaccine (except in emergency vaccination programmes);
4   Immunosuppression (e.g. immunodeficiency states, malignancy, cytotoxic treatment, radiotherapy, steroids).

N.B. Being human immunodeficiency virus (HIV)-positive is not a contraindication to measles, mumps, rubella and polio (but yellow fever and BCG should not be given).

Points of importance individual to particular vaccines
1   *Diphtheria*. A safe vaccine. May cause transient local tenderness/

Table 8.3 A common immunisation schedule.

Age	Vaccination	Route
2 months	DTP	0.5 ml i.m./deep s.c.
	Hib	0.5 ml i.m./deep s.c.
	Plus polio	Oral (3 drops)
3 months	As above (2nd dose)	As above
4 months	As above (3rd dose)	As above
12–15 months	MMR	0.5 ml i.m./deep s.c.
3–5 years	DT plus polio (booster)	As above
	MMR (2nd dose)	
10–14 years	BCG (it tuberculin negative)	0.1 ml i.d.
13–18 years	Td and polio (boosters)	As above
	MMR*	

*If not previously vaccinated.
DTP, diptheria/tetanus/pertussis; DT, diptheria/tetanus; Td, adsorbed tetanus/ low dose diphtheria vaccine for adults; MMR, measles/mumps/rubella.

redness. A low dose booster has been introduced for school leavers, to counter the resurgence of infection in Eastern Europe.

2 *Tetanus.* Also causes occasional local reactions of a minor nature. Rarely a hypersensitivity response when injections are too frequent. A reinforcing dose 10 years after the primary course, and another 10 years later maintains levels of protection that are probably life-long.

3 *Pertussis.* Causes local reactions and mild fever/irritability. Encephalopathy and convulsions are very rare (about 1 in 300000 vaccinations). Guidelines on the vaccine have recently been re laxed.

A severe local/general/neurological reaction last time is still an absolute contraindication, and so is an evolving neurological problem; but the former restrictions in children with a personal or close family history of epilepsy, and children with neonatal cerebral damage have been lifted. Stable neurological conditions such as cerebral palsy and spina bifida do not contraindicate the vaccine either, and it can be given despite a history of febrile fits with appropriate advice on fever control. It has been estimated that 3.5% will receive an incomplete course due to problems arising from the first or second injection (Jelley & Nicoll 1984).

4 *Polio.* Contraindicated in cases of allergy to penicillin, streptomycin, neomycin and polymyxin, but only in cases of extreme hypersensitivity. Very rarely causes vaccine-related paralysis in recipients or contacts (a risk perhaps of one per million doses).

5 *Hib.* Vaccine efficacy exceeds 95%. In up to 10% of first doses redness and swelling occur at the injection site, but resolve within a day. Rarely a severe local or general reaction occurs, and this precludes a booster dose. Hib is not a live vaccine. There is no present information on its safety in pregnancy.

6 *BCG.* Sometimes causes local reactions, including discharging skin ulcers and subcutaneous abscess formation. Contraindicated when there is local sepsis.

7 *Rubella.* May give a mild rubella-syndrome around day 9, arthralgia in women, and rarely thrombocytopenia. Contraindicated when there is a history of anaphylaxis to polymyxin or neomycin. There is a risk of fetal damage in the first trimester, so pregnancy is contraindicated and effective contraception advised for 2 months.

8 *Measles, mumps and rubella (MMR).* The vaccine may cause irritability (1–6%), fever (5–15%), conjunctivitis (2%) or a rash (1–5%) after about a week, lasting about 2–3 days. Parotid swelling occurs in 1% in the third week. This condition is not infectious. Anaphylaxis or serious allergic reaction can occur (1 in 65000). Thrombocytopenia (1 in 30000) and arthopathy have also rarely been described, and older MMR vaccines were rarely linked with mumps meningitis. Contraindications are those for live vaccines; also, allergy to neomycin or kanamycin, and a history of anaphylaxis after eating egg products (milder egg allergy is not a contraindication). If MMR is given to adult women, pregnancy should be avoided for 1 month.

The recent national immunisation campaign, which covered 8 million children aged 5–16 (92% coverage), reduced susceptibility to measles in the target population by 85%, so few confirmed cases now occur. The rate of mumps infection (formerly the cause of 1200 hospital admissions a year, and of permanent sensorineural deafness, meningitis and encephalitis) also fell dramatically.

Recently evidence has begun to accrue about a potential link between MMR and Crohn's disease. So fas this has not been considered sufficient to halt planned immunisation programmes, but there is some concern and plans to evaluate the link more thoroughly.

Vaccination for foreign travel

Recommendations
Recommendations change from time to time, so it is important to keep abreast of the latest ones, which are published regularly in the medical press. The current Red Book vaccination recommendations (accepted for reimbursement) are listed in Table 8.4.

Reimbursement
Reimbursement comes from two sources:
1   *The Health Authority*: for vaccinations given in accordance with the Red Book recommendations (as above).
2   *The patient* for:
    (a) vaccines and the service (if outside the HA guidelines);
    (b) private prescriptions related to foreign travel (prescriptions issued solely for the purpose of foreign travel, as distinct from normal maintenance prescribing, should be *private* prescriptions);
    (c) summary certificates.

Vaccination schedules
Vaccination schedules depend on the countries being visited, the

Table 8.4 Red Book vaccination recommendations.

Area	Vaccinations
Northern Europe, Southern Europe (excluding Turkey), North America, Australia, New Zealand and Japan	No specific needs Update standard domestic vaccinations, e.g. tetanus For special high-risk groups ('living rough') polio, typhoid, tetanus or human immunoglobulin
Turkey	Polio
Central and South America, Central Africa	Polio, typhoid, yellow fever (mandatory)
Middle East, North Africa, South Africa, India, South-East Asia and China	Polio, typhoid

Table 8.5 Full and rapid vaccination schedules for foreign travel.

Time	Vaccination
Full schedule	
First visit	Typhoid 0.5 ml deep s.c./i.m* *plus*
	Tetanus 0.5 ml deep s.c./i.m.
	Polio 3 drops p.o.
3 weeks (if visiting a yellow fever area)	Yellow fever 0.5 ml s.c. (from specialist centre)
4–6 weeks (must be 6 if yellow fever given)	Typhoid 0.1 ml i.d.† (booster)
	(Polio 3 drops p.o. —if part of a primary immunisation course)
7–9 weeks (and 2–4 days before travel)	Human normal immunoglobulin 0.5 ml deep i.m.
(6–8 months later)	(Further tetanus and polio boosters if part of a primary immunisation course)
Rapid schedule	
Day 1	Typhoid, tetanus and polio (as above)
Day 5	Yellow fever (as above—if applicable)
Day 13	(polio booster if part of a primary immunisation course)
Day 28	Typhoid booster† (and tetanus/polio if part of a primary immunisation programme)

(In a true emergency, even the last visit can be omitted, since one typhoid injection gives reasonable immunity)

*Oral vaccine also available for patients over 6 years. One capsule alternate days for 3 doses (spaced 3 weeks from oral polio).
†Whole cell vaccine (the Vi polysaccharide antigen vaccine is a single dose).

Table 8.6 Details relating to specific vaccines used in foreign travel.

Vaccine	Spacing	Side-effects	Contraindications	Efficacy
Polio	If visiting polio-endemic countries	Rarely paralysis in recipients or contacts	Those for any live vaccine	Excellent
Tetanus	5- to 10-yearly	Rare hypersensitivity reactions with too frequent boosters	A tetanus injection within the last year	Excellent
		Transient local pain		
Typhoid	If 3 years or more since last one (*not* after age 35 years)	Local redness and swelling; malaise, nausea, fever, headache—36 h Rare neurological complications	Not under the age of 12 months	70–90% effective for 3–7 years
Yellow fever	10-yearly (certificate valid from 10 days to 10 years)	Rare—sometimes redness/ swelling; myalgia and headache (5–10 days) Rare encephalitis in the under-1-year-olds	Not under the age of 12 months; those for any live virus; egg hypersensitivity	Very good

degree of risk of contracting the disease and the amount of time left before travel. Full and abridged schedules appear in Table 8.5. (Abridged schedules are a compromise, affording reasonable protection when time is short.)

Table 8.7 Incubation and infectivity periods of communicable diseases.

(a) Incubation periods

Disease	Range: max. (days)	Usual (if different)
Short incubation (<7 days)		
Bacillary dysentery	1–7	2–4
Gonorrhoea	1–12	2–6
Influenza	18h to 3 days	18–36h
Anthrax	1–7	1–3
Cholera	Hours to 6 days	2–3h
Diphtheria	2–5	1–7
Scarlet fever	1–3	—
Intermediate incubation (7–21 days)		
Chickenpox	10–21	14–17
Measles	7–14	9–11
Mumps	12–21	18
Whooping cough	7–10	7
Tetanus	1–14	4–13
Rubella	14–21	18
Amoebiasis	14–28	21
Malaria	10–14	—
Polio	3–21	7–14
Typhoid	7–21	10
Long incubation (>21 days)		
Infectious mononucleosis	4–6 weeks	—
Hepatitis A	2–6 weeks	4 weeks
Hepatitis B	6 weeks to 12 months	12 weeks

(b) Infectivity periods

Disease	*Infectivity period*
Scarlet fever	10–21 days after rash onset (but only 1 day if penicillin given)
Chickenpox	5 days before rash until 6 days after the last crop
Measles	From onset of prodromal illness to 4 days after the rash onset
Mumps	3 days before salivary swelling to 7 days after
Whooping cough	7 days after exposure to 3 weeks after onset of symptoms (but only 7 days if antibiotics given)
Rubella	7 days before onset of rash to 4 days after

(c) Interval between disease onset and rash

Disease	*Interval in days*
Scarlet fever	1–2
Chickenpox	0–2
Measles	3–5
Rubella	0–2
Typhoid	7–14

Points of importance relating to specific vaccines
See Table 8.6.

Incubation and infectivity periods of communicable diseases
For details see Table 8.7.

8.2 ADVICE

Medical advice to travellers

Medical contraindications to flight

Physiological problems produced by air flights include:

1 Reduced atmospheric pressure: aircraft cabins are not pressurised to sea level, and cabin pressure drops with ascent until about 7000 feet, hence gas trapped in body cavities *expands*.

2 Hypoxia: reduced atmospheric pressure means a reduced partial pressure of oxygen (Po_2). At 6000 feet oxyhaemoglobin is reduced by 3–4% — a small amount if you are healthy, but not if you are an unhealthy hypoxia-sensitive individual.

3 An upset in the normal circadian rhythms (jet lag).

Other problems can arise from the risk of spreading contagious disease in a confined space, and the impossibility of providing anything other than the most basic medical care during travel.

Most of the contraindications can be remembered by applying these principles in a common sense way. The following is a simple *aide-mémoire*

This problem . . .	*. . . may exacerbate these conditions*
Expansion of gas trapped in body cavities	Asthmatic attack
	Recent middle ear disease, middle ear surgery, and sinusitis with catarrh
	Unresolved pneumothorax
	Recent chest surgery (within 3 weeks)
	Recent abdominal surgery (within 10 days)
	Diving (if within 12 h for aqualung divers or 24 h if diving depth is more than 100 feet)
Hypoxia	Recent myocardial infarction (within 3–6 weeks)
	Uncontrolled cardiac failure
	Severe anaemia (e.g. haemoglobin less than 7 g/dl)
	Severe respiratory disease
	Recent cerebrovascular accident (within 3–6 weeks)
	Sickle cell disease
Spread of infection in a confined space	Contagious diseases in their infectivity period
Remoteness from medical care	Recent gastrointestinal haemorrhage
	Pregnancy (after 35 weeks for long flights and after 36 weeks for domestic ones)
	Acute mental illness (unless the patient is escorted and sedation is to hand)

Motion sickness

1 *Who?* One-third of the populus, especially children (peak age 10 years).

2 *What?* Various symptoms, including: pallor; cold sweats; nausea and vomiting; malaise; yawning; headaches; drowsiness.

3 *Why?* Probably multifactorial, but a mismatch between motion information from the eyes and vestibular apparatus/proprioceptors is the main stimulus.

4 *Advice?*

    (a) sit children up high, so they can see out;

    (b) provide good ventilation;

    (c) provide activities (e.g. games), but no reading;

    (d) limit alcohol intake;

    (e) if severe, lie down with eyes closed;

    (f) choose the most stable part of the vehicle to sit (car—front seat; boat—the middle; plane—between the wings).

5 *Drugs?*

    (a) take preparations 1–2 h prior to travel (otherwise absorption may be impaired).

    (b) either an anticholinergic or antihistamine. Anticholinergics are very effective, but associated with more side-effects. The antihistamines offer a choice in the duration of action (e.g. cyclizine—short-acting; promethazine — once-daily preparation). Tailor the time course of the drug to the duration of travel.

Jet lag

1   *What?* An upset in the circadian rhythms (e.g. sleep cycle; hunger pattern; bowel and urinary habits). Occurs if the time difference is greater than 5 h. *Less* marked when the day *lengthens* (i.e. going westwards).

2 *Advice?*

    (a) avoid unnecessary stress (e.g. arrive in good time);

    (b) avoid smoking, food and alcohol;

    (c) maintain a good fluid intake (non-diuretic beverages);

    (d) sleep on the plane if you can;

    (e) allow an easy first 24 h to adjust after arrival. Remember that performance may be impaired for a week after travel (businessmen beware!).

Food hygiene

1 *The problem.* Food-borne and water-borne infections, e.g.:

    (a) contaminated drinking water may transmit *Escherichia coli*, *Shigella*, cholera, typhoid, hepatitis A, amoebic dysentery or giardiasis;

    (b) poultry are notorious sources of *Campylobacter* and *Salmonella*;

    (c) shellfish may transmit typhoid;

(d) unpasteurised milk is a possible source of tuberculosis, brucellosis, and Q fever.

2 *Advice?*

(a) boil drinking water or chlorinate it (remember—all water);

(b) avoid unpasteurized milk;

(c) do not buy food or ice-cream from street vendors;

(d) avoid salads and unpeeled fruit and vegetables;

(e) eat only food that has been recently cooked (and is hot and steaming);

(f) be wary of seafood, especially shellfish.

Other precautions for travellers

Table 8.8 summarises some of the more common hazards and strategies for reducing the risk.

Table 8.8 Common holiday hazards and how to avoid them.

Problem	Advice
Sunburn	Limit the exposure in very hot climates to 15 min at first, doubled each day thereafter (longer if sunscreens are used, less if fair-skinned and sun-sensitive) Avoid the midday sun Reapply sunscreens after bathing
Prickly heat (a pinhead itchy rash due to keratin plugs blocking sweat ducts which extravasate sweat into the tissues). Mainly in areas of non-evaporation (chest, back, axillae and groins)	Maintain a high fluid and salt intake Reduce sweating, e.g.: • wear loose cotton clothes • swim and shower often • keep in the shade and limit exertion • use the room-fan, if one is provided Dust with talc or apply calamine. Antihistamines for the itching
Insect-borne infections (many problems from local reactions through to rickettsial infections and leishmaniasis!)	Wear long-sleeved shirt and long trousers after dark Do not walk barefoot Use any mosquito net provided Apply insect repellent to *all* exposed skin
Sexually transmitted diseases	Barrier contraception and post-coital douching or micturition offer some partial protection. The high prevalence of AIDS in parts of Central and East Africa and North America makes causal sex very risky: it should be avoided
Accidents	Common sense precautions (e.g. do not drink to excess; do not approach stray animals; drive with extra care) Take important spares (contact lenses, dentures, asthma inhaler, diaphragm, etc.) Arrange adequate medical insurance. Leaflet T1 (DSS) lists countries with reciprocal health care arrangements
Travel vaccinations	Covered separately in Table 8.5, but remember: • consult the latest guidelines • allow adequate time to complete the course

1 *General advice.* The standard insect bite avoidance advice (Table 8.9) is appropriate. Also:

(a) start tablets 1 week before departure and continue for at least 4 (possibly 6) weeks after return;

(b) if you omit any doses, you are taking a risk;

(c) drugs are prophylactic, not curative; furthermore protection is probably only 60–90%, so report fevers within 2 months of return.

2 *Drugs.* The appropriate choice is not straightforward. Recommendations change frequently, so get up-to-date information from an expert source. Two currently favoured preparations are compared in Table 8.9.

Traveller's diarrhoea

1 *Where?* World-wide, but most commonly in Africa and Asia.

2 *What?* 70% of cases are due to enterotoxic *E. coli* strains; other culprits include *Campylobacter*, rotavirus, *Salmonella*, *Shigella*, *Amoeba* and *Giardia*.

Symptoms, which usually only last a few days, include:

(a) nausea and vomiting;

(b) colic;

(c) watery diarrhoea.

3 *Drugs?*

(a) *Prophylactic antibiotics* (e.g. Streptotriad and doxycycline) have been shown to be beneficial but consideration of possible side-effects and drug resistance suggests they are best reserved for the elderly, infirmed and high-risk cases.

(b) *In treatment.* Lomotil or Imodium will reduce stool frequency and abdominal pain, and Septrin/trimethoprim reduces symptoms considerably if taken early. The mainstay of treatment, however, is fluid replacement. Electrolyte mixtures are very useful.

Table 8.9 Two common antimalarial preparations.

Preparation	Form	Availability	Contraindications	Efficacy	Side-effects
Chloroquine	300 mg base/week	No script needed	—	Very good vs. *vivax*, but not *falciparum*	Chronic use can produce corneal and retinal changes
Mefloquine	250 mg T/week	Prescription only	Past neuropsychiatric history e.g. depression, convulsions	90–100%. Effective against *falciparum*	Neuropsychiatric (1 in 10 000), including depression, anxiety, paranoia, hallucinations

(c) *medical advice* may be needed in severe cases (prostration, severe vomiting, fever, and blood per rectum) and for the very young.

Medical advice on fitness to drive

Medical fitness to drive is a favourite examination topic. Some of the more important aspects are summarised in Table 8.10, which is adapted from the definitive and detailed account *Medical Aspects of Fitness to Drive* published by the Medical Commission on Accident Prevention.

Table 8.10 Medical advice on fitness to drive.

Disease or symptoms	Advice to the holder of an ordinary driver's licence	Advice to the holder of an HGV or PSV licence
Cardiovascular system		
Myocardial infarction	Avoid driving within 1 month (no need to notify the DVLA)	Avoid driving for 3 months. Then must be: • symptom-free • able to complete an exercise ECG to a defined standard* • free from angina or heart failure Coronary angiograms are no longer required for licensing
Angina	Avoid driving if angina is easily provoked by it	There should be no anginal pains at all
Arrhythmia	Arrhythmias that distract or affect consciousness must be controlled. After pacemaker implantation driving is allowed (from 1 month) as long as the pacemaker function is checked regularly	Driving is forbidden for persistent or recurrent arrhythmias or conduction defects in the past 5 years *if* these have suddenly impaired consciousness in the last 2 years; *or* there are echocardiography or exercise test* abnormalities
Transient faintness, impaired concentration, syncopal tendency, postural hypotension	If sudden or disabling, avoid driving until the problem is resolved	Depends on the cause but generally driving is not allowed if sudden or disabling syncopal attacks occur
Other problems	Heart surgery, aortic aneurysms, hypertension, cardiomyopathy, peripheral vascular disease, valvular lesions and arrhythmias—no special restrictions (unless they provoke the problems covered above). At least 1 week off after coronary angioplasty	Several conditions cause a ban on driving, e.g. • unrepaired aortic aneurysm • blood pressure $\geqslant 200/110$ mmHg • valvular heart disease with embolism, arrhythmias or ventricular hypertrophy • some exclusions after heart surgery

Continued

Table 8.10 *Continued*

Disease or symptoms	Advice to the holder of an ordinary driver's licence	Advice to the holder of an HGV or PSV licence
Endocrine/metabolic system Diabetes	Notify the DVLA if managed with tablets or insulin. A limited licence will normally be issued in insulin-dependent diabetics, and they particularly should show: • a reasonable understanding • reasonable control of their blood sugar • recognise warning signs of hypoglycaemia	*Insulin treated*: New applicants and existing drivers who become insulin-dependent are barred. Drivers licensed before April 1991 may continue subject to satisfactory annual consultant certification *Other diabetics*: May be licensed unless they develop insulin-dependence or develop eye complications affecting their visual fields or visual acuity
	For all driving diabetics All diabetics must meet visual standards. Driving should be avoided (or carbohydrate taken) at times when hypoglycaemic risk is greatest. Drive by the clock and stop for regular meals. Carry sugar lumps or glucose tablets and at the first hint of hypoglycaemia pull over, switch off, take the ignition key out and vacate the driving seat (then take the sugar)	Advice to the holder of an ordinary driver's licence applies
Neurological system Epilepsy	Notify the DVLA. Under the Road Traffic Act 1988 a limited duration licence (usually 3 years) is granted, providing: • the patient has been fit-free during the previous year, or • has only had attacks while asleep for the last 3 years, *and* • is not likely to be a source of danger to the public	Road Traffic Act regulations bar a vocational licence if there is 'a liability to epileptic seizures'. The Honorary Medical Advisory Panel recommends that a driver would need to be fit-free and off treatment for at least 10 years, and have no continuing seizure vulnerability to qualify again.
1 If a further daytime fit occurs after a licence is granted	Another whole fit-free year must elapse	
2 During treatment changes	Epileptics are advised not to drive for 6 months	
3 The patient with a single fit (diagnosis in doubt)	One year off driving, with medical review before returning to the wheel	
4 After severe head injuries or intracranial haematomas	6–12 months off driving	Not recommended without specialist assessment (the epilepsy risk should not exceed 2%)
Craniotomy	Depending on cause, up to 1 year off driving	Depends on cause

Continued on p. 254

Table 8.10 *Continued*

Disease or symptoms	Advice to the holder of an ordinary driver's licence	Advice to the holder of an HGV or PSV licence
Migraine	Do not drive from the onset of the warning period	(No additional restrictions)
Sudden disabling giddiness/syncope (e.g. due to Meniere's disease, vertebrobasilar insufficiency)	Notify the DVLA which insists on control of symptoms, and may issue a short period licence	These patients are debarred from holding a vocational licence, unless their condition is stable and they have been symptom-free at least 1 year
Muscle weakness, post-CVA, TIAs, sensory defects, multiple sclerosis, Parkinson's disease	Individual assessment of competence and disability. At least 1 month off driving after a CVA	Persistent or recurrent deficits and most disorders of a progressive disabling nature result in a driving ban
Vision	All drivers must pass the standard number plate test: 3.5" figures at 25 yards in daylight: this is a visual acuity of about 6/10 (glasses are allowed). Significant disabilities (e.g. poor visual acuity, diplopia, impaired night vision) will normally debar. Special assessment and review are needed for prospective disabilities (e.g. field defects, cataracts, glaucoma, macular degeneration, diabetic retinopathy)	Uncorrected visual acuity must be at least 3/60 in each eye, and corrected must be 6/9 or better in one eye, and 6/12 in the other. Applicants with any field defect, or diplopia, or a single eye will be banned
Psychiatric aspects		
Psychosis	Should not drive until the illness is controlled; for 6 months after inpatient care; and not unless compliance with treatment is satisfactory and there is evidence of insight	Suspension of a licence for at least 3 years. May be possible then if stable, symptom-free, off treatment (except lithium), and assessed fit by a consultant psychiatrist
Neurosis	Should avoid driving in the early stages of a severe acute illness	Caution is advised. If severe, should be symptom-free for 6 months and not affected by drug therapy. Psychiatric reports may be required
Mental handicap	Depends on the severity of the handicap	If severe, an absolute ban. If slight, would need to demonstrate capability at the wheel
Alcoholism	The law on drinking and driving is clear: the legal blood alcohol limit is 80 mg/100 ml. In many road accidents alcohol plays a part, so do not drink and drive!	Not allowed within 1 year of significant alcohol abuse, or 3 years of alcohol dependency
Personality disorders	Together with drinkers account for more accidents than the other categories combined. Unlikely to accept advice	

Continued

Table 8.10 *Continued*

Disease or symptoms	Advice to the holder of an ordinary driver's licence	Advice to the holder of an HGV or PSV licence
Locomotor system	Largely a matter of common sense and individual assessment. Even amputees can drive safely in adapted vehicles. Prospective disabilities must be notified to the DVLA	The same is true, but assessment is likely to be more stringent
AIDS	Short period licence (1,2 or 3 years)	Barred from vocational driving. (No restriction for HIV, and no need to notify the DVLA)
Drugs CNS depressants (e.g. hypnotics, sedatives, neuroleptics, many antidepressants, antihistamines, anticholinergics, narcotic analgesia)	Impair motor skills and reaction time. Patients should exercise special care, especially when starting drugs for the first time. Sedation is potentiated by alcohol	In general, driving is excluded because of the medical condition for which the drug is taken. Also in general, taking CNS-active drugs, insulin and most hypotensive drugs is felt to be incompatible with vocational driving
Stimulants and appetite suppressants	Avoid driving: they promote risk-taking behaviour	
Anaesthetics	Patients should not drive for 24–48 h after anaesthesia for minor outpatient surgery	
Antihypertensives	May cause hypotension, sedation and fatigue. Exercise care at the outset of treatment	
Age	Drivers over 70 years have to renew their licence and make a health declaration every 3 years, but their insurance companies may demand annual medicals. Common diseases rendering the elderly unfit to drive include: TIAs, vertigo, syncope, arrhythmias, severe angina, Parkinson's disease and senile dementia. (Elderly drivers are advised to avoid peak traffic periods, overlong journeys and a lot of night-time driving)	Vocational drivers must reapply with medical confirmation of fitness at 45 years of age, 5-yearly to 65 years, then annually

HGV, Heavy goods vehicle; PSV, public service vehicle; DVLA, Driver and Vehicle Licensing Agency; TIAs, transient ischaemic attacks; CVA, cerebrovascular accident; CNS, central nervous system.

Note that according to the law:

1   It is the duty of the *applicant* (not his doctor) to declare:

(a) prescribed (relevant) disabilities, e.g. epilepsy and subnormality;

(b) intermittent or progressive disabilities which may become relevant (prospective disabilities).

2   Licence-holders are also obliged to notify the Driver and Vehicle Licensing Agency (DVLA) as soon as they develop relevant or prospective disabilities, and if a previously notified disability becomes worse.

3   Temporary disabilities (e.g. fractures) are excluded, if they are expected to last less than 3 months.

Failure of the licence-holder to notify the DVLA places the doctor in an awkward position, as he may regard the physical safety of other road users to be at risk. This is one of the acknowledged circumstances under which breach of confidentiality may be justified (see Section 7.10).

The Transport Act 1981 states that drivers and front-seat passengers must wear a seatbelt; children must sit in the back and wear seatbelts if fitted. Exemptions are allowed:

1   for drivers who have to get in and out frequently (e.g. from a milk float);

2   while carrying out manoeuvres (e.g. reversing);

3   for holders of medical exemption certificates. Since wearing a seatbelt reduces fatalities and injuries by 50%, very few conditions genuinely justify an exemption and very few exemptions have been approved. The following are *not* generally accepted:

(a) pregnancy;

(b) colostomies (seatbelts are adjustable);

(c) recent abdominal surgery (if a scar prevents the wearing of a seatbelt the person should not be driving).

Advising the person with epilepsy

Epilepsy is a very common problem. It is estimated that one in 20 people have a non-febrile seizure at some stage and one in 200 will have chronic epilepsy. In a practice list of 2000 this means 100 patients with a non-febrile seizure and 10 with epilepsy.

The psychological and social impact of the diagnosis may pose more problems than simple stabilisation to a fit-free state. Advice will be required on drugs and compliance, the likely restrictions on activity and employment, the genetic implications, and to the carers in the first-aid situation. Epileptics will need intensive education and emotional support. Some of these points are now considered.

Driving

Epileptics cannot legally drive until entirely fit-free for 1 year (or experiencing fits only while asleep for 3 years). People who have a 'liability to seizure' are ineligible to hold a vocational licence (to qualify they would need to be fit-free and off medication for 10 years; and have no underlying pathology). After a single fit it is recommended not to drive for a year, and not to resume until medically reviewed. Epileptics should not drive while treatment is being altered (see Table 8.10).

Work

Certain occupations exclude epileptic patients, for example air traffic controllers, the armed forces and police, those debarred by driving restrictions.

Activities

Most young epileptics risk being cocooned in a restrictive environment by overprotective relatives. Activities should be as free as possible with the exception of a few common sense guidelines:
- do not swim alone;
- do not climb trees/ropes or take up mountaineering;
- do not bathe babies whilst alone, etc.

Bicycle riding is generally felt to be an acceptable risk, and little restriction is advised on games and school activities.

Genetic advice

If one parent is epileptic the chance of producing an affected child is about 3% although there are some variations. The risk is higher if the epilepsy is idiopathic or generalised, and lower if focal or structural. However, it is still less than 5%, and therefore no reason to advise against child-bearing. The incidence of congenital malformation is increased from about 2.7 to 7.5% (though abnormalities are often mild).

Epileptics should continue taking their drugs in pregnancy. Although there is a small teratogenic potential, the risk to pregnancy is greater from uncontrolled epilepsy.

Some of the drugs used in treatment (e.g. carbamazepine, phenytoin, phenobarbitone) are potent inducers of liver microsomal enzymes and may interact with oral contraceptives, reducing their effectiveness (a high dose pill or barrier method may be required to avoid pregnancy).

First-aid advice

Simple guidelines are required to help carers cope with a frightening situation, e.g.:
- restrain the patient and prevent him from hurting himself;
- try to prevent him biting his tongue, by putting something in his mouth—this may not be possible in the tonic phase so do not force the issue (you may break his tooth!);
- if possible, try and move the patient into the recovery position;
- if in doubt, and particularly if the fit is prolonged, phone for medical assistance.

Emotional support and education

The patient should be treated as normally as possible. Remember that he (and especially his family) may be experiencing a variety of emotions, e.g.:

- anger and rejection;
- anxiety;
- a sort of bereavement reaction (following loss of health, job, etc.):
- shame or embarrassment.

Offer easy access and a sympathetic ear. Educate at every opportunity: referral to the British Epilepsy Association and books like *Epilepsy—the Facts* may help.

Follow-up

Well organised GPs are armed with a checklist of areas to cover (perhaps a flow sheet or co-operation card) and this may include such aspects as:

- drugs and compliance;
- side-effects;
- blood levels of drugs;
- control;
- social and psychological problems.

Treatment withdrawal

Patients who become seizure-free often want to discuss drug withdrawal. A prospective randomised study of 1013 patients has compared withdrawal with continued treatment. After 2 years 41% of those off treatment had suffered at least one further fit, as compared with 22% of those still taking medication. Recurrence was more likely in those who had previously required multi-drug therapy; those who had previously suffered tonic–clonic seizures; and those who had a shorter fit-free interval prior to treatment withdrawal. A recurrence probability model has been developed to help counsel patients contemplating drug withdrawal (MRC 1993).

Febrile convulsions

Febrile convulsions are very common. It has been estimated that 30 per 1000 children under 7 years have a seizure associated with a fever. (About 5 per 1000 have recurrent non-febrile seizures.) Febrile convulsions are very alarming for parents, who naturally suspect the unpalatable diagnosis of epilepsy or worse.

Characteristics of febrile convulsions include:

- association with fever;
- rarity after age 6 years;
- a strong genetic element (25% in siblings and 50% in identical twins).

The association seems to be with the *rise* in temperature rather than its absolute height.

First-aid measures designed to lower temperature include taking clothes off, sponging with tepid water, fanning and administering antipyretic drugs. Fits can be controlled with diazepam 0.2–0.3 mg/ kg i.v. or rectally. Many authorities would admit to hospital on the first occasion to rule out meningitis.

Parents' major concerns will be with the likelihood of recurrence and of the child being a long-term epileptic. The following information may be given:

1 About 30–40% have a recurrence.
2 Prophylactic medicines are generally disappointing; they may have significant side-effects and do not reduce the risk of subsequent epilepsy. Attempted prophylaxis during a febrile episode is worth trying but often too late.
3 There is an increased risk of epilepsy in adulthood (increased about four-fold compared with the general population) but the risk is still only about 2 or 3 in 100. The risk is higher (perhaps 10%) if seizures:
   (a) are focal;
   (b) are prolonged (more than 15 min);
   (c) run in the family;
   (d) start before age 1 year;
   (e) are associated with developmental or neurological abnormalities.

Advising the person with diabetes

In the complicated and common metabolic disorder of diabetes much ground needs to be covered by way of education and information. There are several important areas.

General information
1 Explanation of the disorder (the underlying principles of the disorder and its management).
2 The dangers if neglected (hypoglycaemia, hyperglycaemia, long-term complications).
3 The range of treatment (diet, drugs, insulin).
4 The need to learn self-monitoring and to make it a way of life.
5 The relevance of follow-up to health.
6 If insulin is prescribed, specific help with needles, syringes, self-injection, dose adjustments, etc.
7 Important 'dos and don'ts', e.g. do:
   (a) always carry a readily absorbable glucose store (e.g. sugar lumps);
   (b) carry a medic-alert bracelet in case of collapse;
   (c) seek medical advice when ill with persistently raised urine or blood tests (more than 1% sugar in the urine or finger-prick blood tests $\geq$13 mmol/l);
   (d) develop a regular routine;

(e) take extra sugar if extra exertion is planned;

(f) contact your doctor in the event of persistent vomiting;

(g) contact your doctor at the earliest opportunity if pregnancy is suspected (or better still see him before conception to plan management);

(h) have your feet and your eyesight checked regularly.

Do not:

(a) smoke;

(b) miss meals;

(c) drive if you feel a hypoglycaemic episode coming on;

(d) walk barefoot;

(e) reduce insulin when unwell and taking a reduced diet — it generally needs increasing, so increase the frequency of self-monitoring and seek advice.

Pregnancy

1 Diabetes is associated with an increased perinatal mortality (PNM) due to an increase in the incidence of:

(a) congenital abnormalities;

(b) long difficult labours (because of big babies);

(c) unexplained intrauterine death in late pregnancy;

(d) respiratory distress syndrome;

(e) neonatal hypoglycaemia;

(f) hydramnios;

(g) pre-eclampsia;

(h) urinary tract infections.

Some of these problems can be ameliorated by stringent control of the blood sugar. However, in gestational diabetes (which is symptomless) the PNM is about 5%, and in full-blown diabetes, even with excellent control, it is around 10%, rising significantly in the poorly controlled diabetic and the diabetic with vascular complications.

2 Pre-conceptual counselling and planning are important:

(a) because of her decreased life expectancy and because of the relationship between PNM and complications, the diabetic woman should be encouraged to start her family earlier rather than later in life;

(b) her diabetic control should be perfected prior to conception (as there is evidence that the incidence of congenital abnormalities can be reduced);

(c) she should be warned of the likely sequence of events (shared care with consultant unit delivery; the need for insulin, and frequent fetal and blood sugar monitoring throughout pregnancy; induction of labour around 38 weeks, etc.).

3 The chance of a child developing diabetes is about 0.5%; the chance of a woman with gestational diabetes developing the full-blown condition is about 20% at 5 years.

Driving
See Table 8.10. Basically, *ordinary licence holders* need to notify the
DVLA and are given a restricted licence if they require insulin, and
may be barred if:
- they do not understand their condition and act sensibly;
- they are poorly controlled;
- they default on follow-up;
- they have major complications.

For *vocational drivers* the rules are more stringent: fresh applicants
will be refused if they are insulin-dependent, as will existing holders
who become insulin-dependent. Non-insulin-dependent diabetics
may hold a vocational licence unless they develop significant eye
complications.

Psychological and social problems
In addition to the practical problems of diabetes there are common
psychological and social problems (many of which can be overcome
with preparation and education). These may include:
- fear of diabetes;
- fear of coping with all the complicated facets of management;
- mourning for lost health, shortened life-span, increased risk of
complications in later life, restricted freedom, etc.;
- fear of needles and self-injection;
- bewilderment (diabetes does take a long time for patients to
understand);
- resentment ('Why me?');
- the stigma and embarrassment of being different from every one
else;
- overprotective instincts shown by parents, relatives and friends;
- the inconvenience of regular attendance for medical follow-up;
- vocational problems;
- interference with normal social activities and rituals (e.g. eating
what your guests eat; eating when your host eats).

Follow-up
Doctors need to be well organised because they have much ground to
cover at follow-up. Flow sheets may help; computer check lists certainly will. Points to consider include:
- quality of control (symptom episodes, self-monitoring results, urinalysis, blood sugar, glycosylated haemoglobin);
- physical examination (fundoscopy, visual acuity, foot pulses, foot
care, weight, etc.);
- discussing problems and reinforcing understanding.

Prescription exemption
Diabetics are exempt from prescription charges and can obtain a prescription charge exemption certificate.

Sources of information

1   Many Health Authorities provide diabetic district nurses to help with problems, especially relating to the use of insulin.

2   Education leaflets of various kinds are available from the British Diabetic Association.

3   Some drug companies produce flow charts and co-operation cards to assist doctors and diabetics in the task of systematic follow-up; the Royal College of General Practitioners also offers a comprehensive information folder.

Advice for women with frequency and dysuria

To counsel individuals with the symptoms of frequency and dysuria, the GP must have an overview of the problem.

The size of the problem

1   500 consultations per GP per year;

2   One survey of 3000 women aged 20–60 years indicated that 50% had experience of dysuria.

The causes

Two-thirds of patients do not have a significant bacteriuria but a urethral syndrome (?traumatic urethritis,?infective organisms that are hard to culture). Among the bacterial causes, *Escherichia coli* is the most common (80–90%); others include *Staphylococcus*, *Proteus* and *Klebsiella*, and the frequency of chlamydial infection is increasing. Occasionally a chemical cystitis develops due to allergy (e.g. to rubber, foams, jellies, soaps and vaginal deodorants).

Mechanical factors come into play, since women are more often affected than men, sexually active individuals more than the celibate, and highly parous women more than those of lower parity. A short urethra, sexual intercourse and the pelvic changes that follow childbirth are implicated in the aetiology.

Natural history

The natural history depends on the sex and age of the patient, and for women on their gestational state. Four different situations can be defined:

1   *The usual situation* (frequency dysuria in a sexually active, non-pregnant adult woman). About 5% of women have asymptomatic bacteriuria, and in any 1-year period about 30% of these go on to suffer an attack of cystitis. Less than 2% then get acute pyelonephritis, and although cystitis is very common, chronic renal failure from pyelonephritis is very rare (20 per million per year). Long-term studies in sexually active young women, in the absence of an abnormal urinary tract or pregnancy, show that both asymptomatic bacteriuria and cystitis are benign, common and self-limiting.

2   *In pregnancy.* Perhaps 5% have asymptomatic bacteriuria and this

tends not to resolve spontaneously. Some 30–40% of pregnant women with this condition go on to develop a pyelonephritis (with increased risk of abortions, small-for-dates babies and premature deliveries), but the risk is substantially reduced (say by 80–90%) if antibiotics are given.

3 *In children.* Some 25% of children with urinary tract infections (UTIs) have grossly scarred kidneys and about 30% show vesico-ureteric reflux on investigation. Chronic renal failure due to pyelonephritis is clearly related to UTIs and reflux in the first 5 years of life, so UTIs in children, as in pregnant women, cannot be dismissed as benign.

4 *In adult males.* Because of the low incidence of UTIs in this group, the strong possibility is either that the man has a sexually transmitted disease (e.g. non-specific urethritis) or a structural abnormality of his renal tract.

Advice
The advice to the groups listed above is clearly different. Groups 2–4 need to see their doctor, have their urine cultured and receive treatment and/or investigation whereas, in the common situation outlined for group 1, self-help has much to offer. Suitable advice for the sexually active, non-pregnant young woman with symptoms of dysuria and frequency might therefore be as follows:

1 *In an attack*:
    (a) drink copious fluids to flush the bladder, dilute the infection and prevent stasis;
    (b) alter the pH of the urine to discourage bacterial growth (using, for example, lemon barley, mixture of potassium citrate or 2 teaspoons of sodium bicarbonate 2-hourly);
    (c) otherwise, consult the GP regarding antibiotic treatment, and take a urine specimen along.

The clear advantage of the first two approaches is that they do not require a medical appointment and possible delay, and offer over-the-counter remedies available without prescription from the chemist. Self-help also benefits the woman without easy access to medical care (e.g. the foreign holidaymaker).

2 *In prophylaxis—in women prone to recurrent attacks:*
    (a) urinate after intercourse;
    (b) ensure adequate lubrication in intercourse;
and in particularly difficult recurrent cases:
    (c) pay close attention to perineal hygiene (use a separate perineal flannel, regularly boiled; wash the perineum twice a day; wipe from the front to the back);
    (d) wash the genitalia before sex, urinate beforehand, drink copious amounts and urinate again afterwards;
    (e) avoid tight clothes and nylons;
    (f) double micturition;

(g) consult a doctor regarding a prophylactic antimicrobial.
(Not all these measures have been strictly validated, but the latter
approach is certainly effective in stubborn cases.)
3   *In general*:
(a) this is a common, benign, nuisance condition—very unpleasant, but not dangerous;
(b) self-help tips may alleviate or palliate, or prevent attacks.

Advice to women with a vaginal discharge

For advice to be appropriate, the diagnosis must be clarified. Is the
discharge physiological, pathological or blood-stained?
1   *Physiological discharges* are:
(a) clear;
(b) odourless or non-offensive;
(c) non-irritant;
(d) associated with the contraceptive pill, the mid-cycle pre-ovu-
latory cascade, pregnancy, the coil or sexual excitement.
2   *Pathological discharges* are:
(a) purulent;
(b) odiferous and offensive;
(c) irritating;
(d) a significant and abrupt change from normal;
(e) associated with the contraceptive pill, recent antibiotics, recent
delivery or abortion, or possible contact with venereal infection.
3   *Blood-stained discharges* may be due to all manner of problems from
retained tampons and atrophic vaginitis, through to salpingitis,
endometritis and cancer of the cervix or uterus.
4   *Thrush* is likely if the discharge is white and scanty with intense
itching, and predisposing factors are present (the contraceptive
pill, broad-spectrum antibiotics, possibly tight-fitting clothing and
nylons). Women who have had the characteristic symptoms on
several occasions usually know their own diagnosis.

Advice
1   If the discharge has physiological characteristics and the predisposing factors are plain, patients can be reassured.
2   If the discharge is pathological, and especially if bloody, they
should see their doctor, who will examine, investigate and treat as
appropriate.
3   Patients with *recurrent thrush* can be advised on self-help. Possible
measures include:
(a) regular or cyclical prophylactic antifungal pessaries (e.g. at
mid-cycle);
(b) simultaneous treatment of any bowel reservoir of organisms
with oral antifungal in stubborn cases;
(c) simultaneous treatment of the male partner, even if asymptomatic (again to clear any possible reservoir of infection);

(d) exclusion of diabetes via the doctor;

(e) avoidance of precipitants (e.g. broad-spectrum antibiotics; the pill as a method of contraception; tight-fitting clothes and nylons);

(f) natural yoghurt orally or intravaginally (apparently the bacteria in natural yoghurt produce favourable pH changes discouraging the growth of pathogens).

9 Allied Services

The primary health care team is only one cog (albeit a central one) in the complex machinery of the country's medical services. Many other bodies provide support for primary care and for patients directly or indirectly, through administration, fiscal planning, resource provision and other activities. Table 9.1 attempts to list some of the principal agencies whose main characteristics will now be described.

Tiers of management
The Secretary of State for Health is responsible to Parliament for effecting national policies for the NHS. In this role he is supported by a two-tier NHS management structure.

Department of Health and Regional Offices
The Department of Health (DOH) represents the first tier, and assists the Secretary of State through the NHS Executive (NHSE) and its Policy Board, and the NHS Regional Offices. The DOH's principal role is planning, budgeting and health service management at a national level; it implements Government policy and advises ministers. (Its sister department, the DSS, administers the large, complex and important Welfare Benefits System.)

Prior to 1996 the Regional Health Authorities (RHAs) represented the next tier, acting as purchasers of health care services at a regional level. However, the 14 Regions have been replaced by 8 Regional Offices, centralised within the DOH tier. Regional Directors are accountable to the NHS Chief Executive and sit alongside him on the Management Board. The Regional Offices have a number of key roles concerned with health care management:
- to manage the performance of Health Authorities (HAs), Trusts and doctors);
- to ensure compliance with national guidelines and the regulatory framework;
- to arbitrate in contractual disputes between purchasers and providers;
- to develop the centre's work on policy and resources.

Health Authorities
The second tier of the NHS consists of *purchasers* and *providers*. HAs are the main commissioners of patient services at the local level. One essential role of the HA is to secure adequate inpatient, day-patient and outpatient hospital services.

These include a number of services from community trusts and local authorities e.g.:
- key health care personnel (district nurses, midwives, community

Indirect patient services
1 Department of Health
    (a) NHS Executive and Policy Board
    (b) Regional Offices

Direct patient services
1 Health Authority services
2 NHS trusts
3 Primary care teams
4 County Council and County District Council services
5 Voluntary services
6 Others—including private medicine, industrial and occupational health
services and alternative medicine

psychiatric nurses, stoma specialists, health visitors, diabetic nurses,
etc.);
•   open-access services for primary care (e.g. physiotherapy, occupational therapy, direct-access investigative facilities);
•   special clinics (e.g. child health, child and family psychiatry, chi-
ropody and dental care, psychosexual counselling);
•   special services (e.g. clinical psychology, cervical cytology, family
planning, health education, medical referee services, school health).

Until recently the main purchasers of primary care medical services, Family Health Service Authorities (FHSAs), existed autono-
mously. But the latest round of NHS reforms abolished FHSAs and
DHAs and created unitary HAs that have subsumed the old functions
of both. Merger has created economies of scale and a single authority
in each locality responsible for implementing national policy. It also
means that HAs have powers:
•   to enter into service contracts with medical, dental and ophthalmic practitioners and pharmacists;
•   to supervise their payment;
•   to ensure practice premises and services meet basic minimum
standards;
•   to deal with disputes and ensure contractual obligations are
fulfilled;
•   to administer (or devolve) a budget to cover primary care
expenditure
•   to maintain a register of local practitioners;
•   to compile lists of doctors eligible to offer maternity, paediatric
surveillance and minor surgery services;
•   to vet and license health promotion clinics;
•   to vet indicative prescribing budgets;
•   to co-ordinate audit in primary care through Medical Audit Advisory Groups (MAAGs).

The HA has a budget out of which hospital, primary care and other community services are jointly funded. The money can be deployed directly or devolved to other purchasers. Under the terms of a new White Paper HAs are required to draw up a 'Health Improvement Programme', based on a local health needs assessment, to establish local commissioning groups (Primary Care Groups (see below)), and to enter into contractual agreements with PCGs to deliver the planned programme from available funds.

The HA is served by four professional committees who advise on matters concerning their own field of experience:

1   The Local Medical Committee (LMC), representing local doctors.
2   The Local Dental Committee (LDC).
3   The Local Pharmaceutical Committee (LPC).
4   The Local Ophthalmic Committee (LOC).

Primary Care Groups

By 1999, according to a Government White Paper, all GPs in England and Wales will have to belong to a local commissioning group, called a Primary Care Group (PCG). Each PCG will represent about 50 GPs. PCG Boards will have nursing and community, as well as GP representatives, and may be advisory to the HA, or act as free-standing purchasers of primary and secondary care services. They will operate within the framework of a HA action plan (Health Improvement Programme) and a cash-limited budget. The proposal is discussed more fully on p. 51. (In Scotland, the arrangements vary. GPs will be invited to form Local Health Care Co-operatives with budgets for primary care, but not hospital services. As the scheme is voluntary, in areas where there is no take up existing fundholders will be able to retain their community service budgets).

NHS trusts

The NHS Act allowed hospitals and community care units to assume managerial independence from HA control and to assume 'trust' status. In the first wave (1990) 57 hospitals or units made the transition. Ninety-eight per cent of eligible units have followed in their wake. As health care providers, trusts now enter into service contracts to deliver hospital services; while service purchasers (HAs and GPs) have some freedom to shop around for the best deals.

Local authorities

Local authority responsibilities include the promotion of social care and a healthy environment for daily living. Provision includes:

•   social services (meals on wheels, social workers, home helps, childminding and fostering services, etc.);
•   special educational facilities for the handicapped;
•   environmental health services;
•   rented housing for general needs, sheltered housing for the elderly, and residential homes for children in care.

Table 9.2 Some well known voluntary associations.

Problem	Voluntary body
AIDS	Terrence Higgins Trust
Alcoholism	Alcoholics Anonymous
	Alanon (self-help group for relatives and friends)
	Alateen (for teenagers with alcoholic relatives)
Alzheimer's disease	Alzheimer's Disease Society
Asthma	Asthma Research Council
Arthritis	Arthritis and Rheumatism Council
Blindness	Royal National Institute for the Blind
Bereavement	Compassionate Friends (bereaved parents)
	Cruse (for the widowed and their children)
Cancer	Cancer relief (MacMillan Cancer Relief Foundation)
	Marie Curie Memorial Foundation
Child cruelty	NSPCC
Coeliac disease	Coeliac Society
Deafness	Royal National Institute for the Deaf
Diabetes	British Diabetic Association
Down's syndrome	Down's Syndrome Association
Drug Abuse	Turning Point
	Drug Line
Dyslexia	British Dyslexia Association
Elderly	Age Concern
	Help the Aged
Epilepsy	British Epilepsy Association
Gambling	Gamblers Anonymous
Haemophilia	Haemophilia Society
Ileostomies	Ileostomy Association
Leukaemia	Leukaemia Care Society
Marriage guidance	Relate
Mental illness	Depressives Anonymous
	National Association for Mental Health (MIND)
	Samaritans
Migraine	British Migraine Association
Multiple sclerosis	MS Society of Great Britain and N. Ireland
One-parent families	Gingerbread
Parkinson's disease	Parkinson's Disease Society
Rape	Rape Crisis Centre
Smoking	ASH
Spastics	Spastics' Society
Tinnitus	British Tinnitus Association

Voluntary associations

There are numerous voluntary associations. The best known include the Red Cross and St John Ambulance Brigade, the Samaritans, Alcoholics Anonymous and the MacMillan Nursing Service. However, voluntary associations have been formed to provide support and advice for families and individuals with a wide range of problems. Table 9.2 illustrates the breadth of support available.

Referral to a voluntary association is a valid, often valuable adjunct to other treatment, and in the MRCGP examination it is well worth rounding off the answer to a management question with a reference to this.

Health education services

At a *national* level the principal responsible agency (other than the DOH) is the *Health Education Authority (HEA)*. This replaced the Health Education Council (HEC) in 1987, forming in its own right a new authority of regional status accountable to the Secretary of State.

Functions

• To organise and institute health education campaigns (in concert with HAs).

• To promote training schemes for health education workers (recently, for example, it announced a health promotion helpline for GPs).

• To offer a consultative service with special expertise in all relevant matters.

• To promote related research.

At a *local level* health education has become the responsibility of HAs. They employ full-time health education and health promotion officers, but health education is offered in addition by health visitors, social workers and community physicians. Many of the functions of the HEA at a national level are reflected by the HA at a local level, but with special emphasis on local needs.

Medical Audit Advisory Groups (MAAGs)

Established in 1991 by FHSAs acting in co-operation with their LMCs.

Role

A local body charged with the task of directing, co-ordinating and monitoring medical audit activities in general practices and hospital services.

Each MAAG is accountable to its HA, which is in turn accountable to its RHA. The aim is to demonstrate, through programmes of audit, professional commitment to securing the highest quality of service within available resources.

Composition

Although the precise size and composition are locally determined and flexible, a MAAG would normally comprise no more than a dozen members, including:

• representatives from the LMC and local Royal College of General Practitioners faculty;

• GP principals with special experience of audit (e.g. regional or associate GP advisers, academic staff of the local medical school's department of general practice);

• a public health physician;

• HA representatives.

Prescription Pricing Authority (PPA)

Within the NHS the PPA has the status of a special health authority. Its functions include:

1 Feedback to prescribers:
  (a) annual PD2s;
  (b) detailed PD8s on request;
  (c) quarterly PACT reports;
  (d) monthly reports to assist drug budget planning.

2 Information for the DOH on high prescribers and prescribing patterns and costs.

3 Pricing arrangements which enable pharmacists and dispensing doctors to be paid.

4 Assistance in research, post-marketing surveillance and even police investigations!

Composition

The PPA is a large organisation with 2000 employees and one of the largest computer systems within the NHS—it processes a million prescriptions a day. Its board has a chairperson, chief executive and representatives from the DOH, HAs, Community Health Councils, as well as pharmacists and GPs.

The General Medical Council (GMC)

Prior to 1858 the regulation of medical practice in the UK was chaotic: 19 separate licensing bodies conferred various professional titles after tests of competence whose standards varied widely, and more than one-third of UK practitioners were not qualified. The Medical Act of 1858 laid down minimum standards of medical education and established a new regulatory body called the General Council of Medical Education and Registration of the UK. In later years this body became known as the GMC, but did not receive its first major overhaul until more than a century had passed. These changes (in composition, size, structure and function) came with the Medical Act 1978 and left the GMC in its present form.

Composition

The GMC has approximately 95 members:
• more than half are elected by the profession;
• about one-third are chosen by universities and other bodies empowered to grant registrable qualifications;
• a few others are nominated by Her Majesty on the advice of her Privy Council.

The Council is served by various professional and disciplinary committees including:
• the Preliminary Proceedings Committee (PPC);
• the Professional Conduct Committee (PCC);
• the Health Committee.

Functions

The GMC is the watchdog for professional standards.

1 It maintains a medical register.

2 It provides guidelines on expected standards of care.

3 It judges on cases of professional misconduct and disciplinary matters, and decides in such cases on fitness to remain registered.

4 It is empowered to vet overseas doctors for linguistic competence prior to registration.

5 The Professional Performance Act 1995 gave the GMC new powers to investigate doctors' poor professional performance, and to discipline them, help them or require them to undergo remedial training.

The Royal College of General Practitioners

The College of General Practitioners was founded in 1952 and obtained 'Royal' status in 1967. In 1992 it had a membership of about 17 000 doctors.

Function

Its main function since inception has been to serve as a think-tank for the setting of standards and the improvement of general practice. The Royal College of General Practitioners seeks to achieve this broad aim through its main activities, important among which are:

• the setting of a postgraduate examination as a benchmark of expected standards;

• the organisation and conduct of general practice research;

• the publication of an academic journal based on original research and frequent special reports;

• the provision of reference and advisory material to aid good practice;

• the stimulation of debate through policy statements and its national and local educational meetings;

• the promotion of continuing medical education (CME);

• direct influence on the structure of vocational training.

The Royal College represents the academic voice of general practice. Although it does not speak for the whole of the medical profession, and critics level against the membership the charge of elitism, it has contributed significantly to the state of improved esteem and morale that exists within general practice. It has proved a successful breeding ground for fresh and innovative thinking (see Section 4.11), and is likely to remain at the forefront when it comes to future developments within the profession.

10 The MRCGP Examination

10.1 THE SYLLABUS

The MRCGP examination has no strictly defined curriculum, just as the discipline of general practice has few fixed boundaries. However, the Royal College recently has provided information on the 'domains of competence' that constitute a blueprint for assessment by examination (Table 10.1).

Of course the interpretation of the blueprint is a subjective exercise, but it is important to note that pure clinical medicine (symptoms, signs, investigations, treatment, etc.) comprises only a small part of what is being tested. Candidates should also be able to show competency in:

- *business methods*: the GP as policymaker and manager, as the organiser of practice services, as a self-employed business person;
- *the handling of people*: communication, attitudes, appreciation of human behaviour, teamwork;
- *the global view*: ethics, the law, consumer rights, resources, epidemiology;
- *a critical approach*: dogma or fact? What are the alternatives? What do my colleagues do?
- *the application of principles:* translating knowledge and research findings into problem-solving and case management;
- *personal development*: self-awareness, professional growth, etc.

This book has tried directly to address these areas. Broadly speaking, practice matters are discussed in Chapters 1 and 3; communication in Chapter 2; the wider issues in Chapters 5, 6, 7 and 9; research methods, statistical methods, and critical reading in Chapter 11; and matters of debate throughout, but with specific emphasis in Chapter 4.

In general, pure clinical material has been passed over, because experience suggests that candidates with several years of training and exams behind them have least difficulty with this part of the test. It is also true to say that greater emphasis is placed in the examination on the non-clinical areas of general practice than on classical medical school teaching.

In deciding how to allocate his revision time the candidate would do well to remember this. Revising the whole broad canvas of clinical medicine is a disheartening business, and may not be rewarded proportionately. Given a reasonable level of clinical competence, the candidate would do better devoting the majority of his time to the sorts of issues and areas that this book covers.

Table 10.1 Domains of competence tested in the modular MRCGP examination.

A	Factual knowledge
B	Evolving knowledge: uncertainty, 'hot topics', qualitative research
C	The evidence base of practice: knowledge of literature, quantitative research
D	Critical appraisal skills: interpretation of literature, principles of statistics
E	Application of knowledge: justification, prioritising, audit
F	Problem-solving: general applications
G	Problem-solving: case-specific, clinical management
H	Personal care: matching principles to individual patients
I	Written communication
J	Verbal communication: the consultation process
K	The practice context: 'team' issues, practice management, business skills
L	Regulatory framework of practice
M	The wider context: medico-political, legal and societal issues
N	Ethnic and trans-cultural issues
O	Values and attitudes: ethics, integrity, consistency, *caritas*
P	Self-awareness: insight, reflective learning, 'the doctor as a person'
Q	Commitment to maintaining standards: personal and professional growth, continuing medical education

10.2 EXAM ELIGIBILITY AND QUALIFYING REQUIREMENTS

In addition to sitting all parts of the modular MRCGP exam, candidates must demonstrate proficiency in two qualifying areas, namely:

1 simple cardiopulmonary resuscitation; and
2 child health surveillance.

Certificates of proficiency in each area *must* be provided when applying to take the consulting skills assessment module (see Section 10.6, p. 286).

The cardiopulmonary resuscitation certificate

The Royal College provides a list of regional centres at which this cardiopulmonary resuscitation (CPR) skills can be formally tested. Training is available too (though candidates would have to bear the costs of this). A certificate signed by an A & E consultant will also suffice. Candidates who hold a Diploma in Immediate Medical Care, a certificate in Pre-hospital Emergency Care, or a certificate in Advanced Life Support are exempted. Certificates and Diplomas are considered valid for 3 years.

The CPR certificate is reproduced in Fig. 10.1. The text on the certificate specifies the requirements, so candidates should read it with some care. The test criteria are based on the 1997 guidelines of the Basic Life Support Working Party of the European Resuscitation Council.

It is worth considering how CPR skills need to be adapted because of the unique position GPs are in, providing immediate care in the surgery and the home rather than a hospital:

- What resuscitation facilities should be available in surgeries?
- What equipment and drugs should GPs carry around with them?

It is conceivable that a question or two on this theme might arise in the viva.

The child health surveillance requirement

A certificate of proficiency in basic child health surveillance is also required on application for the consulting skills module. Again the certificate (reproduced in Fig. 10.2) identifies the skills that must be demonstrated. There are no exemptions from certification. It may be counter-signed by a GP principal on a Health Authority (HA) child health surveillance list, a community paediatrician or clinical medical officer active and competent in the field (but not by a health visitor alone). Certificates are considered valid for 3 years from the date of the last test.

Other eligibility criteria are described in the documentation the Royal College supplies to prospective candidates. Applications need to be supported by a photograph, photocopy evidence of full GMC registration, and occasionally evidence of eligibility to practice.

10.3 THE FORMAT

Prior to 1998 the examination comprised five main elements: a Multiple Choice Questionnaire (MCQ); a Modified Essay Question (MEQ); a Critical Reading Question Paper (CRQ); two vivas, and a videotape assessment of consulting skills. A rearrangement of these elements has led to the present four module examination:

1 Paper 1—a written prose paper derived from the old MEQ and elements of the former CRQ;

2 Paper 2 — a machine marked paper based on the existing MCQ formats together with some CRQ material;

3 An assessment of consulting skills (video tape or simulated surgery); and

4 Two vivas of somewhat shorter length.

These changes have a largely cosmetic appearance, and the Royal College has provided assurance that the difficulty of the examination, and the steps required for successful preparation are unaltered.

One important difference, however, is that the modules can be taken separately, together or in any order: success in any one section is not a qualifying requirement for passage to any other. The result in each module will be graded as 'fail', 'pass' or 'pass with merit' (roughly the top 25% of those taking the module). To achieve the MRCGP, a pass is required in all four modules within a 3-year period from first application. Three attempts are allowed at each module; thereafter the candidate is deemed to have failed overall, and must re-sit. Conversely, for high-flyers, a pass with merit in two modules may

THE ROYAL COLLEGE OF GENERAL PRACTITIONERS
EXAMINATION FOR MEMBERSHIP

CARDIO-PULMONARY RESUSCITATION PERFORMANCE TEST
REVISED JULY 1997
Candidates must obtain a pass in each activity

Candidate's Name _____ Date _____

Activity	Ideal Performance	Acceptable Variables	Pass	Fail
1. Check for personal safety before treating the casualty	Shake gently by shoulders - ask loudly "are you alright?"	None		
2. Call for help	Call for help immediately	None		
3. Open airway and check mouth	Head tilt and chin lift	Jaws thrust in case of trauma		
4. Determine whether casualty is breathing or not	Look, listen and feel for breathing for up to 10 seconds	None		
5. Activate 999 system		None		
6. Breathe	Give two effective, slow ventilations 400 -600 mls. Inspiratory time per ventilation 2 seconds	Up to 5 attempts until 2 breaths are effective		
7. Determine whether a pulse is present or not	Palpate carotid artery and look for other signs of life for up to 10 seconds	None		
8. Cycles of chest compressions and ventilations	15 chest compressions to a depth of 4-5 cms over the mid and lower part of the sternum avoiding pressure on the ribs or abdomen

Alternate 15 compressions at a rate of 100 per minute with 2 ventilations

At least 70% correct ventilations
At least 70% correct compressions
At least 4 cycles of compressions and ventilations must be performed | None | | |
| 9. Timing of activitiy | Step 1 to the completion of 4 cycles of compressions/ventilations to be performed within 1 minute and 45 seconds | Performed within 2 minutes | | |

Examiners Signature _____ Result: Pass _____ Fail _____

Professional Status _____

Name _____

Address _____ *Candidates who fail the test may he re-tested after instruction*

ATTACH MANIKIN PERFORMANCE RECORD IF AVAILABLE
THIS CERTIFICATE REMAINS VALID FOR THREE YEARS FROM DATE OF THE TEST

Figure 10.1 The cardiopulmonary resuscitation certificate (reproduced by permission of the Royal College of General Practitioners).

earn an overall Pass with Merit, and a pass with merit in three, a Pass with Distinction.

Candidates in training can start at any stage from hospital GP registrar jobs through Vocational Training, although the modules are designed for candidates with active general practice experience.

Each section will now be considered in detail.

10.4 PAPER 1

Time allowed
3 h.

Format

A loose-leaf book with questions fairly evenly spread over the pages. After each question blank spaces are left for the answers. Sometimes this may involve a structured response (such as entering the response in a table). There are about 12 questions. Expanded note form is encouraged, rather than lengthy prose. All questions must be answered.

Marking scheme

Each page covers one question and is independently marked. The questions all contribute equally to the final mark. Each has a series of themes, and the examiners are looking to see whether you can identify the main concepts, and how clearly you understand them. You score points for covering all the concepts and for grasp of each one. A marking grid specifies the points you are expected to make. This is fairly rigid: if you do not make those particular points, a mark cannot be allocated.

Content

Paper 1 questions focus on three principal areas:
1 knowledge and interpretation of general practice literature;
2 evaluation of written material; and
3 ability to apply theoretical knowledge and professional values to the UK primary care setting.

The College provides broad guidance on the scope and emphasis of the questioning:

1 Questions in the first category will normally involve discussing/evaluating a major topic, and the evidence underlying current views. They test the candidate's familiarity with current issues, 'hot topics', and the key literature in general practice. Topics are generally common and important. Examples include the evidence for the effectiveness of post-hospital drug treatment after myocardial infarction, and the prevention and management of common viral illnesses (areas of controversy, and the underlying evidence).

2 Questions in the second category will involve published papers or extracted material from papers, such as summaries, methods and results (without the discussion), or a systematic review: candidates will be asked to appraise the material critically (methods, strengths and weaknesses, sources of bias, validity and practical implications). They may also include an interpretation of the meaning of common statistical measures, such as P values and confidence intervals. Alternatively, the written material may be a problem-solving scenario, for which the strength of evidence is sought. Extra time is allowed to read the supplied material.

3 Questions in the third category test the candidate's practical approach to primary care problems, and often take the form of a possible practice problem (either patient-focused or practice-focused), or wider medical issues.

ROYAL COLLEGE OF GENERAL PRACTITIONERS
EXAMINATION FOR MEMBERSHIP
CERTIFICATE OF COMPETENCE IN CHILD HEALTH SURVEILLANCE

CANDIDATE'S NAME: ....

1   I have observed this doctor undertaking satisfactorily the examination of a child aged 6 - 8 weeks in each of the appropriate surveillance tasks listed overleaf.

Signature:.................................   Date:...............................

Name (Block Capitals please):   ....

Address: ....

....

....

Professional Status ....   FHSA/Health Board/
Employing Authority..........................

2   I have observed this doctor undertaking satisfactorily the examination of a child aged 6 - 9 months in each of the appropriate surveillance tasks listed overleaf.

Signature:.................................   Date:...............................

Name (Block Capitals please):   ....

Address: ....

....

....

Professional Status ....   FHSA/Health Board/
Employing Authority..........................

3   I have observed this doctor undertaking satisfactorily the examination of a child aged 36 - 48 months in each of the appropriate surveillance tasks noted overleaf.

Signature:.................................   Date:...............................

Name (Block Capitals please):   ....

Address: ....

....

....

Professional Status ....   FHSA/Health Board/
Employing Authority..........................

THIS CERTIFICATE REMAINS VALID FOR THREE YEARS FROM THE DATE OF THE LAST TEST

Figure 10.2 (*Above and opposite*) The child health surveillance certificate of competency (reproduced by permission of the Royal College of General Practitioners).

Please tick each box as appropriate

GENERAL	6-8 WEEKS	6-9 MONTHS	36-48 MONTHS
1. Seeks parents concern re: health, development and behaviour			
2. Handling and approach to child			
3. Makes adequate record			
CHECK			
4. Weight			
5. Length/Height	✕	✕	
6. Head Circumference			✕
CHECK			
7. General behaviour			
8. Appearance			
9. Skin			
10. Fontanelles			✕
11. Palate		✕	
12. Motor tone			✕
13. Reflexes		✕	
14. Co-ordination (fine motor)	✕		
15. Vision/Eyes		*	*
16. Squint			
17. Ears			
18. Hearing	*	*	*
19. Language/Vocalisation			
20. Heart		✕	
21. Femoral Arteries		✕	✕
22. Spine		✕	✕
23. Hips		✕	
24. Feet		✕	✕
25. Hernia		✕	✕
26. Testes			✕
27. Genitalia		✕	✕
28. Bladder Control	✕	✕	*
29. Bowel Control	✕	✕	*
ADVICE RE:			
30. Health Education			
31. Immunisation			

*Check parents perceptions and refer if concerned. ✕ = not essential

Ref (i): Child Health Surveillance - A District Core Programme (BPA) 1990
(ii): Handbook of Preventive Care for Pre-School Children (GMSC/RCGP) 1988
(iii): Royal College of General Practitioners and British Paediatric Association - Guidelines for the training and accreditation of general practitioners - Child Health Surveillance, December 1989.

Figure 10.2 (*Continued*).

(a) Patient-focused problems often entail problem patients and awkward situations (the liberated rebel demanding natural childbirth in a swimming pool or caravan; the patient who demands tranquillisers, and insists your colleague has always prescribed them 'without this bother'; 'unreasonable' patient requests, etc.).

(b) Practice-focused problems may involve such matters as the development of patient services, quality standards, liaison (and potential conflicts) with colleagues, team-building, practice dynamics and alternative ways of organising and running a practice.

(c) The wider issues' encompass socio-political matters, ethical dilemmas, professional values and the doctor in society. For example, is commissioning a good or a bad thing for patients, doctors, the NHS and society? What problems does it create? What implications does it have? It may also include aspects of personal and professional development.

Past papers

Sample questions are provided on exam application. In addition, past papers are reprinted from time to time in the *British Journal of General Practice*. (At present candidates may need to look at old-style MEQ and CRQ papers, until more examples of the new format appear in print.)

General points of technique

1 Read the questions very carefully.

2 Write in note form: it takes less time, allows you to write more, and is easier for the examiner to mark. It may help to structure the reply into logical subdivisions, but an essay-style sentence construction is not required.

3 Be prepared to repeat yourself from one answer to the next: the answers are marked independently, so the same point may score in more than one question.

4 There is less time than you think for this exam. Practise some mock papers and time yourself. Allot the time roughly equally between questions—you have about 15 minutes per question, as a rough guide.

5 Answer all the questions, as they carry an equal weighting in the final score.

Specific pointers

Questions in the different categories pose different problems to the candidate.

1 Those in the **first category** require careful advanced preparation. It is helpful to start with a list of the common problems and themes in general practice. Earlier chapters of this book cover a part of this mate-

rial, but it would be wise during the course of training (and certainly in the course of exam preparation), to assemble a list of target areas; and to find out what the main evidence is in each. These areas can be identified during training, because they commonly arise in surgery, and they feature frequently in the mainstream journals. Keep a running list of topics; have a 'brain-storming' session with colleagues, and write your best guesses down.

2 'Hot topic' items concern matters of current interest to GPs, the emphasis being on British general practice and British journals. A careful study of the last 2 years of major editorials and reviews in the *Lancet, British Medical Journal* and *British Journal of General Practice* is likely to yield a useful list of study items. Look for topics with some factual background, which are both important and controversial.

3 In assembling the evidence, start with recent reviews and relatively recent textbook accounts. These will provide an overview. By skimming forwards through the journals it should then be possible to see whether and how views have recently changed. Awareness of recent literature is an important aspect. Guidelines of national status should also be identified, and mark a useful point of reference.

4 These questions test more than knowledge. They test:
   (a) appraisal of what is accepted and what is controversial;
   (b) where the limits of knowledge lie;
   (c) the strength of evidence in favour of alternative views;
   (d) the clinical relevance of research. (If true, would it change what I do? How should the knowledge be applied in the surgery and in particular clinical problems?)

5 Questions in the **second category** require some appreciation of epidemiology and statistical methods. This is an area that candidates sometimes find conceptually difficult, and it is worthy of some independent reading. Chapter 11 provides an introductory overview; other suggestions are provided under **Further reading**.

6 It is worth practising some questions in this category. Choose a selection of original papers from recent copies of the *British Medical Journal* or *British Journal of General Practice*, and begin by reading only the introduction and the methods. Then test yourself:
   (a) Can you fit the methods into one of the models described in Chapter 11?
   (b) What was done, and why?
   (c) Are there any potential weaknesses and biases?
   Then look at the results:
   (d) If true, how does it affect your practice?
   (e) Write down what you consider to be the main discussion points; then check what the authors of the paper said.

7 Discuss papers in a regular journal club, and thereby familiarise yourself with the process of critical analysis.

8 Critical assessment of common written material from general practice may form part of Paper 1. Likely issues can readily be anticipated, e.g.:

This material . . .	*. . . may well raise these issues*
Letters between colleagues	Confidentiality
	Communication
	Interprofessional relationships
	Hidden agendas
Practice protocol or audit	Defining objectives and standards
	Defining valid methods
	Colleagues' attitudes to peer review
Advertising or promotional material	Worthwhile question asked
	Valid study method and analysis
	Context established
	Credibility
	Practical importance

9 In **patient-focused questions**, the ingredients of a comprehensive answer may include psychological and social aspects, implications for the primary health care team, the law, society and the NHS, and not merely the physical aspects of the case.

(a) You must think and write from all aspects: see it from the doctor's point of view, from the patient's, from that of the primary health care team, society and any other viewpoint you can think. Don't waffle, but *if it might be relevant write it down*.

(b) This is easier to do if you memorise a checklist of areas to consider. You can then scribble down in rough the main headings of your *aide memoire*. These might be for example:

- physical, psychological, social;
- options, implications, choice;
- doctor's angle, patient's view, profession's view, other view (e.g. society, solicitor, defence union);
- pros and cons (to all relevant parties);
- evidence (Any relevant studies?).

(c) Regarding management it is easy to construct a similar *aide mémoire*, e.g.:

- clarify the problem (in physical, psychological and social terms);
- investigate if necessary;
- treat (counsel and advise; prescribe drug and/or appliance; carry out a procedure, e.g. intrauterine device fitting, vaccination, injection of tennis elbow, minor surgery, etc.);
- refer:
  within the primary health care team (e.g. health visitor, midwife, practice nurse, district nurse);
  to hospital services (e.g. inpatient, outpatient, day hospital, consultant, domiciliary visit, physiotherapy);
  to the social services (e.g. social worker, social services day

centre, part 3 accommodation, meals on wheels, home help, orange badge, welfare benefits department);

to the community services (e.g. dentist, optician, chiropodist);

to other agencies (self-help, voluntary, local authorities, etc.);

- follow up;
- preventive action desirable? health education possible?;
- liaison needed (e.g. with colleagues, school, community physician, solicitor, etc.)?

10 By practising a few past papers you can identify questions with a common theme; for example, if a patient asks you to do something that could be construed as controversial, your options are: agree, disagree, refer, bargain/counsel/educate—and each has predictable implications. Advance planning allows you to offer polished and comprehensive answers.

11 Be honest and say what you would really do, not simply give the textbook answer. We do not X-ray all children who are chesty for a week because general practice requires a modified and pragmatic approach, and your answer should reflect this (although it is reasonable to consider and reject alternatives). Similarly, differential diagnoses must list common things first and rarities in passing.

10.5 PAPER 2

Time allowed
3 h.

Format
This is a machine-marked paper. Answers are transferred to a computer card by colouring in the appropriate lozenges with a pencil; marking can then be performed automatically by computer-scanning of the answer sheet.

Questions are of three kinds:

1 *Simple true/false questions.* Most questions are of this sort. A stem statement is followed by 3–6 completion statements of the true/false variety. Each complete statement can be answered 'True' or 'False'. A maximum of 400 true–false items is offered.

2 *Extended matching questions.* These typically present a scenario ('item') that needs to be matched to one answer from a list of possibilities ('options'). For each item the single best option needs to be selected. The list contains more possibilities than scenarios, so not all options will be relevant; by the same token, a given option may represent the best answer to a number of 'items'.

3 *Single best answer questions.* A statement or stem followed by a number of items, one of which represents the single best answer (the best treatment, the most likely diagnosis, etc.). This item needs to be selected from the available choices.

Extended matching and single best answer questions appear in their own separate section, which may include up to 100 items.

Marking scheme
- Correct answers each score 1 mark.
- No penalty for incorrect answers.

(Trial questions may also be included, and these do not count towards the candidate's final score.)

Content
Paper 2 tests the candidate's knowledge base. It contains questions on:
- critical appraisal—knowledge of statistics, research methods and the evaluation of published papers;
- general medicine and surgery;
- medicine of the specialities (ENT, dermatology, orthopaedics, etc.)
- women's health;
- child health;
- service management.

There is no set quota of questions from each field. New items derive from review articles and commonly read medical journals such as the *British Medical Journal*, *The British Journal of General Practice* and *Drugs and Therapeutics Bulletin*. Graphs and photographs may be used in the questioning.

Past papers
Past papers are not available, but many practice papers are, including: *The MRCGP Study*, Butterworth-Heinmann; *MRCGP Practice Exams*, Pastest; *MRCGP MCQ Practice Papers*, Pastest; *The Multiple Choice Question in Medicine*, Pitman; and regular MCQs in general practice magazines. Never let a practice paper pass by without trying it!

Points of technique

For true/false questions
1   Read the stem and *the item in question*, and consider them in isolation: they have nothing to do with the stem and any other completion. Always go back and read the stem as well as the completion so it makes *a complete sentence*, otherwise by item six you may have forgotten the exact sense of the stem statement.
2   The exact wording is important; indeed, a paper published on the linguistic significance of questions in MCQ exams (Slade & Dewey 1983) suggests that by attention to this alone a candidate with little knowledge of the subject can pass. I will leave the reader to make up his own mind on this, but the importance of wording cannot be

overemphasised. To take a typical example, 'always' and 'never' are in most cases wrong, because in medicine there are usually exceptions. Expressions like 'is associated with' cause more problems, because able candidates can often construct a tenuous link between even the most distantly related events. In Table 10.2 guidelines are given on the interpretation of some common question wordings.

3   The most important thing is to trust the examiner and to accept questions at face value: the obvious meaning of the statement is the intended one. Slightly more difficult is the situation in which you know both the commonly accepted answer, and the exceptions and qualifications to it. Consider in this case what the examiner intended you to answer: in most cases the straightforward answer is the intended solution, and the questioner did not spot the ambiguity (or anticipate your sophistication!).

4   Answers can be subdivided into:
   (a) those you are *confident* you know;
   (b) those you have *a feeling* are true or false for some reason, but cannot swear to;
   (c) those you feel you can *rationalise* the answer to, without knowing;
   (d) those you have *no clue about at all*;
   (e) those you find *ambiguous*.
These should be tackled differently.

Table 10.2 Interpretation of the wording in Paper 2 (MCQ type) questions.

Wording	Interpretation
Always	Invariably and without a single exception (usually the answer to this is false)
Never	Not in one single person nor on one single occasion (again usually false)
The majority	More than 50%
A minority	Less than 50%
Usually	In the majority of cases (see above)
Pathognomonic, diagnostic, characteristic, in the vast majority	In at least 90%
Typically, frequently, commonly, significantly, in a substantial majority	In at least 60% of cases
In a substantial minority	In up to 30%
Recognised, reported, has been shown, is associated with	Can be found in an authoritative text on the subject (NB no implication about how commonly the feature occurs)
In 25% of cases	When figures are quoted they are usually 'true' or very wide of the mark. (Thus, some studies may say 24% of cases, some 26%, and so on. When examiners quote a figure there must be some leeway, so if you think the answer is 30% of cases, the answer is probably true; if you think 50%, it is probably false)

(a) The answers you are confident about are probably right, assuming you read the question carefully. They may not all be right but the vast majority should be, so answer them with confidence.

(b and c) Questions you have a feeling about, or believe you can rationalise, are not usually guesses at all. They usually relate to something you know or have heard, but cannot freshly recall. It has been shown that these 'guesses' are more often right than wrong. (Try this for yourself—practise some mock papers noting your performance in this category). In the absence of a negative marking scheme it would be a serious mistake not to attempt such questions. However, another mistake would be to guess before trying to *work out* the answer—this too is giving up too early!

(d) When you have no clue at all, the question is best guessed. You lose nothing, but have everything to gain.

(e) Ambiguous questions are answered as described in 4, but must be attempted. Again you are likely to be right more often than wrong.

For extended matching questions
• Since questions in this category take longer to answer, it may be helpful from the point of view of time planning to attempt them first.
• Read the instructions carefully, as there is scope for misunderstanding. Don't forget that several scenarios (items) can theoretically point to the same diagnosis (option); and don't try to make every option fit an item—they won't, as there are more answers than questions.
• Read the item, and before looking at the option list try to work out the differential diagnosis, and which of these is the most likely diagnosis. Remember the truism: *'common things are common'*.

For all questions
• Read the question carefully. This is mundane advice but many mistakes are made by answering what it was thought the examiner asked, not what was asked.
• *Answer every question.* Don't waste time trying to tot up your score, but answer each and every question to the best of your ability.

10.6 ASSESSMENT OF CONSULTATION SKILLS

The candidate's consulting skills can be assessed by one of two methods:
1 *either* by submitting a video tape of surgery consultations;
2 *or*, by taking part in a 'simulated surgery' in which actors role-play a series of consultations.

Video recording is regarded as the normal method of assessment (the alternative is only made available if a candidate can convince the examiners that there are insuperable difficulties in making a video). This account is restricted to the normal video tape method of assessment, but details of the alternative can be obtained on application to the College.

Format and content of the video tape

Candidates need to submit a video tape containing 15 of their surgery consultations, together with a workbook containing details of each consultation and some self-assessment proformas. (See also Section 10.2).

In producing a technically adequate tape, a number of practical points need to be observed:

1   The recording should be made on a standard normal-play VHS tape. Some camcorders use a smaller format cassette (VHS-C), or record in 'slow play', or in the more exacting Super VHS format. These will not be acceptable. The recordings should also indicate the elapsed time for each consultation, to enable each consultation to be readily located by the examiners. All recorded consultations must be in English and should not be more than 15 minutes each in length.

2   Recordings cannot be assessed unless they achieve reasonable sound and picture quality. Of these, sound quality is generally more problematic. If the built-in microphone gives poor reproduction an external microphone may be needed. Background noise (e.g. telephones, computer printers) should be avoided. The camera must be positioned on a tripod or stable platform, in such a way that both doctor and patient are visible; and not directed towards a source of light immediately behind the parties (this will darken the picture). It makes sense to do some trial recordings to iron out these problems before trying to assemble a portfolio.

3   Intimate physical examinations should be held off camera (or with the lens cap placed over the lens). The camera need not be stopped, and it may be helpful to the examiners to give a running commentary on the findings. Less sensitive examinations may be recorded, if they can be adequately performed without the patient leaving his seat.

4   Recording requires patient consent. The GMC advises that before a recording is made the patient should understand its intended use and who will see it; whether copies will be made (this is a sensible precaution, given the effort and the risk of tape damage or loss); when the tape will be destroyed; and that they can refuse without prejudice to their care, or change their minds later. The College provides a consent form which will need to be copied. Explanations should be given and written consent obtained when patients make their appointment. This will mean instructing the receptionists on the procedure and its purpose. Patients should sign a second consent form after the consultation to confirm that they have not changed their mind. They have a right to expect that the recording will be stored securely and confiden-

tially, as with other personal records. Evidence of consent for each recording must be included when the tape is submitted to the examiners.

5 Fifteen consultations are required, in the normal surgery setting. The recording can be a *pot-pourri* of consultations spaced widely in time, and does not need to be made in a single surgery. The tape must include at least two consultations with children under 10 years, and at least two consultations involving chronic disease in adult patients. The candidate is asked to highlight five consultations for more intensive scrutiny by the examiners.

6 The candidate has to complete a workbook describing the portfolio case by case, including the elapsed time. For the five highlighted consultations a separate proforma must be completed, with a minute by minute reflection on the content and progress of the consultation.

Marking

The tape will be viewed by two examiners. They will look through the workbook and agree seven consultations to view, including at least three of the five highlighted by the candidate. Typically these will represent a spectrum of patient contacts. The examiners will decide whether or not the required competencies have been consistently met (it is expected that 70% of tapes will fall into this camp). If they do not consider this to be so, the tape will be referred to a second pair of examiners who will view the remaining consultations; the candidate will only be failed if these too prove unsatisfactory.

Points of technique

1 Make sure the video complies in *content* and *technical quality* with the stipulated requirements. Examiners cannot give credit for omitted items and consultations they cannot hear or see properly.

2 As consultations need not be consecutive ones, you can choose when and what to submit. You should wait until you can assemble a recording that meets the standard, and portrays you in a favourable light. Knowing when you have reached the standard is part of the educative process. Canvass the opinion of your trainer, a fellow trainee or other colleague; watch other peoples' consultations, including those of your mentors.

3 Take particular care in choosing the five consultations for in-depth analysis: examiners will assume that these are your best efforts, so a weak performance will seriously undermine your credibility.

4 'Safe' consultations, such as a succession of sore throats, may appear an attractive option, but they give little scope to impress the examiners and show them your skills. Try to show more confidence than this.

5 The areas in which you are required to demonstrate competence are identified in Table 10.3. Before submission look critically through your portfolio and workbook. Do they meet the performance criteria?

Table 10.3 Performance criteria* in the videotape assessment of consulting skills.

289

*Chapter 10
The MRCGP
Examination*

Units of competence
- Discovering the reasons for a patient's attendance
- Defining the clinical problem(s)
- Explaining the problem(s) to the patient
- Addressing the patient's problem(s)
- Making effective use of the consultation (e.g. for health promotion)

The candidate should be seen to:
- develop a rapport with the patient
- encourage the patient's contribution to the consultation
- recognise at least some of the cues present in the consultation
- elicit details that place the complaint(s) in a social and psychological context
- obtain enough information to ensure no serious condition is overlooked
- perform a physical examination which helps confirm/refute a reasonable working hypothesis (or which addresses the patient's concern)
- reach a clinically appropriate working diagnosis
- explain the diagnosis, proposed management and effects of treatment in language and content appropriate to the patient's need
- select an appropriate management plan, consistent with a good understanding of modern accepted practice
- share management options with the patient
- prescribe appropriately

* Units of competence are broken down into a series of subsidiary performance criteria—e.g. 'discovering reasons for attendance' includes the patient's account, the cues he presents, the impact on his work and home life, his health understanding and his continuing problems.

Are the main issues addressed? If not, why not? Again canvass the views of your peers, and practice regularly throughout the final training year.

6   Reflections on the content of consultations should be more than a simple minute by minute description of the tape ('then I shook his hand . . . then I examined his chest.', etc.). A safer bet is to talk about the dynamics of the consultation and the hidden agenda; and to paint the whole-patient picture, and set the consultation in its psychological and social context.

7   It may help to read Chapter 2 of this book, and a textbook on consultation techniques such as those listed under further reading. These will highlight the issues at the forefront of the examiners' minds.

10.7 THE VIVAS

Time allowed
Two successive vivas each 20 min long.

Format
Each oral examination is conducted by a pair of examiners (and

possibly a third, or a video camera, invigilating not on your performance but that of the examiners). After the first viva you will be conducted to an ante-room, and then, after a break of around 5 min, introduced to a new pair of examiners. They will have an indication of the areas covered in the first viva, so there is no accidental duplication of questioning.

Content

This part of the exam is intended to assess decision-making and professional values. There is no planned difference in emphasis between the two vivas. The reason that there are two short orals rather than one long one is simply to ensure that the candidate's performance is evaluated by a number of different assessors.

Each viva will explore several question areas (about five). The questions may be loosely based on the experiences of the examiners who are practising GPs. Cases may be clinical or may be widened to include any issue that impinges on general practice. There is free rein: examples from my own viva (including the legal requirements for prescribing to addicts, the problem of a partner propositioned by means of a love letter, the counselling of a patient demanding inappropriate emergency referral, and the role of the family in schizophrenic illness) illustrate this point very well!

No significant reference will be made to the candidate's own practice or patients, although different approaches to the delivery of primary care (the pros and cons of a high list size, or a surgery-based endoscopy clinic, or a hospital assistantship, etc.) may feature.

The vivas provide the chance to test areas that are not readily tested elsewhere, such as ethical values and ideas of professional development (how to keep up to date; how to avoid burn-out; how to handle friction and dissension within a partnership, or a poorly performing practice manager).

Marking scheme

Because of the nature of the viva it is difficult to employ a rigid marking scheme. However, examiners have some general guidelines. In particular they seek to determine whether candidates:

- are competent, safe and reasonably well read;
- consider reasonable alternatives;
- can present a coherent argument;
- tolerate alternative attitudes;
- behave in an ethical and sensitive way;
- are aware of their own limitations;
- display appropriate professional values.

Points of technique

1 Usual points of viva technique (dress conservatively, be courteous, do not argue, be punctual, sit up, do not mumble) are particularly

valid in this exam, since GPs are innately conservative, and often entertain quite stereotyped views of the fitting dress, deportment and manner of prospective College members.

2   Do not raise a topic unless you are prepared to talk about it. The converse is to bait the examiner into asking you a question that you have thoroughly prepared. Although the battleground is chosen by the examiner, it is still possible with care to lead the questioning into the relative calm of prepared backwaters.

3   Quote-dropping is useful in small amounts. Examiners read the same journals as you, so scrutinise the main ones in the lead-up to the exams. 'Hot topics' are likely to be in the forefront of their minds and may well surface in some form.

4   Do not express your view too early in proceedings. You may be left defending only one side of the argument! In this exam you score best by teasing out the reasonable alternatives, so introduce the pros and cons first, talk about them at some length, support them with evidence if you can, and then give your qualified view. Remember the emphasis should not be so much on facts but options, alternatives and implications: your chances of success will be enhanced if you keep this firmly in mind every time you speak.

5   As always, thorough preparation pays dividends: although you cannot anticipate every question, with wide preparation you should be able to say *something* about most topics. It then becomes an exercise in organising packets of knowledge into a sensible argument. Practise your viva technique regularly with a colleague.

6   Make sure that you have your own common sense limited prescribing policy which you can justify and cost.

10.8 SUMMATIVE ASSESSMENT

Summative assessment concerns the satisfactory completion of vocational training and eligibility to practice as an accredited, fully trained GP. It is different from passing the MRCGP, but the points of overlap are now many.

Formerly, doctors entering practice needed only to complete a 4-year approved training programme and to emerge with a satisfactory trainer's report. The Joint Committee on Postgraduate Training for General Practice (JCPTGP) has now developed a process of summative assessment, that more formally evaluates the endpoint skills. GP registrars are expected to pass this assessment before completing their training (although the legal imperative for this remains somewhat ambiguous).

The earlier ingredients remain, but trainees must also satisfy the JCPTGP that they have:

1   adequate knowledge;
2   adequate problem-solving skills;

3   adequate clinical competence;

4   adequate consultation skills; and

5   have completed a written report of practical work in general practice (specified by the UK Regional Advisers in General Practice).

The relation of summative assessment to the MRCGP examination is still a matter of negotiation. Under a preliminary agreement between the Royal College and JCPTGP, those who passed the College exam were deemed to have demonstrated adequacy in the first three of the test areas. The UK advisers in general practice were required to make their own assessment of a video tape of consultation skills, but it was possible for candidates to submit their MRCGP video, or a copy of it, for assessment. The Royal College hopes that in future a Membership pass will become accepted (together with the trainer's report) as sufficient evidence of adequacy, removing the need for a second assessment. But at the time of writing the issue is not resolved, and the candidate is advised to consult the JCPTGP for the latest position.

11 Epidemiology and Statistics

Paper 1 in the new style MRCGP examination often requires candidates to read a published paper (or some parts of a paper), on a general practice topic, and to offer a critical evaluation. This may encompass: summarising the study, commenting on the strengths and weaknesses of its design, the validity and meaning of the data, and its relevance to practice. The ability to read, comprehend, appraise and digest new findings is an important life-long skill for aspiring general practitioners, and may also be assessed in other exam sections too.

This chapter begins with some brief advice on critical reading, and then proceeds to a simple overview of statistics and epidemiology for the uninitiated. Other tips for coping with this aspect of the syllabus, are offered in Section 10.4, and suggestions for further reading on p. 311.

Digesting scientific material

An orderly approach to critical reading has much to commend it. Many journals organise their abstracts in a semi-structured manner, and a similar model can conveniently be used by candidates for analysing and summarising published material. For example:

- *Introduction*: why did the author start?
- *Methods*: what did the author do?
- *Results*: what did the author find?
- *Discussion*: what does it mean?

In the same vein, the abstracts of recent papers in the *British Medical Journal* contain the following structured headings: objectives; design; setting; subjects; interpretation; end-points; measurement and main results; and conclusions.

The findings need to be placed in context, and three useful supplementary questions will help:

1 What is the message?
2 Do I believe it?
3 If true, how does it affect what I do at present?

Candidates should be able to discuss their reading at this level, particularly as this relates to common, important and topical themes. Some suggestions on *selective* reading are provided later (see Further Reading, p. 309).

11.1 EPIDEMIOLOGY: BASIC DEFINITIONS

1 *Epidemiology* is the study of the distribution and determinants of disease and other indices of health in human populations.
2 A *population* is a circumscribed group of individuals sharing one or

more defined characteristic in common. Several groups may exist, e.g.:

These groups . . .	. . . are	. . . for example
The target population	All people everywhere who share the characteristic(s) defined	Men aged 40–50 years with diastolic blood pressures >100 mmHg
The study population	A fraction of the target population selected for study	All such men in region X
A study sample	The fraction of the study population sampled when the numbers are large	All such men in practice Y from region X

Epidemiology seeks to infer from the *particular* (study sample or population) to the *general* (target population). Whether it can do so depends critically on whether the study population is *typical* of the target population.

3   A *measuring instrument* means (speaking epidemiologically) any technique used to collect data.

(a) Examples might equally include:
- blood samples;
- X-rays;
- spirometric graphs;
- questionnaires;
- agreed sets of diagnostic criteria.

(b) Good measuring instruments must be:
- *valid*, i.e. provide a true assessment of what they purport to measure;
- *repeatable*, i.e. provide the same result when remeasured under the same conditions.

(c) Validity is measured in terms of *sensitivity* and *specificity*, as compared with the gold-standard of all measuring instruments (see Table 3.2, p. 91).

(d) Repeatability may be less than perfect because of:
- *within-observer* variation (e.g. although the blood pressure is the same, I read it differently after a coffee break than I did before it);
- *between-observer* variation (e.g. I tend to make the same blood pressure higher than you do);
- *within-subject* variation (his blood pressure changes anyway).

(e) Measuring instruments should be chosen, refined or tested by pilot study to ensure that they are as valid and repeatable as possible. (The best existing ones, e.g. the Medical Research Council Respiratory Questionnaire, have been developed in this way and should be used where appropriate and possible.)

Longitudinal vs. cross-sectional

1   A study in which events evolve and are enumerated over a period of time is said to be *longitudinal*—case control and cohort studies are of this type.

2   A study which takes a snap-shot picture of the state at a particular point in time is said to be *cross-sectional*, and is also known as a survey.

Some examples should make the difference clear:

Longitudinal study

In a study from general practice, patients with backache were randomised between receiving an education leaflet or not. Over the next year the numbers presenting with backache were counted for the two groups.

Cross-section study

In another study doctors from practice, X examined a randomly chosen selection of patient records to establish the proportion of patients currently being treated for backache.

Cohort vs. case control

1   The cohort study (also called a prospective study) is a longitudinal study which follows forwards over a fixed period of time two groups of people who have different exposures to an agent of interest (e.g. contraceptive pill-takers and non-pill-takers), but are otherwise matched. The incidence of disease is compared in the two groups.

2   In practice two basic approaches are possible:

(a) we could start today and count events occurring over the next 10 years (a so-called *truly* prospective design);

(b) we could finish today and look at disease in contraceptive pill- and non-pill-takers over the last 10 years (a so-called *historically* prospective design).

3   The case control study (or retrospective study) compares people who have a specific disease (cases) with those who do not (controls) to establish whether their past exposure to possible disease risk factors (e.g. contraceptive pill-taking) differed.

The essential difference between cohort and case control studies is illustrated in Fig. 11.1. Note particularly that groups in a cohort study are compared with respect to *disease*, while those in a case control study are compared with respect to *exposure*.

Randomisation, placebos and blind trials

1   If the purpose of a study is to compare two groups receiving different treatments (e.g. chemotherapy vs. placebo), patients would ideally be randomised between the groups. This design would be called a randomised controlled trial.

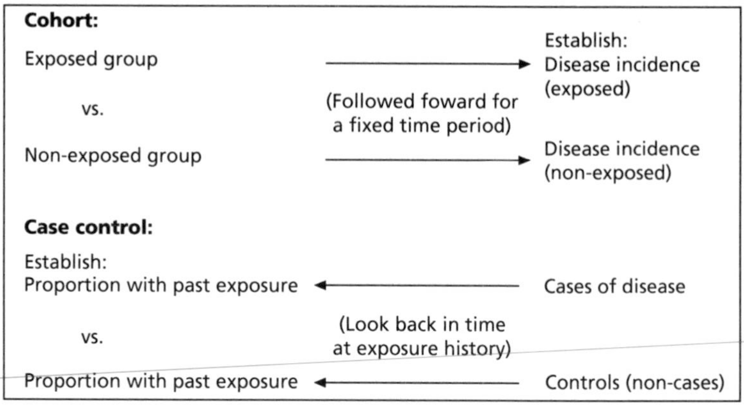

Figure 11.1 Cohort and case control study designs.

2 If the patient does not know which treatment he is receiving but the doctor does, this is called single-blind randomisation.
3 If neither the patient nor the doctor knows which treatment is being given, this is called double-blind randomisation.

The purpose of randomisation is to iron out any chance differences that exist between the groups. The double-blind design removes one source of bias—that due to patient and doctor expectation.

Error and bias

These terms have distinct and separate meanings. *Bias* is a form of systematic error, leading to consistent over- or under-recording of the true situation. *Random error*, because of its chance nature, leads to neither.

This is a more important distinction than it seems. Random error leads to a less precise estimate of the study parameter, but the degree of imprecision can be statistically estimated, and the effect can be offset by making the study larger. The effect of bias is harder to estimate and its magnitude cannot be reduced simply by including more subjects. A study beset with random error may be salvaged; a biased study may not, unless the bias is recognised and removed.

Designing questionnaires

Designing a good questionnaire is an art—bad questions beget bad answers. There are a few cardinal rules:
• keep questions short, clear and concise;
• use language which is unambiguous but intelligible to its readership;
• ensure that possible answers are restricted in choice and can be objectively interpreted (e.g. yes/no, or a number);
• do not seek too much information from one question (it often confuses).

It is important too to get a good response rate (inevitably when studies are incomplete there is suspicion that the participants differed from the non-responders in important ways — 'they had an axe to grind'). Response rates can be improved by making the survey more acceptable to the target group:
- by prior publicity;
- by convenient timing;
- by polite and full explanation of the use that will be made of the information;
- by assurance of confidentiality.

11.3 MEASURING RATES

1 *Incidence*—the rate of occurrence of new cases. (Note that you need to exclude old cases at the outset of the study, as they must not be counted.)

2 *Prevalence*—the proportion of the population at risk affected at a given time (point prevalence = at a given point in time; period prevalence = within a stated period).

3 *Age standardisation* — age is such an important determinant of ill health that it would be very misleading to compare two study populations with different age structures. Suppose, for example, we suspected that the medical standards exercised in preventing cerebrovascular accidents differed in Bournemouth and Milton Keynes. We could attempt to test this hypothesis by comparing the incidence of cerebrovascular accidents in each population, but the comparison would be meaningless unless some account was taken of the age groups found in each community. Age standardisation is a technique that allows the comparison to be made (the details need not concern us). It is from this technique that the standardized mortality ratio (SMR) is derived.

4 *Expressing results*—in comparing the incidence rates of disease in exposed (Ie) and non-exposed (In) populations we are asking, what is the risk in the one population compared with the other? This comparison can be expressed in several ways, e.g.:
  (a) the absolute difference between the rates (Ie−In);
  (b) the proportionate difference in rates [(Ie−In)/Ie];
  (c) the ratio of the rates (Ie/In).
  The latter is usually chosen. It is called the *relative risk*.

The SMR is an important example. It is also a product of convenience: because of the expense and difficulty of following groups through a cohort study, convention allows the control group in mortality studies to exist only on paper, a reference population whose mortality experience can be looked up in tables of national statistics. After age standardisation the rates are compared:

$$\text{SMR} = \frac{\text{Observed deaths in study population}}{\text{Expected deaths in study population}} \times 100$$

Expected is understood in the sense of 'the number of deaths that would occur in the study population if it experienced the same age-specific mortality as the reference population'.

A mortality experience equivalent to that of the reference population gives an SMR of 100. If >100, the mortality experience was greater, and so on.

Because the starting point in the design of a case control study is quite different, we cannot calculate relative risk in quite the same way. The *odds ratio* (OR) is an approximation to relative risk suitable in interpreting the findings of case control studies.

$$\text{OR} = \frac{\text{Odds of developing disease in the exposed}}{\text{Odds of developing the disease in the unexposed}} \times 100$$

Its interpretation is broadly similar to that of the SMR.

11.4 BASIC PRINCIPLES OF MEDICAL STATISTICS

Definitions

1 Statisticians divide their field into:
   (a) *descriptive statistics*—the summarising, enumerating and presenting of data in meaningful forms;
   (b) *inferential statistics*—the use of data from study groups to draw inferences concerning target populations.
2 Statistical data can be:
   (a) *quantitative*—data to which an exact number can be ascribed (blood pressure, episodes of backache);
   (b) *qualitative*—data to which a quality can be ascribed but not an exact member (sex, blood group).
   Quantitative data may be:
   (a) *discrete*—assuming only certain discrete values (e.g. number of children);
   (b) *continuous*—assuming any value along a continuum (e.g. serum cholesterol).
   It is subject to the normal rules of arithmetic.
   Qualitative data may be grouped into categories that have an order (ordinal data, e.g. clinical severity grading scales for breathlessness), but cannot be treated in a simple arithmetic way.
3 Data can be summarised in tabular or graphical form by means of contingency tables, bar charts or frequency histograms.
4 It is conventional in describing statistical data to measure central tendency and distribution or dispersion of the data points.
   (a) Measures of central tendency include:
   • the *mean*—the average value;

- the *mode*—the most commonly occurring value;
- the *median* — the middle observation when all the values are ranked in ascending or descending order.

The mean is the most widely used of these measures, because it can be mathematically manipulated. In a normal distribution all three have the same value.

(b) The most important measure of dispersion around the mean is called the *standard deviation* (SD).

(The square of the deviation from the mean is taken for each data point. The results are summed and averaged. The square root of this value is the SD.)

The SD has convenient properties where values are normally distributed (as in many biological systems):
- 66% of values lie within the range of $X \pm 1$ SD;
- 95% of values lie within the range of $X \pm 2$ SD;
- 99% of values lie within the range of $X \pm 3$ SD.

Correlation and regression

If we wished to assess the association between two quantitative variables (say height and blood pressure) we might start by plotting height against the blood pressure for each of the individuals studied. The variables height and blood pressure would be X and Y co-ordinates on the graph and each subject would be represented by a single point. An immediate visual inspection of this graph (which is called a *scatter diagram*) might give the impression that a linear association existed. Correlation is the mathematical verification of this impression.

A *correlation coefficient* is a measure of the strength of linearity between two quantitative variables. It has a value on a scale of −1 to +1:
- +1 indicates a perfect direct association;
- −1 indicates a precise inverse association;
- 0 (and values close to it) indicate no association.

The process is a descriptive one.

Regression, by contrast, is a predictive process. The line of best fit in the scatter diagram is found mathematically, and used to *predict* the value of one variable given the value of another.

Notes

1 The processes are complementary. Regression can always find a line of best fit — even if the fit is very poor and in all probability no linear relationship exists. A high correlation coefficient tells us that there probably *is* a line there, so the regression result is credible.

2 Strictly speaking this is *linear* regression. Non-linear regression is also possible, but here the association is assumed to be non-linear and calculations are based on formulae describing the form of relationship between the variables.

Sampling statistics: standard error of the mean

If we take a study sample and ascertain its mean and standard deviation we have an approximation of the true population mean and standard deviation. If we took another sample and repeated the exercise we would probably end up with a slightly different estimate.

According to the theory of sampling statistics, if we take an infinite number of samples our estimates of the population mean would show a normal distribution around the true mean. The standard deviation of this sampling distribution could in turn be described and is called the *standard error of the mean*.

This standard deviation of the sampling means gives us an idea of the dispersion of our estimates around the true value, and a better statement of the range in which the true value is likely to lie.

Significance tests

1   Tests of statistical significance, though varied, are based on a common line of reasoning. The so-called *null hypothesis* contends that no true differences exist between population groups in a study and that any apparent difference is due to the effects of chance alone. This results, for example, in their sample means lying at different points on a single normal distribution of sample means.

2   The probability (P) of getting values as far apart as those observed, while still belonging to the same family of sampling means, can be deduced.

3   If the probability appears extremely small we would contend that the null hypothesis is unlikely and that the two populations are indeed different; if the probability does not appear small enough we would contend that the null hypothesis could still be true and the differences observed could be due to chance alone. The value of P at which we make this distinction is chosen arbitrarily, and is called the *significance level* of the test. Usually: $P < 0.05$ leads to rejection of the null hypothesis and a *significant difference*, and $P < 0.01$ is regarded as *highly significant*.

Notes

1   Even if $P > 0.05$, the difference could still be genuine, but such a study would have failed to prove it so.

2   A statistically significant difference may not be a *clinically* significant one: while it is likely to be a genuine difference, the magnitude of effect may be small and the consequences clinically unimportant.

Type I and type II errors

Significance testing only indicates the balance of probabilities. A conclusion based on it can still be wrong:

1   A *type I error* occurs if the test leads us to conclude that there is a difference when one does not actually exist. The risk of this occurring depends on the significance level we choose for the test: the lower it is,

the more convinced we require to be, the lower the risk of a false positive.

2   However, if we are too strict we may miss a genuine difference between compared groups. Because we insisted on a value of $P < 0.0001$ when we could only demonstrate $P < 0.01$, we draw a false-negative conclusion. This is a *type II error*.

3   Type II errors can be reduced by increasing the size of the study. They are not normally quoted, but they are used beforehand by statisticians in this way to establish the minimum size worthy of study.

Confidence intervals

Many published articles now report their findings using *confidence intervals* rather than tests of statistical significance.

1   A confidence interval is a range of values within which it can be stated, with a certain degree of confidence, that the population statistic lies.

2   A 95% degree of confidence is often chosen, though this is arbitrary and could be higher or lower.

3   The confidence interval is preferred because it contains useful additional information: the likely upper and lower limits of the range in which the statistic is to be sought.

4   The value of this can be illustrated by reference to a fictitious study of relative risk: suppose that a study suggests the relative risk of a cerebrovascular accident in Bournemouth compared with Basingstoke is 1.5:

> (a) if the 95% confidence intervals are 1.0–2.0 this is consistent with a two-fold increase in risk (relative risk = 2) but also with no increase in risk at all (relative risk = 1)!
>
> (b) if the 95% intervals are 1.3–2.0 we can at least say that an increased risk exists (assuming we have designed and conducted the study properly and compared age-adjusted figures). (Table 3.8, p.119 provides examples of confidence intervals used in this way in major mammography screening trials.)

11.5 THE ROLE OF THE STATISTICIAN

If the reader is confused by my explanations, I hope it will at least be clear that it is worth consulting a statistician or epidemiologist from the outset in a planned study worth its salt. This would help in:

- selecting appropriate controls (often the most difficult exercise);
- choosing the right numbers;
- eliminating important sources of bias;
- applying the statistical tests appropriate to the circumstances in question.

This chapter has been difficult to write and, if unfamiliar, the concepts make for difficult reading. If you feel at sea but out of your depth, do not lose heart! The objective is to pass the MRCGP and in this context more information has been provided than is strictly necessary. If you find the material straightforward it may earn you an extra mark or two; it may even have stimulated your interest; if not there are other more important fish to fry!

12 Facts and Figures

This chapter lists some of the major statistics relating to the clinical and administrative content of general practice and the provision of health care under the NHS. It is not essential to memorise all the figures, but it may well be useful to quote one or two statistics in support, or to provide perspective for your arguments. (Most of these figures are derived from the meticulous records that John Fry has kept over many years in general practice.)

Levels of care
1   75% of ill health is dealt with by 'self-care', made up roughly as follows:
   - (a) 25% upper respiratory infections;
   - (b) 20% aches and pains;
   - (c) 20% emotional upsets;
   - (d) 10% gastrointestinal upsets;
   - (e) 5% rashes.
2   20% dealt with by GPs.
3   10% by hospitals.

Vital statistics of workload

List sizes
The trend is towards smaller list sizes. The averages have been, respectively:
- 1969   2495;
- 1981   2200;
- 1995   1887.

Consultation rates
1   Average consultations per patient each year: approximately 5 (men 4; women 6).
2   Average home visits per patient each year: approximately 0.5. In 1994 10% of consultations were at the patient's home (compared with 22% in 1971), and 8% by telephone (4% in 1971).
3   Average surgery consultation time: approximately 5–6 min.
4   Average time per home visit: approximately 15 min.
5   75% of the practice consults over a 1-year period, and 90% over 5 years. 15% consult a GP within any 2-week period.
6   Doctors with a list of 2000 patients provide on average 6000–8000 consultations per year (115–154 per week).
7   The average GP works 69 h/week (including 43 h on general medical services)

Practice size

The trend is towards bigger practices with fewer 'single-handers', e.g.

	1969	1994
1 doctor	22%	11%
2 doctors	25%	14%
3 doctors	26%	17%
4 doctors	15%	18%
5 doctors	7%	16%
≥6 doctors	5%	24%

Areas are categorised according to the average list size within them:

Category	Mean list size
Restricted	0–1700
Intermediate	1701–2100
Open	2101–2500
Designated type 1	2501–2999
Designated type 2	3000+

In 1991 only 5% of areas were under-doctored (designated or open).

Provision of staff and premises for primary care

In the UK there are approximately:

34 000 GPs (81 000 doctors);

9000 surgeries (25% of which are Health Centres);

3200 dispensing GPs;

20 000 district nurses;

10 000 practice-employed nurses;

9000 health visitors;

35 000 secretarial staff;

2000 trainees per year (25% of practices undertake training);

10 400 GP fundholders in 2600 practices (1995).

Clinical content of general practice

Each year, in an average list of 2000 patients, the following clinical events would typically be seen.

Births and deaths

26 births.

23 deaths made up of:

    10 coronaries

    5 cancers

    3 strokes

    2 respiratory diseases

    2 others

25% of deaths at home, 65% in hospital, 10% in other places, e.g. nursing homes, public places.

Minor and major illnesses
400 upper respiratory tract infections
110 middle ear infections
325 emotional upsets
200 gastrointestinal upsets
120 acute backs
50 urinary tract infections
12 pneumonias
10 coronaries
8 new cancers
6 acute abdomens
1 suicide per 4 years

Chronic illness, consultations per year
450 chronic mental illness
100 chronic rheumatism
150 hypertension
50 coronary artery disease
50 asthma
35 chronic bronchitis
30 diabetes
20 peptic ulcers
10 thyroid disease
7 epilepsy
2 multiple sclerosis
>1 chronic renal failure
    Overall:
65% of disease is minor/self-limiting
15% of disease is major/life-threatening
20% of disease is chronic with permanent disability

Social pathology
200 patients receiving welfare benefit
90 unemployed patients
70 physically handicapped patients
30 mentally handicapped patients
30 single-parent families
25 deaf patients
10 blind patients
10 alcoholics
5 schizophrenics

New cancers
1 lung every 6 months
1 breast every 12 months
1 colorectal every 18 months
1 skin every 18 months

1 stomach every 18 months to 2 years
1 prostate every 2 years
1 cervix every 6 years
1 leukaemia every 6 years
1 ovary every 6 years
1 larynx every 6 years
1 uterus every 7 years
1 brain every 10 years
1 lymphoma every 15 years
1 thyroid every 25 years

Congenital disorders
1 cardiac disorder every 5 years
1 spina bifida every 5 years
1 pyloric stenosis every 7 years
1 mongolism every 10 years
1 cleft palate every 15 years
1 congenital hip dislocation every 20 years
1 phenylketonuria every 200 years

Non-illness events
Contraception   100 per year
Immunisation   100 per year
Smears   120 per year

Reasons for consulting

According to the fourth National Morbidity Study in General Practice, the most common reasons for consulting in 1991–2 were:

Respiratory diseases	31%
Ear problems	17%
Musculoskeletal conditions	17%
Skin conditions	15%
Injuries/poisonings	14%
Infections/parasitic conditions (mainly thrush)	14%
GU disorders (mainly cystitis)	11%

The special demands of the young and old

• *Children* (under 15 years) are 15–20% of the population, but 25% of GP consultations; 90% of the under-5s are seen each year.
• *The elderly*: 16% of the population are over 65 years (12% 65–79 years, 4% 80 years or over), but 40% of GP consultations are for this age group. As the proportion of very elderly in the population rises, the workload will rise.

Obstetric and gynaecological trends

1   Delivery in hospital is increasing and home confinements are far

less common; for example, in 1962 65% of deliveries were in hospital, whereas in 1994 the figure was 98%.

2   The average family size is 2.3 children.
3   In 1994 178000 terminations occurred in England, the majority of these in non-NHS hospitals.
4   Since 1950 the perinatal mortality rate has fallen from 35 to 9 per 1000 live births.
5   The maternal mortality rate is about 6 per 100000.
6   10% of couples are involuntarily infertile, the mean number of cycles to conception is 6, and 80% of couples achieve a pregnancy in 12 months.
7   Contraceptive methods are used to the following degrees:
  (a) the pill   25%;
  (b) sheath   16%;
  (c) withdrawal   4%;
  (d) intrauterine device   6%;
  (e) diaphragm   1%.
8   66% of single women and 53% of married women are said to show a preference for the Family Planning Clinic over their own GP.

Referral rates and the use of hospital facilities

1   One in three people visit hospital outpatient departments each year, comprising:
  (a) 1 in 6 referred by their GP;
  (b) 1 in 5 self-referred to casualty.
2   Each elective outpatient department referral generates 4.2 follow-up visits (8.5 for psychiatry).
3   Referral rates vary greatly between doctors: one study (Last 1967) suggests that two-thirds of doctors refer 10–35 per 1000 each month, but this varies from 5 to 115 per 1000 each month.
4   The provision of hospital beds is 9 per 1000 populus.
5   One in nine of the population is admitted to hospital (i.e. 11%) over a 1-year period.
6   This admission risk rises 10-fold over age 65 years.

Prescribing

Each GP issues 13000 scripts per year; over 60% of consultations end in prescription and 60% of the populus takes medicine each day; the average person receives 8.7 scripts per year (compared with 10–11/year in France, Germany and Italy).

The annual cost to the NHS is about £120000 per GP each year, or £4 billion (still less than 8% of the total NHS budget).

Complaints against doctors

In 1994 a total of 1862 complaints against GPs were investigated by service committees and 25% were upheld. The major cause of complaint was delay in or failure to make a diagnosis (25%). The number of complaints has doubled over the last decade.

NHS facts and figures

NHS expenditure (1993–4) was £36 billion total, i.e. £800 per head. This is nearly 7% of the gross national product (one of the lowest costs per capita in the world — OECD average 10.4%). The funding is derived mainly from Government (88%) with only small contributions from National Insurance (9%) and direct payments (3%). Nearly two-thirds of this money is spent on hospitals, 10% on drugs and only 6% on general practice.

Further Reading

Recommendations for further reading can be divided into two categories: there are those books and articles which (like the claim forms of the same name) are immediately necessary and emergency 'treatments' in the urgent run-up to the examination. These are deliberately thin, concise texts that cover the bones of their subject in a straightforward and direct way, perhaps suitable in each case for a weekend's intensive study. Then there are the more expansive texts which are desirable supplementary reading for those with more time to spare. I have concentrated, in producing this reading list, for the most part on the former type of reading material, and also focused on clinical topics which constraints of space have prevented me from including elsewhere in the text.

Recommendations have been listed according to subject and are arranged in order of mention in the text. Those who have rather more time for independent reading should consult the reference list that follows.

In preparing for exams there is always more material available to read than time in which to read it. This is especially true when it comes to *journal work*, where the dramatic proliferation of published material requires doctors to acquire strategies for selective reading, weeding out the relevant and discarding the rest. Newell (1988) has provided an excellent step-by-step catechism which should help the busy physician:

1 Does the title describe something in which I have the slightest interest?
2 Are the conclusions of limited application?
3 If true, would they alter the way in which I work?

And only then:

4 Are the aims clearly stated?
5 Is the context clear?
6 Are the methods appropriate?
7 How complete are the data?
8 Is the result credible, rationally or intuitively?

The ruthless application of such an approach will help examination candidates in the endless, seemingly impossible task of cramming their quarts into pint pots!

Practice management

Ellis N. (1994) *Employing Staff* (5th edn). BMA, London.
Jones R.V.H., Bolden K.J., Pereira Gray D.J. & Hall M.S. (1990) *Running a Practice: Manual of Practice Management* (4th edn). Croom Helm, London.

Consulting

Pendleton D. & Hasler J. (eds) (1993) *Doctor–Patient Communication*. Academic Press, London.

Pendleton D., Schofield T., Tate P. & Havelock P. (1984) *The Consultation: an Approach to Learning and Teaching*. Oxford Medical Textbooks, Oxford.

Prevention

Fry J., Jeffree P., Scott K. (1990) *The Screening Handbook: a Practitioner's Guide*. Kluwer Academic Publishers, Lancaster, UK.

Clinical

Paediatrics

Illingworth R.S. (1987) *The Normal Child: Some Problems of the Early Years and their Treatment* (9th edn). Churchill Livingstone, Edinburgh.

Hall D.M.B. (ed.) (1996) *Health for All Children. Report of the Joint Working Party on Child Health Surveillance*. 3rd edn. OUP, Oxford.

Pharmacology

British National Formulary. British Medical Association and the Pharmaceutical Society of Great Britain, London (published annually).

ENT

Ludman H. (1993) *ABC of ENT* (3rd edn). BMA, London.

Ophthalmology

Banks J.L.K. (1994) *Clinical Opthalmology: A Text and Colour Atlas* (3rd edn). Churchill Livingstone, Edinburgh.

AIDS

Adler M.W. (ed.) (1993) *ABC of AIDS* (3rd edn). BMA, London.

Psychiatry

Puri B.K. (1995) *Saunders Essentials of Psychiatry*. W.B. Saunders, London.

Dermatology

Callen J.P. (ed.) (1995) *Current Practice of Dermatology*. Current Medicine, Philadelphia.

Obstetrics and gynaecology

Anthony J. & Kaye P. (1995) *Notes for the DRCOG* (3rd edn). Churchill Livingstone, Edinburgh.

Community medicine

Donaldson R.J. & Donaldson L.J. (1993) *Essential Public Health Medicine* (3rd edn). Kluwer Academic Publications, London.

Legal and ethical

Taylor J.F. (ed.) (1995) *Medical Aspects of Fitness to Drive* (5th edn). Medical Commission on Accident Prevention.

Phillips M. & Dawson J. (1985) *Doctors' Dilemmas: Medical Ethics and Contemporary Science*. Harvester Press, Brighton.

The General Practitioner's Yearbook. Winthrop, Winthrop House, Surbiton on Thames, Surrey.

Epidemiology and statistics

Gore S.M. & Altman D.G. (1982) *Statistics in Practice*. BMA, London.

Newell D. (1988) Reading scientific articles, or how to cope with the overload. *Practitioner* 232, 720–5.

Swinscow T.D.V. (1996) *Statistics at Square One* (9th edn). BMA, London.

Exam study books

Gambill E., Moulds A, Fry J., Brooks D. (1988) *The MRCGP Study Book* (2nd edn). Butterworth-Heinmann Publications, London. (Sample exam papers with worked answers.)

Sandars J.E. (ed.) (1992) *MRCGP Practice Exams* (2nd edn). Pastest, Knutsford.

Elliott P. (1993) *MRCGP MCQ Practice Papers*. Pastest, Knutsford.

Moore R. (1994) *The MRCGP Examination: A Guide for Candidates and Teachers*. Royal College of General Practitioners, London. (A College guide on the format of the exam and what the examiners are looking for.)

Facts and figures

Fry J. & Sander G. (1993) *Common Diseases* (5th edn). Kluwer Academic Publishers, London.

Fry J. (1993) *General Practice: The Facts*. Radcliffe Medical Press, Oxford.

Topical information

Consult the last 1–2 years' editorials and major review articles in *Update* magazine and the *British Journal of General Practice*.

Select Bibliography

Acres (1979) In: Edwards G. & Grant M. (eds) *Alcoholism: New Knowledge and New Responses*, pp. 324–5. Croom Helm, London.

Anderson P. (1984) What are safe alcohol levels? *Br. Med. J.* **289**, 1657–8.

Andersson I., Aspegren K., Janzon L. *et al.* (1988) Mammographic screening and mortality from breast cancer: the Malmo mammographic screening trial. *Br. Med. J.* **297**, 943–8.

Anonymous (1987) Management of hyperlipidaemia. *Drug Ther. Bull.* **25**, 89–92.

Argyle M. (1972) *The Social Psychology of Work.* Penguin, Harmondsworth, Middlesex.

Atkin W.S., Cuzick J, Northover J.M.A. & Whymer D.K. (1993) Prevention of colorectal cancer by once-only sigmoidoscopy. *Lancet* **341**, 736–40.

Audit Commission (1996) *What the Doctor Ordered: A Study of GP Fundholders in England and Wales.* HMSO, London.

Austoker J. (1990) Breast cancer screening and the primary care team. *Br. Med. J.* **300**, 1631–4.

Austoker J. (1994) Screening for cervical cancer. *Br. Med. J.* **309**; 241–8.

Australian National Board (1980) The Australian Therapeutic Trial in Mild Hypertension. *Lancet* **i**, 1261–7.

Bain D.J. (1984) Deputising services: the Portsmouth experience. *Br. Med. J.* **289**, 471–3.

Bain J. (1985) Developmental screening for preschool children: is it worthwhile? *J. R. Coll. Gen. Pract.* **39**, 133–7.

Balint M. (1957) *The Doctor, his Patient and the Illness.* Pitman Medical, London.

Banks M., Beresford S., Morrell D., Wailer J. & Watkins C. (1975) Factors influencing demand for primary care in women aged 20–64 years: a preliminary report. *Int. J. Epidemiol.* **4**, 189–95.

Bateman D.N., Campbell M., Donaldson L.J., Roberts S.J. & Smith J.M. (1996) A prescribing incentive scheme for non-fundholding general practices: an observational study. *Br. Med. J.* **313**, 535–8.

Baum M. (1995) Screening for breast cancer, time to think — and stop? *Lancet* **346**, 436–7.

Beardon P.H.G., Brown S.V., Mowat D.A.E. *et al.* (1987) Introducing a drug formulary to general practice — effects on prescribing costs. *J. R. Coll. Gen. Pract.* **37**, 305–7.

Beardow R., Oerton J. & Victor C. (1989) Evaluation of the cervical cytology screening programme in an inner city health district. *Br. Med. J.* **299**, 98–100.

Bernadt M.W., Mumford J., Taylor C., Smith B. & Murray R.M. (1982) Comparison of questionnaire and laboratory tests in detection of excessive drinking and alcoholism. *Lancet* **i**, 325–8.

Berne M.D. (1964) *Games People Play.* Penguin, Harmondsworth, Middlesex.

Berquist-Ullman M. & Larsen U. (1977) Acute low back pain in industry. *Acta Orthop. Scand. Suppl.* **170**.

Bertakis K.D. (1977) The communication of information from physician to patient. *J. Fam. Pract.* **5**, 217–22.

Birmingham Research Group of General Practitioners (1978) Practice activity analysis. 6: visiting profiles. *J. R. Coll. Gen. Pract.* **190**, 316–17.

Black D.G. *et al.* (1994). Non-fundholding in Nottingham: a vision of the future. *Br. Med. J.* **309**; 930–2.

Bloom J.R. & Monterossa S. (1981) Hypertension labelling and sense of well-being. *Am. J. Public Health* **71**, 1228–32.

Bogle S.M. & Harris C.M. (1994) Measuring prescribing: the shortcomings of the item. *Br. Med. J.* **308**; 637–40.

Bradley C.P. & Bond C. (1995) Increasing the number of drugs available over the counter: arguments for and against. *Br. J. Gen. Pract.* **45**; 553–6.

British Heart Foundation (1987) *Screening for Ischaemic Heart Disease Risk in General Practice*. British Heart Foundation, London. (Factfile.)

Brody D. (1980) An analysis of patient recall of their therapeutic regimens. *J. Chron. Dis.* **33**, 57–63.

Brown G. & Harris T. (1978) *Social Origins of Depression*. Tavistock Publications, London.

Brown G.W., Birley J. & Wing J.W. (1972) Influence of family life on course of schizophrenic disorders: a replication. *Br. J. Psychiatry* **121**, 241–58.

Brumfitt W. & Slater J.H.D. (1957) Treatment of acute sore throat with penicillin. *Lancet* **i**, 8.

Butler-Sloss E. (1988) *Report of the Inquiry into Child Abuse in Cleveland*. HMSO, London.

Buxton M.J. & Klein R.E. & Sayer J. (1977) Variations in GP night visiting rates, medical organisation and consumer demand. *Br. Med. J.* **i**, 827–30.

Byrne P.S. & Long B.E.L. (1976) *Doctors Talking to Patients*. HMSO, London.

Cambell R., Macdonald Davies I., Macfarlane A. & Beral V. (1984) Home births in England & Wales, 1979: perinatal mortality according to intended place of delivery. *Br. Med. J.* **289**, 721–4.

Capewell S. (1996) The continuing rise in emergency admissions. *Br. Med. J.* **312**, 991–2.

Cartwright A. (1964) *Human Relations and Hospital Care*. Routledge & Kegan Paul, London.

Cartwright A. & Anderson R. (1967) *Patients and their Doctors: a Study of General Practice*. Routledge & Kegan Paul, London.

Cartwright A. & Anderson R. (1981) *General Practice Revisited: a Second Study of General Practice*. Tavistock Publications, London.

Cartwright A. & O'Brien M. (1976) The sociology of the NHS. In: Stacey M. (ed.) *Sociology Review Monograph no. 22*. University of Keele, Keele.

Central Statistical Office (1984) *Social Trends* no. 14 HMSO, London.

Central Statistical Office (1989) *Social Trends* no. 19, HMSO, London.

Chen E. & Cobb S. (1960) Family structure in relation to health and disease. *J. Chronic Dis.* **12**, 544–67.

Chick J., Kreitman N. & Plant M. (1981) Mean cell volume and gammaglutamyltranspeptidase as markers of drinking in working men. *Lancet* **i**, 1249–51.

Clark E.M. & Forbes J.H. (1979) *Evaluating Primary Care*. Croom-Helm, London.

Clinical Standards Advisory Group (1995). *Back pain: Report of a CSAG Committee on Back Pain*. HMSO, London.

Cobbe S.M. (1992) ISIS 3: the last word on thrombolysis? *Br. Med. J.* **304**, 1454–5.

Cockburn J., Gibberd R.W., Reid A.L. & Sanson-Fisher R.W. (1987) Determinants of non-compliance with short-term antibiotic regimens. *Br. Med. J.* **295**, 814.

Cohen J. (1986) Diagnosis and management of problem patients in general practice. *J. R. Coll. Gen. Pract.* **36**, 51.

Coleman P. (1989) The value of screening the elderly. *Family Pract. Service* **16**, 424.

Collier J. (1988) The case for and against prescribing generic drugs: generic prescribing benefits patients. *Br. Med. J.* **297**, 1596–8.

Colling A., Dellipiani A.W., Donaldson R.J. & MacCormack P. (1976) Teesside coronary survey: an epidemiological study of acute attacks of myocardial infarction. *Br. Med. J.* **2**, 1169.

Committee on Medical Aspects of Food Policy (COMA) (1987) *The Use of Very Low Calorie Diets in Obesity: Report on Health and Social Subjects*. no. 31. HMSO, London.

Costello R. (1975) Alcoholism treatment and evaluation, I & II. *Int. J. Addict.* **10**, 251–75, 857–67.

Court Report (1976) *Fit for the Future*. Report of the Committee on Child Health Services, Cmnd 6680. HMSO, London.

Cruickshank J.M. (1988) The case for and against prescribing generic drugs: don't take innovative research-based companies for granted. *Br. Med. J.* **297**, 1597–8.

Cumberledge Report (1986) *Neighbourhood Nursing: A Focus for Care*. Report of the Community Nursing Review. HMSO, London.

Dahl-Jorgensen K., Brinchmann-Hansen O., Hanssen K.F., Ganes T. *et al.* (1986) Effect of near normoglycaemia for 2 years on progression of early diabetic retinopathy, nephropathy and neuropathy: the Oslo study. *Br. Med. J.* **293**, 1195–9.

Davey A., Smith G., Barley M. & Blane D. (1990) The Black report on socioeconomic inequalities in health 10 years on. *Br. Med. J.* **301**, 373–7.

Davey Smith G. (1996) Income inequality and mortality: why are they related? *Br. Med. J.* **312**, 987–8.

Davis M.S. (1968) Variation in patients' compliance with doctors' advice: an experimental analysis of patterns of communication. *Am. J. Public Health* **58**, 274–88.

Delamonthe T. (1991) Social inequalities in health. *Br. Med. J.* **303**, 1046–50.

Department of Employment (1977) *New Earnings Survey*. HMSO, London.

Department of Health (1992) *Health of the Nation: a Strategy for Health in England*. HMSO, London.

Dickerson J.E.C. & Brown M.J. (1995) Influence of age on general practitioners' definition and treatment of hypertension. *Br. Med. J.* **310**, 574.

Dillane J.B., Fry J. & Kalton G. (1966) Acute back syndrome—a study from general practice. *Br. Med. J.* **2**, 82–6.

Dixon J., Hodson D., Dodd S., Rice P., Doncaster I. & Williams M. (1994) *Br. Med. J.* **309**, 30–4.

Dixon R.A. & Williams B.T. (1988) Patient satisfaction with general practitioner deputising services. *Br. Med. J.* **297**, 1519–22.

Doran D.M.L. & Newell D.J. (1975) Manipulation in treatment of low back pain: a multicentre study. *Br. Med. J.* **2**, 161–4.

D'Souza M.F., Swan A.V. & Shannon D.J. (1976) A long-term controlled trial of screening for hypertension in general practice. *Lancet* **i**, 1228–31.

Dunnell K. & Cartwright A. (1972) *Medicine Takers, Prescribers and Hoarders*. Routledge & Kegan Paul, London.

Eachus J., Williams M., Chan P., Davey Smith G., Grainge M., Donovan J. & Frankel S. (1996) Deprivation and cause, specific morbidity: evidence from the Somerset and Avon survey of health. *Br. Med. J.* **312**, 287–92.

Edwards G., Orford J., Egbert S., Guthrie S., Hawkes A., Hensman C., Mitcheson M., Oppenheimer E. & Taylor C. (1977) Alcoholism: a controlled trial of 'treatment' and 'advice'. *J. Stud. Alcohol* **38**, 1004–31.

Egbert L.D., Battit G.E., Welch C.E. & Bartlett M.K. (1964) Reduction of postoperative pain by encouragement and instruction of patients. *N. Engl. J. Med.* **270**, 825–7.

Ellman R. & Chamberlain J. (1984) Improving the effectiveness of cervical cancer screening. *J. R. Coll. Gen. Pract.* **267**, 537–42.

Elwood J.M., Cotton R.E., Johnson J., Jones G.M., Curnow J. & Beaver M.W. (1984) Are patients with abnormal cervical smears adequately managed? *Br. Med. J.* **289**, 891–4.

Engelhard D., Cohen D. & Strauss N. (1989) Randomised study of myringotomy, amoxycillin/clavulanate or both for acute otitis media in infants. *Lancet* **ii**, 141–3.

Epstein A.M., Hall J.A., Fretwell M. *et al.* (1990) Consultant geriatric assessment for ambulatory patients. *J.A.M.A.* **263**, 538–44.

European Myocardial Infarction Project Group (1993) Prehospital thrombolytic therapy in patients with suspected acute myocardial infarction. *N. Engl. J. Med.* **329**, 383–9.

European Working Party on High Blood Pressure in the Elderly (1985) Mortality and morbidity results from the European Working Party on High Blood Pressure in the Elderly Trial. *Lancet* **i**, 1349–54.

Fahey T.P. & Peters T.J. (1996) What constitutes controlled hypertension? Patient based comparison of hypertension guidelines. *Br. Med. J.* **313**, 93–6.

Forrest P. (1987) *Breast Cancer Screening*. HMSO, London.

Fowler G. (1982) Smoking: practising prevention. *Br. Med. J.* **284**, 1306–8.

Fowler G. (1988) Coronary heart disease prevention: a general practice challenge. *J. R. Coll. Gen. Pract.* **38**, 391–2.

Francis V., Korsch B.M. & Morris M.J. (1969) Gaps in doctor–patient communication: patient's response to medical advice. *N. Engl. J. Med.* **280**, 535–40.

Friedman M. & Rosenman R. (1974) *Type A Behaviour and your Heart*. Knopf, New York.

Froom J., Gilpeper L., Crob P. *et al.* (1990) Diagnosis and antibiotic treatment of acute otitis media: a report from the International Primary Care Network. *Br. Med. J.* **300**, 582–6.

Fry J. (1958) Antibiotics in acute tonsillitis and acute otitis media. *Br. Med. J.* **2**, 883.

Fry J. (1973) *Present State and Future Needs of General Practice* (3rd edn). Royal College of General Practitioners, London.

Fry J. (1979) *Common Diseases: their Nature and Incidence*. MTP Press, London.

Fulton M., Kellett R.J., MaClean D.W., Parkin D.M. & Ryan M.P. (1979) The management of hypertension—a survey of opinions among general practitioners. *J. R. Coll. Gen. Pract.* **29**, 583–7.

General Medical Council (1996) *Duties of a Doctor*. GMC, London.

Gerrard T.J. & Riddell J.D. (1988) Difficult patients: black holes and secrets. *Br. Med. J.* **297**, 530–2.

Gill O.N., Adler M.W. & Day N.E. (1989) Monitoring the prevalence of HIV: foundations for a programme of unlinked anonymous testing in England and Wales. *Br. Med. J.* **299**, 1295–8.

Glover J.R., Morris J.G. & Khosla J. (1974) Back pain: a randomized clinical trial of rotational manipulation of the trunk. *Br. J. Indust. Med.* **31**, 59–64.

GMSC & Royal College of General Practitioners (1984) *Handbook of Preventive Care for Pre-school Children*. GMS Defence Fund & RCGP, London.

Goldberg D. (1981) The recognition of psychological illness by general practitioners. In: Edwards G. (ed.) *Psychiatry in General Practice*. University of Southampton, Southampton.

Grampian region early antistreplase trial (GREAT) group (1992). Feasibility, safety, and efficacy of domiciliary thrombolysis by general practitioners: Grampian region early antistreplase trial. *Br. Med. J.* **305**, 548–53.

Gray M. & Fowler G.H. (eds) (1983) *Preventative Medicine in General Practice*. Oxford University Press, Oxford.

Grol R., Whitfield M., De Maesener J. & Mokkink H. (1990) Attitudes to risk taking in medical decision making among British, Dutch and Belgian general practitioners. *Br. J. Gen. Pract.* **40**, 134–6.

Groves J.E. (1951) Taking care of the hateful patient. *N. Engl. J. Med.* 298, 883–5

Gruppo Italiano per lo Studio delta Streptochinasi nell' Infarto Miocardico (GISSI) (1987) Long-term effects of intravenous thrombolysis in acute myocardial infarction: final reports of the GISSI study. *Lancet* **ii**, 871–4.

Hall D.M.B. (ed.) (1996) *Health for All Children. Report of the Third Joint Working Group on Child Health Surveillance* (3rd edn). Oxford University Press, Oxford.

Hall M.H., Chng P.K. & MacGillivray I. (1980) Is routine antenatal care worth while? *Lancet* **ii**, 78–80.

Hallam L. (1992) *Out-of-hours Care in General Practice: Further Analysis of Data*. Centre for Primary Care Research, University of Manchester, Manchester.

Halstead C., Lepow M.L., Balassarian N., Emmerick J. & Wolinsky E. (1968) Otitis media. *Am. J. Dis. Child.* **115**, 542.

Hampton J.R., Morris G.K. & Mason C. (1975) Survey of general practitioners' attitudes to management of patients with heart attacks. *Br. Med. J.* **4**, 146–8.

Hardcastle J.D., Chamberlain J.O., Robinson M.H.E., Moss S.H., Satya S.A., Balfour T.W., James P.D. & Mangham C.M. (1996) Randomised controlled trial of faecal occult blood testing for colorectal cancer. *Lancet* 348, 1472–7.

Harris A.I., Cox E. & Smith C.R.W. (1971) *Handicapped and Impaired in Great Britain.* OPCS Social Survey Division, HMSO, London.

Harrison A.T. (1987) Appointment systems: Feasibility study of a new approach. *Br. Med. J.* **294**; 1465–6.

Hart J.T. (1986) Reduction of blood cholesterol in the population: can it be done? *J. R. Coll. Gen. Pract.* **36**, 538–9.

Haverkorn M.J., Valkenburg H.A. & Goslings W.R.O. (1971) A controlled study of streptococcal pharyngitis and its complications in the Netherlands. *J. Infect. Dis.* **124**, 339.

Haynes R.B., Sackett D.L., Taylor D.W., Gibson E.S. & Johnson A.I. (1978) Changes in absenteeism and psychosocial function due to hypertension screening and therapy among working men. *N. Engl. J. Med.* **299**, 741–4.

Health Education Council (1983) *That's the Limit.* HMSO, London.

Health Survey for England 1994 (1996) HMSO, London.

Hellman G.C. (1981) Disease vs. illness in general practice. *J. R. Coll. Gen. Pract.* **31**, 548–52.

Hendriksen C., Lund E. & Stromgard E. (1984) Consequences of assessment and intervention among elderly people: a three year randomised controlled trial. *Br. Med. J.* **289**, 1522–4.

Hill J.D., Hampton J.R. & Mitchell J.R.A. (1978) A randomized trial of home-vs-hospital management for patients with suspected myocardial infarction. *Lancet* i, 837.

Hill D., White V., Jolley D. & Mapperson K. (1988) Self examination of the breast: is it beneficial? Meta-analysis of studies investigating BSE and the extent of disease in patients with breast cancer. *Br. Med. J.* **297**, 271–5.

Hinton J. (1980) Whom do dying patients tell? *Br. Med. J.* **281**, 1328–30.

Holme I. (1995) Relation of coronary heart disease incidence and total mortality to plasma cholesterol reduction in randomised trials: use of meta-analysis. *Br. Heart J.* **69** (supplement); S42–S47.

Holmes T. & Masuda M. (1974) Life change and illness susceptibility. In: Dohrenwend B.S. & Dohrenwend B.P. (eds) *Stressful Life Events: Their Nature and Effects.* John Wiley, New York.

Holmes T. & Rahe R. (1967) The social readjustment rating scale. I. *Psychosom. Res.* **11**, 213–18.

Houston H.L.A. & Davis R.H. (1985) Opportunistic surveillance of child development in primary care: Is it feasible? *J. R. Coll. Gen. Pract.* **35**, 77–9.

Howie J.G.R., Porter A.M.D. & Forbes J.F. (1989) Quality and the use of time in general practice: widening the discussion. *Br. Med. J.* **298**, 1008–10.

Howie J.G.R., Porter A.M.D., Heaney D.L. & Hopton J.L. (1991) Long to short consultation ratio: A proxy measure of quality of care for general practice. *Br. J. Gen. Pract.* **41**, 48–54.

Hypertension Detection and Follow-up Cooperative Group (1979) Five years findings of the Hypertension Detection and Follow-up Programme. *J.A.M.A.* **242**, 2562–71.

ISAM study group (1986) A prospective trial of intravenous streptokinase in acute myocardial infarction (ISAM). Mortality, morbidity and infarct size at 21 days. *N. Engl. J. Med.* **314**, 1465–71.

ISIS-2 (Second International Study of Infarct Survival) Collaborative Group (1988) Randomised trial of intravenous streptokinase, oral aspirin, both or neither among 17 187 cases of suspected myocardial infarction: ISIS2. *Lancet* ii, 349–60.

Isles C.G., Hole D.J., Gillis C.R., Hawthorne V.M. & Lever A.F. (1989) Plasma cholesterol, coronary heart disease and cancer in the Renfrew and Paisley survey. *Br. Med. J.* **298**, 920–4.

Jelley D.M. & Nicoll A.G. (1984) Pertussis: what percentage of children can we immunize? *Br. Med. J.* **288**, 1582–4.

Kales A. (1974) Treating sleep disorders. *Am. Fam. Physician* **8**, 158–68.

Keeble B.R., Shivers C.A. & Muir-Gray J.A. (1989) The practice annual report: postmortem or prescription? *J. R. Coll. Gen. Pract.* **39**, 467–9.

Kenny R.A., Brennas M., O'Malley K. & O'Brien E. (1987) Blood pressure measurements in borderline hypertension. *J. Hypertension* **5** (suppl), 483–5.

Keys A., Aravanis C., Blackburn H., van Buchem F.S.P., Buzina R., Djordjeuik B.S. *et al.* (1972) Coronary heart disease: overweight and obesity as risk factors. *Ann. Intern. Med.* **117**, 15–27.

Kholer L. (1984) Early detection and screening programmes for children in Sweden. In: McFarlane J.A. (ed.) *Progress in Child Health.* Churchill Livingstone, Edinburgh.

Kincey J., Bradshaw P. & Key P. (1975) Patient's satisfaction and reported acceptance of advice in general practice. *J. R. Coll. Gen. Pract.* **25**, 558–62.

Kinlay S. & Heller R.F. (1990) Effectiveness and hazards of case finding for a high cholesterol concentration. *Br. Med. J.* **300**, 1545–7.

Kjekshus J. & Pedersen T.R. (1995) Reducing the risk of coronary events: Evidence from the Scandinavian Simvastatin Survival Study (4S). *Am. J. Cardiol.* **76**, 64c–68c.

Knowles H.C. (1970) Control of diabetes and the progression of vascular disease. In: Ellenberg M. & Rifkin H. (eds) *Diabetes Mellitus: Theory and Practice.* McGraw-Hill, New York.

Korsch B.M. & Negrete V.F. (1972) Doctor–patient communication. *Sci. Am.* **227**, 66–74.

Kubler Ross E. (1970) *On Death and Dying.* Tavistock Publications, London.

Laing R. & Esterson A. (1964) *Sanity, Madness and the Family.* Penguin, Harmondsworth, Middlesex.

Lancet, Editorial (1990) Taking risks in general practice. *Lancet* **336**, 541.

Last J.M. (1967) Quality of general practice. *Med. J. Aust.* **i**, 780–4.

Lauritzen T., Frost-Larsen K., Larsen H.W., Deckert T. and the Steno Study Group (1983) Effects of 1 year of near normal blood glucose levels on retinopathy in insulin-dependent diabetes. *Lancet* **i**, 200–4.

Law M.R., Wald N.J. & Thompson S.G. (1994) By how much and how quickly does reduction in serum cholesterol concentration lower risk in ischaemic heart disease? *Br. Med. J.* **308**, 367–72.

Law SAT & Britten N. (1995) Factors that influence the patient centredness of a consultation. *Br. J. Gen. Practice* **45**, 520–4.

Laxdal O.E., Merida J. & Trefor Jones R.H. (1970) Treatment of acute otitis media. *Can. Med. Assoc. J.* **102**, 263.

Leach J., Ridsdale L. & Smeeton N. (1993) Is there a relationship between a mother's mental state and consulting the doctor by the family? *Fam. Pract* . **10**, 305–11.

Leitch D. (1989) Who should have their cholesterol concentrations measured? What experts in the United Kingdom suggest. *Br. Med. J.* **298**, 1615–6.

Ley P., Whitworth M.A., Skilbeck C.E., Woodward R., Pinsent R., Pilce L.A., Clarkson M.G. & Clark P.B. (1976) Improving doctor–patient communication in general practice. *J. R. Coll. Gen. Pract.* **26**, 720–4.

Lieberman D. & Sleisenger M.H. (1996) Is it time to recommend screening for colorectal cancer? *Lancet* **348**, 1463–4.

Little P., Smith L., Cantrell T., Chapman J., Langridge J. & Pickering R. (1996) General practitioners' management of acute back pain: a survey of reported practice compared with clinical guidelines. *Br. Med. J.* **312**, 485–8.

Lowenthal L. & Bingham E. (1987) Length of consultation: how well do patients choose? *J. R. Coll. Gen. Pract.* **37**, 498–9.

Lynge E. (1981) Occupational mortality in Norway, Denmark and Finland (1971–5). In: Committee for International Cooperation of National Research in Demography (ed) *Socio-economic Differential Mortality in Industrialised Societies.* Paris, WHO.

Mant D. & Fowler G. (1990) Screening in practice: mass screening — theory and ethics. *Br. Med. J.* **300**, 916–8.

Marinker M. (1988) The referral system. *J. Coll. Gen. Pract.* **38**, 487–91.

Marsh G.N. (1985) New programme of antenatal care in general practice. *Br. Med. J.* **291**, 646–8.

Marsh G.H. & Dowes M.L. (1995) Establishing a minor illness service in a busy general practice. *Br Med. J.* **310**, 778–80.

Marsh G.H., Horne R.A. & Channing G.M. (1987) A study of telephone advice in managing out of hours calls *J. R. Coll. Gen. Pract.* **37**, 301–4.

Marteau T.M. (1989) Psychological costs of screening. *Br. Med. J.* **299**, 527.

Martikainen P.T. (1990) Unemployment and mortality among Finnish men 1981–5. *Br. Med. J.* **1990**; 301: 407–11.

Mather H.G., Morgan D.C., Pearson N.G., Read K.L.Q., Shaw D.B., Steed G.R., Thorne M.G., Lawrence C.J. & Riley I.S. (1976) Myocardial infarction: a comparison between home and hospital care for patients. *Br. Med. J.* **i**, 925.

Maw A.R. (1983) Chronic otitis media with effusion (glue ear) and adenotonsillectomy: a prospective randomised control study. *Br. Med. J.* **287**, 1586–8.

Mayfield D., McLeod G. & Hall P. (1974) The CAGE questionnaire: validation of a new alcoholism screening instrument. *Am. J. Psychiatry* **131**, 1121–3.

Mazhari M. (1987) Decent paediatric care costs money. *GP Magazine*, Jan 16th, p. 17.

McGayock H.M. (1990) Developing a practice formulary. *Update* **39**, 121–4.

McGhee A. (1961) *The Patient's Attitude to Nursing Care.* E. & S. Livingstone, Edinburgh.

Mead T.W., Dyer S., Browne W., Townsend J. & Frank O. (1990) Low back pain of mechanical origin: randomised comparison of chiropracter and hospital outpatient treatment. *Br. Med. J.* **300**, 1431–7.

Medical Research Council Antiepileptic Srud Withdrawal Study Group (1993) Prognostic index for recurrence of seizures after remission of epilepsy. *Br. Med. J.* **306**, 1374–8.

Miller P. McC. & Plant M. (1996) Drinking, smoking, and illicit drug use among 15 and 16 year olds in the United Kingdom. *Br. Med. J.* **313**, 394–7.

Moore A.T. & Roland M.O. (1989) How much variation in referral rates among GPs is due to chance? *Br. Med. J.* **298**, 500–2.

Morrell D.C., Gage H.G. & Robinson A. (1971) Referral to hospital by GPs. *J. R. Coll. Gen. Pract.* **21**, 77–85.

Morrell D.C., Evans M.E., Morris R.W. & Roland M.O. (1986) The five minute consultation: effect of time constraint on clinical content and patient satisfaction. *Br. Med. J.* **292**, 870–3.

Morton-Jones T. & Pringle M. (1993) Explaining variations in prescribing across England. *Br. Med. J.* **306**, 1731–4.

Moser K.A., Fox A.J. & Jones D.R. (1984) Unemployment and mortality in the OPCS longitudinal study. *Lancet* **ii**, 1324–9.

Moulds A.J. (1985) Making the most of the Lloyd George. *Update*, 15th March.

Mourin K. (1976) Auditing and evaluation in general practice. *J. R. Coll. Gen. Pract.* **26**, 726–33.

MRC Working Party (1992) MRC trial of treatment of hypertension in older adults. *Br. Med. J.* **304**, 405–12.

Multiple Risk Factor Intervention Trial Research Group (1982) Multiple risk factor intervention trial: risk factor changes and mortality results. *J.A.M.A.* **248**, 1465–77.

Murray S.A. & Paxton F. (1993) Nurses or doctors: patient choice in family planning? *Health Bull.* **51**, 394–8.

Nachemson A. (1976) The lumbar spine: an orthopaedic challenge. *Spine* **1**, 59–71.

National Ambulatory Medical Care Survey (1980) 1977 Summary. United States, Jan-Dec 1977. Data from the National Health Survey Series 13, no. 44. Hyattsville, Md: DHEW Publication No. (PHS) 80–1795, April.

Northern Region Perinatal Mortality Survey Co-ordinating Group (1996) Collaborative study of perinatal loss in planned and unplanned home births. *Br. Med. J.* **313**, 1306–9.

Nystrom L., Rutqvist L.E., Wall S., Lindgren A., Lindqvist M., Ryden S. *et al.* (1993) Breast cancer screening with mammography: overview of Swedish randomised trials. *Lancet* **341**, 973–8.

Oboler S.K. & LaForce M. (1989) The periodic physical examination in asymptomatic adults. *Ann. Intern. Med.* **110**, 214–16.

O'Dowd T.C. (1988) Five years of heartsink patients in general practice. *Br. Med. J.* **297**, 528–30.

Office of National Statistics (1996) *Childhood, Infant and Perinatal Mortality Statistics England & Wales, 1993 & 1994*. Series DH3 no. 27. The Stationary Office, London.

Office of Population Censuses and Surveys (1986) *Occupational Mortality: Decennial Supplement, 1979–80, 1982–3*. Series DS no. 2. HMSO, London.

Office of Population Censuses and Surveys (1995) *Morbidity Statistics from General Practice 1991–2*. HMSO, London.

Office of Population Censuses and Surveys (1996) *Living in Britain: General Household Survey 1994*. Series GHS no. 25. HMSO, London.

Parkes C.M., Benjamin B. & Fitzgerald R.G. (1969) Broken heart: a statistical survey of increased mortality among widowers. *Br. Med. J.* **1**, 740–4.

Patterson H.R. (1985) The problems of audit and research. *J. R. Coll. Gen. Pract.* **35**, 118.

Pell A.C.H., Stuart P.C., Stewart M.J. & Fraser D.M. (1990) Home or hospital care for acute myocadial infarction? A survey of GPs' attitudes in the thrombolytic era. *Br. J. Gen. Pract.* **40**, 323–5.

Peto R., Gray R., Collis R., Wheatley K. *et al.* (1988) Randomised trial of prophylactic daily aspirin in British male doctors. *Br. Med. J.* **296**, 313–16.

Pharoah P.D. & Hollingworth W. (1996) Cost effectiveness of lowering cholesterol concentration with statins in patients with and without pre-existing coronary heart disease: life table method applied to health authority population. *Br. Med. J.* **312**, 1443–8.

Pickering T.G., James G.D., Boddie C., Harshfield G.A., Blank S. & Largh J.H. (1988) Flow common is white-coat hypertension? *J.A.M.A.* **259**, 225–8.

Pietroni P. (1976) NVC in the GP surgery. In: Tanner B. (ed.) *Language and Communication in General Practice*, pp. 162–79. Hodder & Stoughton, Sevenoaks.

Ploeckinger B., Dantendorfer K., Ulm M., Baischer W., Derfler K., Musalek M. *et al.* (1996) Rapid decrease of serum cholesterol concentration and postpartum depression. *Br. Med. J.* **313**, 664.

Podell R. (1975) *Physician's Guide to Compliance in Hypertension*. West Point, Merck, Pennsylvania.

Pokorny A.D., Miller B.A. & Kaplan H.B. (1972) The brief MAST: a shortened version of the Michigan Alcoholism Screening Test. *Am. J. Psychiatry* **129**, 342–5.

Polich J.M. (1980) Patterns of remission in alcoholism. In: Edwards G. & Grant M. (eds) *Alcoholism Treatment in Transition*. Croom Helm, London.

Pollak B. (1978) A two-year study of alcoholics in general practice. *Br. J. Alcohol Alcoholism* **13**, 24–35.

Pringle M., Stewart-Evans C., Coupland C., Williams I., Allison S. & Sterland J. (1993) Influence on control in diabetes mellitus: patient, doctor, practice or delivery of care? *Br. Med. J.* **306**, 630–4.

Raine R., Streetly A. & Maryon Davis A. (1996) Variations in local policies and guidelines for cholesterol managment: national survey. *Br. Med. J.* **313**, 1368–9.

Rastam L., Luepker R.V. & Pirie P.L. (1988) Effect of screening and referral on follow-up and treatment of high cholesterol levels. *Am. J. Prev. Med.* **4**, 244–8.

Raw M., Jarvis M.J., Feyerabend C. & Russell M.A.H. (1980) Comparison of nicotine chlewing-gum and psychological treatments for dependent smokers. *Br. Med. J.* **281**, 481.

Reader G., Pratt L. & Mudd M. (1957) What patients expect from their doctor. *Mod. Hosp.* **July**, 19–21.

Report of the British Heart Foundation Working Group (1989) Role of the general practitioner in managing patients with myocardial infarction: impact of thrombolytic treatment. *Br. Med. J.* **299**, 555–6.

Report of the Joint Working Group of the Royal Colleges of Physicians, Psychiatrists & General Practitioners (1996) *Chronic Fatigue Syndrome*. Cr 54. RCP, London.

Risdale L, Morgan M. & Morris R. (1992) Doctors' interviewing technique and its response to different booking times. *Fam. Pract.* **9**, 57–60.

Roberts M.M., Alexander F.E., Andersson T.J. *et al.* (1990) Edinburgh trial of screening for breast cancer: mortality at 7 years. *Lancet* **335**, 241–6.

Roland M.O., Bartholomew J., Courtenay M.J.F. *et al.* (1986) The five minute consultation: effect of time constraint on verbal communication. *Br. Med. J.* **292**, 874–6.

Roland M. & Dixon M. (1989) Randomised controlled trial of an educational booklet for patients presenting with backache in general practice. *J. R. Coll. Gen. Pract.* **39**, 244–6.

Rosenstock I.M. (1966) Why people use health services. *Millbank Memorial Fund Q.* **44**, 94–124.

Rotter J. (1966) Generalised expectancies for internal vs. external control of reinforcement. *Psychol. Monograph* **80**, no. 609.

Royal College of General Practitioners (1972) *The Future General Practitioner: Learning and Teaching.* RCGP, London.

Royal College of General Practitioners (1982) *Healthier Children — Thinking Prevention.* Report from General Practice 22. RCGP, London.

Royal College of General Practitioners (1983) The quality initiative — summary of council meeting. *J. R. Coll. Gen. Pract.* **33**, 523–4.

Royal College of General Practitioners (1985a) *Booking for Maternity Care — A Comparison of Two Systems.* Occasional paper 31. RCGP, London.

Royal College of General Practitioners (1985b) *Towards Quality in General Practice.* Council Consultation Document. RCGP, London.

Royal College of General Practitioners (1985c) *What Sort of Doctor?* Report from General Practice 23. RCGP, London.

Royal College of General Practitioners (1985d) *Quality in General Practice.* Policy Statement 2. RCGP, London.

Royal College of General Practitioners, Office of Population Census Surveys, and Department of Health (1995) *Morbidity Statistics from General Practice. Fourth national study, 1991–2.* HMSO, London.

Royal College of Psychiatrists (1979) *Alcohol and Alcoholism.* Tavistock Publications, London.

Royal Commission on the Distribution of Income and Wealth (1978) *Report 6. Lower Incomes.* Cmnd 7175. HMSO, London.

Royal Commission on the Distribution of Income and Wealth (1980) *Inequalities in Health.* HMSO, London.

Russell M.A.H., Wilson C., Taylor C. & Baker C.D. (1979) Effect of general practitioners' advice against smoking. *Br. Med. J.* **2**, 231.

Sacks F.M., Pfefier M.A., Moye L.A., Rolleau J.L., Rutherford J.D., Cole T.G. *et al.* (1996) The effects of pravastatin on coronary events after myocardial infarction in patients with average cholesterol levels. *N. Engl. J. Med.* **335**, 1001–9.

Sainsbury, Lord (1967) *Report of the Committee of Enquiry into the Relationship of the Pharmaceutical Industry with the NHS.* Cmnd 3410, p. 209. HMSO, London.

Sanderson S. (1996) Hypertension in the elderly: pressure to treat? *Health Trends* **28**, 71–5.

Sawyer L. & Arber S. (1982) Changes in home visiting and night and weekend cover: the patient's view. *Br. Med. J.* **284**, 1531–4.

Scientific and Medical Advisory Committee of the Coronary Prevention Group (1987) *Risk Assessment: its Role in the Prevention of Coronary Heart Disease.* Coronary Prevention Group, London.

Scott T. (1985) Do we need to repeat prescribe? *J. R. Coll. Gen. Pract.* **35**, 91–2.

Secretaries of State for Social Services, Wales, Northern Ireland and Scotland (1986) *Primary Health Care: An Agenda for Discussion.* HMSO, London.

Secretaries of State for Social Services, Wales, Northern Ireland and Scotland (Nov. 1987) *Promoting Better Health: The Government's Programme for Improving Primary Health Care.* HMSO, London.

Secretaries of State for Health, Wales, Northern Ireland and Scotland (1989) *Working for Patients.* HMSO, London (Cmnd 555).

Sempos C., Fulwood R., Haines C. *et al.* (1989) The prevalence of high blood cholesterol levels among adults in the United States. *J.A.M.A.* **262**, 45–52.

Sever P., Beevers G., Bulpitt C., Lever A., Ramsay L., Reid J. & Swales J. (1993) Management guidelines in essential hypertension: report of the second working party of the British Hypertension Society. *Br. Med. J.* . **306**, 983–7.

Shapiro S., Venet P., Strax P. & Roeser R. (1982) Ten to fourteen year effect of screening on breast cancer mortality. *J. Natl. Cancer Inst.* **69**, 349–55.

Sharpe M., Archand L., Banatvala J., Broysiewicz L.K., Clare A.W. & David A. (1991) Chronic fatigue syndrome: guidelines for research. *J. R. Soc. Med.* **84**, 188–121.

Sheldon Report (1967) *Child Welfare Centres. Report of the Subcommittee of the Standing Medical Advisory Committee.* HMSO, London.

Sheldon M.G. & Harris S.J. (1984) Use of deputising services and night visit rates in general practice. *Br. Med. J.* **289**, 474–6.

Shepherd J., Betteridge D., Durrington P. *et al.* (1987) Strategies for reducing coronary heart disease and desirable limits for blood lipid concentrations: guidelines of the British Hyperlipidaemia Association. *Br. Med. J.* **295**, 1245–6.

Shepherd M., Cooper B., Brown A.C. & Kalton G.W. (1966) *Psychiatric Illness in General Practice.* Oxford University Press, Oxford.

Sikorski J., Wilson J., Clement S., Das S. & Smeeton N. (1996) A randomised controlled trial comparing two schedules of antenatal visits: the antenatal care project. *Br. Med. J.* **312**, 546–53.

Slade P.D. & Dewey M.E. (1983) The role of grammatical clues in the MCQ: an empirical study. *Med. Teacher* **2**, 146–8.

Smith D. (1976) *The Facts of Racial Disadvantage.* Political and Economic Planning, London.

Smith R. (1989) NHS Review — words from the source: an interview with Alain Enthoven. *Br. Med. J.* **298**, 1166–8.

Smith W.C.S., Konicer M.B., Davies A.M., Evans A.E. & Yarnell J. (1989) Blood cholesterol: is population screening warranted in the UK? *Lancet* **ii**, 372–3.

Smith W.C.S., Lee A.J., Crombie J.K. & Tunstall-Pedoe H. (1990) Control of blood pressure in Scotland: the rule of halves. *Br. Med. J.* **300**, 981–3.

South East London Screening Study Group (1977) A controlled trial of multiphasic screening in middle-age: results of the South East London Screening Study. *Int. J. Epidemiol.* **6**, 357–63.

Stevenson J.S.K. (1982) Advantages of deputising services: a personal view. *Br. Med. J.* **284**, 947–9.

Stott P. (1989) Value for money. *Med. Monitor*, 9th June, p. 13.

Stott N.C.H. & Davis R.H. (1979) The exceptional potential in each primary care consultation. *J. R. Coll. Cell. Pract.* **29**, 201.

Sullivan F. & Mitchell E. (1995) Has general practitioner computing made a difference to patient care? A systematic review of published reports. *Br. Med. J.* **311**, 848–52.

Tabar L., Fagerberg C.J., Tad A. *et al.* (1985) Reduction in mortality from breast cancer after mass screening with mammography. *Lancet* **ii**, 829

Thomas K.B. (1987) General practice consultations: is there any point in being positive? *Br. Med. J.* **294**, 1200.

Thompson N.F. (1990) Inviting infrequent attenders to attend for a health check: costs and benefits. *Br. J. Gen. Pract.* **40**, 16–18.

Troup R.C. (1989) What influences doctors' prescribing. *J. R. Coll. Gen. Pract.* **39**, 2551.

Tucker J.S., Hall M.H., Howie P.W., Reid M.E., Barbour R.S., Florey C du V. & McIlwaine G.M. (1996) Should obstetricians see women with normal pregnancies? A muticentre randomised controlled trial of routine antenatal care by general practitioners and midwives compared with shared care led by obstetricians. *Br. Med. J.* **312**, 554–9.

Tudor Hart J. (1971) The inverse care law. *Lancet* **i**, 405–12.

Tulloch A.K. (1976) *The design and evaluation of a modern medical record system.* MD Thesis, Aberdeen University.

Tulloch A.J. & Moore V. (1979) A randomised controlled trial of geriatric screening and surveillance in general practice. *J. R. Coll. Gen. Pract.* **29**, 733–42.

Tyrer P., Owen R. & Dawling S. (1983) Gradual withdrawal of diazepam after long-term use. *Lancet* **i**, 1402–6.

Tyrer P., Seivewright N., Murphy S. *et al.* (1988) The Nottingham study of neurotic disorder: comparison of drug and psychological treatments. *Lancet* **ii**, 235–40.

UK Trial of Early Detection of Breast Cancer Group (1988) First results on mortality reduction in the UK trial of early detection of breast cancer. *Lancet* **ii**, 411–16.

Vaillant G.E. (1980) The doctor's dilemma. In: Edwards G. & Grant M. (eds) *Alcoholism, Treatment in Transition*, pp. 13–31. Croom Helm, London.

Van Buchem F.L., Dunk J.H.M. & Van't Hof M.A. (1981) Therapy of acute otitis media: myringotomy, antibiotics, or neither? *Lancet* **ii**, 883–7.

Verbeck A.L.M., Hendricks J.H.C.L., Holland R., Mravunac M., Sturmans F. & Day N.E. (1984) Reduction of breast cancer mortality through mass screening with modern mammography. First results of the Nijmegan Project 1975–1981. *Lancet* **i**, 1222–4.

Veterans Administration Cooperative Study Group on Antihypertensive Agents (1970) *J.A.M.A.* **213**, 1143–52.

Waine C. (1988) *The Prevention of Coronary Heart Disease*. Royal College of General Practitioners, London.

Walker C.H.M. (1986) Child health surveillance. *Update*, 15th Nov., 906–14.

Walker J.H., Stanley I.M., Venables T.L., Gambrill E.C. & Hodgkin G.K.H. (1983) The MRCGP examination and its methods. *J. R. Coll. Gen. Pract.* **33**, 662–5.

Wallace P. & Haines A. (1985) Patients' responses to a self-administered questionnaire. *Br. Med. J.* **290**, 1949–53.

Wallis J.B. & Barber J.H. (1982) The effect of a system of geriatric screening and assessment on general practice workload. *Health Bull. (Edin.)* **40**, 125–32.

Ward A. (1974) Terminal care in malignant disease. *Soc. Sci. Med.* **8**, 233.

Watt G.C.M. (1996) All together now: why social deprivation matters to everyone. *Br. Med. J.* **312**, 1026–9.

Webb E., Ashton C.H., Kelly P. & Karnali F. (1996) Alcohol and drug use in UK university students. *Lancet* **348**, 922–5.

Weed L. (1969) *Medical Records, Medical Education and Patient Care*. Cleveland Press of Case Western Reserve University.

Wessely S., Chalder T., Hirsch S., Pawlikowska T., Wallace P. & Wright D. (1995) Post infectious fatigue: a prospective study in primary care. *Lancet* **345**, 1333–1338

Weston C.F.M., Penny W.J. & Julian D.G. (1994) Guidelines for the early managment of patients with myocardial infarction. *Br. Med. J.* **308**, 767–71.

Whitfield M.J. & Hughes A.O. (1981) Penicillin in sore throat. *Practitioner* **225**, 234.

Wiesel S.M., Cuckler J.M., Deluca F. *et al.* (1980) Acute low back pain. An objective analysis of conservative therapy. *Spine* **5**, 324–30.

Wilkin D. & Smith A.G. (1987) Variation in GPs' referral rates to hospitals. *J. R. Coll. Gen. Pract.* **37**, 350–3.

Wilkin D., Metcalfe D.H.M., Hallam L., Cooke M. & Hodgkin P.K. (1984) Area variations in the process of care in urban general practice. *Br. Med. J.* **289**, 229–32.

Wilkins R.H. (1974) *The Hidden Alcoholic in General Practice*. Chapter 3. Elke Science, London.

Wilson A., McDonald P., Hayes L., Cooney J. (1991) Longer booking intervals in general practice: Effects on doctors' stress and arousal. *Br. J. Gen. Pract.* **41**, 184–7.

Wilson A., McDonald P., Hayes L., Cooney J. (1992) Health promotion in the general practice consultation: A minute makes a difference. *Br. Med. J.* **304**, 227–30.

Wilson J.M.G. (1966) In: Teeling-Smith G. (ed.) *Surveillance and Early Diagnosis in General Practice*. Proceedings of Colloquium, pp. 5–10. Office of Health Economics, London.

Wilson P., Christiansen J., Anderson K. *et al.* (1989) Impact of national guidelines for cholesterol risk factor screening. *J.A.M.A.* **262**, 41–4.

Wynder E.L., Field F. & Haley N.J. (1986) Population screening for cholesterol determination: a pilot study. *J.A.M.A.* **256**, 2839–42.

Zander L.I. (1982) Practising prevention: making a start. *Br. Med. J.* **284**, 1241–2.

Zola I. (1973) Pathways to the doctor: from person to patient. *Soc. Sci. Med.* **7**, 677–89.

Index

(Note: page numbers in **bold** represent tables, those in *italic* represent figures)